The Best
Supplements
for Your
Health

The Best Supplements for Your Health

Donald P. Goldberg, R.Ph.
Arnold Gitomer, R.Ph.
Robert Abel, Jr., M.D.

TWIN STREAMS
Kensington Publishing Corp.
http://www.kensingtonbooks.com

"How Do You Read a Supplement Label?" on page 26 is reprinted by permission from the Council for Responsible Nutrition website (www.crnusa.org).

The quote on page 75 is reprinted by permission from the Council for Responsible Nutrition website (www.crnusa.org).

"Vitamins: Historical Comparison of RDIs, RDAs and DRIs, 1968 to Present" on page 399 is reprinted by permission from the Council for Responsible Nutrition website (www.crnusa. org).

"Minerals: Historical Comparison of RDIs, RDAs and DRIs, 1968 to Present" on page 401 is reprinted by permission from the Council for Responsible Nutrition website (www. crnusa.org).

TWIN STREAM BOOKS are published by

Kensington Publishing Corp.
850 Third Avenue
New York, NY 10022

All Kensington titles, imprints, and distributed lines are available at special quantity discounts for bulk purchases for sales promotions, premiums, fund-raising, educational or institutional use.

Special book excerpts or customized printings can also be created to fit specific needs. For details, write or phone the office of the Kensington Special Sales Manager: Kensington Publishing Corp., 850 Third Avenue, New York, NY 10022. Attn: Special Sales Department. Phone: 1-800-221-2647.

Twin Streams and the TS logo Reg. U.S. Pat. & TM Off.

ISBN 0-7582-0219-9

First Trade Printing: October 2002
10   9   8   7   6   5   4   3   2   1

Designed by Leonard Telesca

Printed in the United States of America

Don Goldberg would like to dedicate this book to his grandparents, Lewis Park and Dora Dobbin, who emigrated to this country from Europe, met while learning English, and taught by example the virtues of hard work and moral integrity. And to my sister, Gloria Anne Ein-Dor, who wanted so much more from life than her ill health allowed.

Arnie Gitomer would like to dedicate this book to his parents, Minnie and Nathan Gitomer. Although formally uneducated, they made sure that I understood the importance of higher education.

Dr. Robert Abel, Jr., dedicates this book to his dad, Robert Abel, Sr., who continues to teach all of us to live, learn, and love.

Contents

Acknowledgments

Don and Arnie would like to thank Dr. Robert Abel, Jr., for initially approaching us to collaborate on this book. We thank Lee Heiman from Kensington Publishing for his support and encouragement. And we want to thank Elaine Will Sparber, Senior Health Editor at Kensington, for her exhaustive editing efforts.

We want to thank Larry Siegel, R.Ph., D.C., for his help in proofreading and for his technical support. Larry is the chief pharmacist at Willner Chemists' midtown store.

We want to thank our wives, Roberta Gitomer and Helen Goldberg, for their support, allowing us to spend evenings and weekends working on this project. And Don wants to thank his two sons, Joshua and Jordan, for forgiving him for not spending more time with them.

Don Goldberg
Arnie Gitomer

Foreword

As a practicing physician and surgeon known for my interest in complementary medicine, I am bombarded by the question, "What vitamins should I take?"

So when I was asked by Lee Heiman of Kensington Publishing what was missing from the current array of self-health books on the market, I knew immediately: People need to learn more about essential supplements, their forms and their uses.

Eighty percent of the world's population continues to use plant-based medical systems. In other words, indigenous people rely on plants and herbs instead of drugs and surgery for their basic health problems. In fact, higher animals have lost the ability to make certain basic nutrients because these nutrients were readily available in the forests and the plains thousands of years ago. So like the leopard on the Serengeti Plain of Africa, which has to eat the liver of his prey to maintain his vision and his health, we, too, are dependent on our food to provide us with the essential building blocks for our bodies.

Americans now consume more food with artificial coloring, hydrogenated fats, processed sugars, and meats with saturated fats. We eat less green leafy vegetables and fish or algae that supply omega-3 oils. We exercise less and are surrounded by pollutants and pesticides in soil and air. In 1937, the Congress of the United States of America declared that the soil in many parts of this country was deficient in certain key minerals and compounds. Weston Price, a dentist who traveled around the world in the 1930s, photographed the mouths of indigenous peoples. He documented the increase in tooth decay and crowding of teeth within one generation of eating a Western diet. Dr. Price also realized that these natives were developing cancer, arthritis, high blood pressure, and tuberculosis, conditions that had not been present with the diets they had consumed for millennia.

I was trained in medical school and residency to treat disease. After ten years of practice, I realized that removing cataracts, treating eye pressure with drops, and lowering blood pressure with pills was focusing on symptoms and not the root causes. As an ophthalmologist, I was treating the part and not the whole. The eye is intimately connected to all the body systems and an imbalance causes deficiency and disease.

Harmony of mind, body, and spirit hinged on a balance of free radicals or oxidants (created by products of oxygen molecules) and antioxidants, which protect our cell membranes throughout the body. Illness occurs when we are in a deficient state. Nutrition and lifestyle and environmental choices must be balanced to maintain our antioxidant bank account.

When a fast-food diet, a hectic lifestyle, and increased stress tip the antioxidant balance in our bodies, deficiencies occur. The word *supplement* means to fill the deficiencies. People need to supplement to fill the void and support the cell membranes in all our body systems.

I have taken numerous courses to learn more about the biochemistry of our bodies and have traveled to places with herbal healers such as India, Nepal, Brazil, Colombia, and Tunisia. But I received a great education about nutritional supplements when I visited the Willner Chemists Pharmacy in New York City in 1994 and met Arnie Gitomer and Don Goldberg.

I was aware that pharmacists knew a great deal about the uses and side effects of current pharmaceutical agents, but I met two outstanding pharmacists who worked in the natural food and supplement field. Arnie and Don had used their extensive scientific training and years in the drug-manufacturing industry to compile a great deal of useful information on vitamins and minerals that were effective in not only treating many of the common diseases (with fewer side effects, I might add), but preventing them as well.

My patients with cataracts, macular degeneration, and glaucoma were getting better naturally, without having to wait for worsening of the vision. My recommendations to colleagues who were managing arthritis, hypertension, coronary artery disease, colitis, elevated cholesterol, and even cancer provided healthy alternatives to a rigid pharmaceutical approach. Numerous controlled scientific studies are validating the facts that vitamin C, E, lutein, DHA, zinc, selenium, magnesium, and others as being important in the prevention and management of a wide variety of medical problems.

People hear the names of all these vitamins and are frankly confused. Some take handfuls of pills, others are content with a daily vitamin, and many just don't know where to seek good advice. I was delighted to learn that Arnie and Don, who publish a quarterly nutrition periodical, would collaborate on such an important undertaking.

The Best Supplements for Your Health will become an indispensable reference on your bookshelf and a daily reminder to evaluate what you need and how supplements can contribute to a lifetime of good health.

Robert Abel, Jr., M.D.

Preface

As pharmacists, we (Don Goldberg and Arnie Gitomer) have a healthy respect for drugs and their benefits. When we were in pharmacy school, however, there was still a great deal of respect for the fact that a large number of the drugs listed in the pharmacopeia were derived from natural sources. A substantial amount of the curricula back then was devoted to subjects such as pharmacognosy, the study of natural substances, particularly plants, that are used in medicine. Over the years, however, courses of this type have been dropped from most pharmacy schools.

Why? Advances in chemistry enabled the pharmaceutical industry to synthesize ever more powerful drugs. We were less dependent on natural products as sources of lifesaving therapeutic agents. Instead, we looked to the chemist's lab bench.

There were good reasons for this movement away from natural products. Supply problems were alleviated. Greater potency could be achieved. The drugs were more easily standardized, and they could often be made available in a more reproducible, convenient form.

And we cannot ignore the economic incentive. A drug derived from a natural substance cannot be patented. A synthesized chemical drug, on the other hand, can be patented, giving the pharmaceutical company an opportunity to recoup the cost of Food and Drug Administration approval, and earn a handsome profit for seven or more years.

As is usually the case, unfortunately, there is no such thing as a free ride. Along with this increased potency comes increased toxicity and the potential for undesirable side effects. When deciding on the treatment for a health problem, a choice has to be made. We have to evaluate the benefit versus the risk of the various options available to us. Killing a fly with a shotgun blast will work, but using a fly swatter might work equally well, without such extensive collateral damage.

In our opinion, the medical establishment became enamored with high-tech, high-powered solutions to many of the health problems facing us today and lost sight of the fact that more gentle, less toxic alternatives were available. There are times when a fly swatter is actually all that is needed.

And even better, put screens on the windows! In other words, prevention—prevent the fly from entering in the first place. Too often, I will hear a patient complaining that "the doctor gave me this prescription, and now I feel worse than I did before." Or the doctor says, "Your blood pressure is a little high—have this prescription filled!"

According to recently released medical guidelines, almost everybody should be taking a "statin" drug to bring their cholesterol levels down to the recommended levels. Is elevated cholesterol or heart disease caused by a deficiency of "statin" drugs? Is arthritis caused by a deficiency of aspirin?

It has been said that we are experiencing an increase in diabetes of almost epidemic proportions. Heart disease, obesity, and cancer are rampant. Is this because we have not yet developed newer or more powerful drugs? Of course not.

Instead, these serious health problems are related to changes in our lifestyles and environment. We do not eat healthy food, we do not get enough exercise, and we are exposed to pollutants and toxins that did not exist in our grandparents' time. We live longer, but not healthier.

It's easy to respond with an admonition to just eat the right foods, prepared properly, get more exercise, and move out of the city. This would be fine, and it is an appropriate goal to strive for, but it's obviously a goal that cannot be achieved by the average person.

We consider nutritional supplements and herbal medicines to be a valuable compromise, or a bridge, between the two extremes—unrealistic lifestyle changes and reliance on miracle drugs. These agents can provide us with the healthy components of foods in quantities that might be difficult or impossible to get through diet alone. They also provide those natural agents that, when ingested at higher levels, exert therapeutic action with fewer side effects than more powerful, synthetic drugs. They offer a convenient and effective way to augment our diet with agents that have been shown to ward off the onset of aging,

cancer, heart disease, Alzheimer's disease, osteoporosis, birth defects—
nearly all health problems.

The benefits of nutritional supplementation are now being recognized not only by the general public, but also by the medical commu-
nity. Interest in these alternative "remedies" is at the highest level ever.
Everybody is looking for more information on which supplements to
use and how to use them. Factual answers to these questions can be
hard to find. Unfounded and exaggerated claims are easy to find. That
is why we are writing this book.

The information we provide is designed to help you distinguish fact
from hype. We want to help you choose the best supplements for your
health.

How to Use This Book

This book is not intended to be used as a replacement for professional medical advice. Instead, it is meant to help you understand the benefits associated with the use of nutritional and herbal supplements and advise you about how best to use these supplements.

The book is divided into two parts. In Part One, we will discuss what nutritional supplements are and the reasons for taking them. First, we will take you through a series of steps that will help you choose the right type of supplement. We will then teach you how to tailor a supplement program to your own unique health needs. And we will review how to best use the supplements you have chosen. We will also teach you how to tell the difference between a good supplement and a bad one, and how to separate unfounded marketing hyperbole from sound nutritional advice. We suggest you read through Part One in its entirety.

In Part Two, we will present information on specific dietary supplements. We have drawn this information from a variety of sources, including those listed in the bibliography. Some of the information is based on recent scientific study and some is based on traditional and historic usage patterns. We have tried to indicate the degree of reliability when appropriate.

In Chapter 5, we provide information on individual nutrients and herbs. Representative products are provided as well, with educational and evaluative annotations when appropriate.

In Chapter 6, we provide a selection of popular combination remedies designed for specific health conditions. Representative products are listed, with ingredient information when possible.

The mention of specific products is for educational purposes only and is not an endorsement. Similar products are available from numerous additional sources. By providing you with examples and pointing out their strengths and deficiencies, we hope to enable you to make better decisions when evaluating which products to purchase on your own. To make it easier for you to find those products and categories that pertain to your personal needs, we have provided a "Therapeutic Cross-Reference" on page 297. Additional references and Internet links can be found on our website, www.bestsupplementsforyourhealth.com.

PART ONE

How to Choose and Use Supplements

CHAPTER ONE

Why Take Supplements

The mention of the term *nutritional supplement* can evoke strong and contradictory reactions from various groups of health professionals. To some, supplements are akin to snake oil, worthless and a total waste of money. Others promote nutritional supplements as the answer to almost every illness we face.

The truth lies somewhere between these two extremes. There was a time when mainstream medicine refused to acknowledge any role for diet in the prevention and treatment of cancer and heart disease. Now, this is a cornerstone of their official positions. There was a time when conventional physicians dismissed any use of supplements with disdain. Now, doctors are being encouraged to learn more about the therapeutic use of vitamins, herbs, and other complementary remedies. There was a time when it was nearly impossible to find well-controlled, scientific studies on the use of supplements in treating health problems. Now, studies are being published in the most highly respected medical journals in America and ongoing research is being funded by the National Institutes of Health. Even the American Dietetic Association, which historically has been vehemently antisupplement, has moderated its position in recent years.

What exactly is a nutritional supplement? A narrow definition might be a nutrient, or nutrients, in a form other than as it occurs in food—that is, in a capsule, tablet, concentrate, and so forth. Thus, a tablet containing vitamin C would clearly fall under the definition of a nutritional supplement. But what about a tablet that contains brewer's-type yeast? Or a soy protein powder? Or amino acids, such as lysine, glutamine, or carnitine? Or acidophilus? Or digestive enzymes?

Obviously, a broader definition is needed, one that includes a wide variety of food factors, nutrients, and other natural agents that support normal body function and contribute to good health. From a regulatory standpoint, any natural substance intended for oral use but not intended to cure, treat, or mitigate disease might be called a nutritional supplement.

In this book, we will adopt the broadest of definitions. This adheres to the common perception and can include everything from vitamins to herbs, and enzymes to homeopathic remedies.

Reasons for Taking Supplements

Why bother with supplements at all? According to some, all we have to do is eat the right foods, properly prepared and selected according to the latest dietary pyramid guidelines. This will provide us with all the nutrients we need. If we get ill, there are drugs that will heal whatever ailment befalls us.

The fact is that few of us are able or willing to follow the recommended dietary guidelines. While it might be theoretically possible for an otherwise healthy person to get all of the nutrients needed from foods, most people do not even come close to achieving this goal. Numerous studies, many sponsored by the government, have confirmed the presence of various nutrient deficiencies in significant segments of the American population.

Nutritional supplements provide a way of alleviating this nutrient shortfall from foods. In some cases, it is now acknowledged that supplements may even be preferable to food. Those who need to increase their calcium intake, for example, may be better off taking an inexpensive, convenient calcium supplement than consuming a large amount of dairy products with their additional calories and fats.

In addition, many people have found that they feel better—have more energy, are more resistant to disease, etc.—when they take supplements. And others have found that supplements can actually provide drug-like therapeutic benefits.

There are three main reasons for taking supplements. First, supplements can help prevent nutritional deficiency diseases such as scurvy, beriberi, pellagra, and rickets. In developed countries, this is more a theoretical point than a practical one. Second, and more important to most of us, supplements can prevent subclinical deficiencies, promote optimal health and function, prevent disease, and retard the aging process. And third, supplements can actually be used therapeutically, like drugs, to treat and reverse various health problems, often without the toxicity and side effects associated with stronger pharmaceuticals. Let's examine each of these reasons in more detail.

Supplements Can Prevent Nutritional Deficiency Diseases

Vitamins are called vitamins because they are essential for life and must be obtained from sources outside the body. In other words, these nutrients—vitamins, minerals, water, amino acids (protein), etc.—cannot be synthesized within the body. They must be obtained from the food we eat. Without an ongoing supply of these essential nutrients, we will die.

When the body is deprived of one or more of these nutrients, the effect manifests itself in various and unique ways. Examples of these nutritional deficiency diseases are scurvy, pellagra, beriberi, and rickets.

The story of the discovery of the role of vitamin C in preventing scurvy is perhaps the best known. The symptoms of this disease include bleeding gums, easy and extensive bruising, wounds that do not heal, lethargy and depression, and joint pain. Before the nineteenth century, this was a disease of significant importance, occurring whenever fresh fruits and vegetables were unavailable for extended periods of time, such as during the winter or long sea voyages. It was not uncommon, for example, for one-half of the crew to die from scurvy on a long sea voyage. At one point, the British lost more sailors to scurvy than to warfare.

What seems obvious to us now—that the disease is caused by a nutrient deficiency—was not at all obvious to the people of that time. According to some accounts, it was explorers like Jacques Cartier who associated eating certain foods with curing these diseases. James Lind, a British physician, is usually credited with the first scientific proposal that scurvy was, in fact, caused by a nutrient deficiency. He reported in the mid-1700s that lemon juice would reverse the progression of the disease. It took some time, but eventually the British Navy provided lime juice to its sailors as a means of warding off this disease. It is for this reason that British sailors became known as "Limeys."

Eventually, the components of food responsible for preventing each of the deficiency diseases were identified and isolated. In the case of vitamin C, it was first identified by Albert Szent-Gyorgyi. In most cases, these essential nutrients can now be synthesized in the laboratory. And they can be provided in supplement form.

In the United States, full-blown nutritional deficiency diseases are now rare. Foods are often fortified with those vitamins and minerals most often lacking in our diets. Fresh foods of all types are available in the neighborhood supermarket throughout the year. And contrary to the way it was a few hundred years ago, we all know about the importance of vitamins and minerals. Taking a daily multivitamin is now an accepted practice, even if only as insurance to make sure we get the necessary levels of these critical nutrients.

But even though we live in a nation of plenty, we also live during a time when most Americans are strongly influenced by outside pressures—marketing, advertising, and the pursuit of pleasure. We know that eating broccoli and fruit is healthy, but we are bombarded with enticing images of meals consisting of a hamburger, fries, and a cola drink. It is difficult for the modern parent to resist the demand by their children for the fast foods and junk foods they see advertised on television. It is also difficult for working people to find the time to properly prepare healthy meals. Eating out is no less of a problem. In many restaurants, it is difficult to find an item on the menu that is not deep fried, full of salt, etc. After all, the more fat in the food, the better it tastes—and taste is what drives us, much more so than health considerations.

Supplements Can Ensure Optimal Health, Vitality, and Longevity

It is naive to think that either you have a deficiency of a particular vitamin or you don't. To exhibit the symptoms of a deficiency disease, you must have experienced a significant lack of intake for an extended period of time. What happens when you get enough of a vitamin to prevent full-blown clinical symptoms of deficiency, but not enough to ensure optimal health?

This lack of optimal intake of essential nutrients is the key problem facing most of us. Sure, we get enough vitamin C even in a poor diet to prevent scurvy. But are we getting enough vitamin C to prevent subclinical scurvy? Might we be less susceptible to periodontal disease, osteoarthritis, heart disease, fatigue, vascular disorders, and a whole range of disorders related directly or indirectly to collagen formation, immune function, metabolism, and oxidative damage if we ingested *optimal* levels of vitamin C (and other nutrients) rather than *minimal* levels?

A COMMENT FROM DR. ABEL

I always refer to what I call the wellness meter. First comes excellent health, then mild deficiency, then moderate degenerative chronic disease, then acute disease, and finally potential death. Western medicine is well prepared for chronic and acute disease, and potential death intervention. Eastern medicine, on the other hand, is used to managing disharmonies from the body and detecting subtle deficiencies. Those mild complaints that are ignored for so long are the same ones that may respond to very simple systems and to the incorporation of supplements into one's health protocol.

What is the optimal level? Nobody knows for sure. Remember, first, that the levels of essential nutrients recommended by the various governmental agencies and used on food labels are the amounts thought to be necessary to prevent deficiency diseases, not the amounts necessary for optimal health. And they are the amounts estimated necessary for groups, or averages, not for each individual.

This is important because each individual is unique and has different requirements for each nutrient. This concept—biochemical individuality—was emphasized by Dr. Roger Williams and is the reason that, whenever possible, an excess of nutrients should be used, allowing the body to utilize as much of each nutrient as it needs, discarding the excess. For the most part, this is easy to do because most nutrients are relatively nontoxic and inexpensive. The few exceptions—such as vitamin A, vitamin D, and iron—are well known, and responsible supplement manufacturers and health professionals are quick to caution consumers and patients about this.

Again, most of us are interested in optimal health, not the prevention of scurvy, beriberi, and pellagra. We want to increase our lifespan. We want not only to live longer, but also to remain healthy and vital as we age. We want to improve our chances of avoiding degenerative diseases such as cancer, Alzheimer's, heart disease, and osteoporosis. We don't want to catch colds so often. We don't want to struggle with arthritic pain, vision loss, and diabetes.

Even in our younger years, we increasingly struggle with problems such as fatigue, infertility, and stress. We want to enhance performance, whether in the workplace, the athletic field, or in the bedroom.

Using nutritional supplements to ensure optimal levels of the essential nutrients is an easy and logical way to achieve this goal. Equally important, of course, is to strive for a healthy, balanced diet, adequate exercise, and avoidance of detrimental practices such as smoking, excessive exposure to sun, and overeating.

Supplements Can Be Used Therapeutically

What is food? It is a substance consisting of protein, fat, carbohydrates, vitamins, and minerals—that is, nutrients, ingested and assimilated by the body to provide energy and to promote the growth, repair, and maintenance necessary for sustaining life. Supplements provide these same nutrients, but in concentrated or isolated form. The nutrients serve the same purpose, preventing life-threatening deficiencies and ensuring optimal function.

What is a drug? There are various definitions, but all of them boil down to "an agent that treats or prevents a disease or condition." Going even further, from a regulatory standpoint, the Food, Drug, and Cosmetic Act considers something a drug merely if there is a claim that it treats, cures, or ameliorates a disease associated with it.

Section 201(g) of the Federal Food, Drug, and Cosmetic Act defines drugs as "articles intended for use in the diagnosis, cure, mitigation, treatment, or prevention of disease in man or other animals" and "articles (other than food) intended to affect the structure or any function of the body of man or other animals (for example, articles intended for weight reduction)."

It is the intended use that determines whether an article is a drug. Thus, foods and cosmetics may also be subject to the drug requirements of the law if therapeutic claims are made for them.

A food, or a dietary supplement, when used to cure, mitigate or treat a disease, is no longer functioning as a food. Instead, at least legally, it is being used as a drug. Theoretically, then, if a doctor prescribes chicken soup to treat a cold, the chicken soup is a drug.

> ## A COMMENT FROM DR. ABEL
>
> Eighty percent of the Earth's human population uses a plant-based medical system. That means most people still use herbs and vitamins to combat their diseases without the benefit of sophisticated diagnostic testing and specific synthetic medications. There remain centuries-old traditions and medical systems. With the world becoming a global village, we are sharing remedies throughout the world and hybridizing our ways of preventing and treating disease. Hybridizing, or integrating, means that we are using the best of both worlds. To do this, we try to pick what is simple and natural as our first option, unless our disease is life threatening.

Interestingly enough, many nutritional supplements can function as drugs or therapeutic agents. When vitamin B_3 (niacin), for example, is taken as a supplement in the usual range of 20 to 50 milligrams, it is functioning as a nutrient. As a vitamin, it will prevent deficiency disease (pellagra), prevent subclinical deficiencies, and promote optimal metabolic function. But what happens when a person takes a dose of 500 milligrams of niacin two or three times a day? At this level, niacin is being used to treat coronary artery disease. It has been shown to be an effective agent in lowering elevated low-density lipoprotein (LDL) cholesterol and triglycerides, and raising high-density lipoprotein (HDL) cholesterol. At that dosage, it is functioning as a drug, not a nutrient.

Today, the therapeutic use of dietary supplements is both exciting and promising, not because this is something new—to the contrary, this is one of the oldest forms of medicine—but because many of these uses are now being validated by modern medicine.

Ginkgo biloba may delay the onset of Alzheimer's disease. Folic acid may prevent birth defects and, in conjunction with vitamins B_6 and B_{12}, lower the risk of heart disease. Saw palmetto has been shown to be an effective treatment for benign prostatic hyperplasia. Niacin is a powerful cholesterol-lowering agent. Alpha-lipoic acid may help in treating diabetic neuropathy. Various antioxidant vitamins and minerals may prevent macular degeneration.

Are Supplements Really Necessary?

Our body is like a machine, a very complex one. Compare it to an automobile engine. We can put high-quality motor oil or cheap oil into the engine. We can change the oil frequently or rarely. Even if we use low-quality oil and change it rarely, the engine will not seize up and fail. It will, on the other hand, wear more rapidly, lose power and efficiency, and most likely require frequent repairs and adjustments. With higher-quality oil, containing additives that enhance its function, changed frequently, the engine will run smoother, more powerfully, and longer.

In this analogy, the seizing up of the engine, or catastrophic failure, is similar to the development of clinical deficiency disease. Low-quality oil and poor maintenance will not cause catastrophic failure in the automobile engine, just as a less than optimal diet will not likely cause a full-blown clinical deficiency disease. But it will cause less than optimal function.

Ensuring that the engine runs well, runs long, and runs efficiently without requiring constant repair is similar to ensuring that our body is not suffering from a subclinical nutritional deficiency. For our body to function as efficiently as possible, for our immune system to function optimally, and for maximum longevity, we have to provide it with optimal levels of essential nutrients, not the minimal levels needed to prevent catastrophic breakdown, or seizing up of the engine.

Nutritional supplementation offers an effective way to provide optimal levels of vitamins, minerals, and all essential food factors that support optimal function. Optimal function, combined with the enhanced protective actions of antioxidant nutrients, leads to prevention.

When disease does strike, the choice of treatment should involve an evaluation of risk versus benefit. If more than one treatment is available, it makes sense to choose the one that is effective yet least toxic. It also makes sense to treat the underlying cause of the disease rather than only the symptoms. The therapeutic use of nutritional and herbal supplements, either alone or as adjuncts to drug treatments, is often more effective and less damaging than drugs alone.

Many of us take greater care of our automobile engine than we do of our own bodies. We are more concerned with what we feed our pets than with what we feed ourselves and our families. We take greater interest in the chemical composition of the fertilizer we spread on our lawns than we do in the composition of the foods we eat.

We are not helpless when it comes to fighting off cancer, Alzheimer's disease, heart disease, diabetes, and other degenerative disorders. A good-quality, balanced multivitamin and multimineral supplement, with adequate amounts of calcium and magnesium and extra antioxidants, is certainly not too difficult a pill to swallow! The potential benefit of even this basic supplement regimen is tremendous. The downside is minimal.

A COMMENT FROM DR. ABEL

I find that there is always a lag time between the introduction of new therapies to my medical colleagues and their acceptance. However, in the case of vitamins and nutrition, this really isn't new therapy. Vitamins have been found to be essential for nearly a century and recommended daily allowances (RDAs) have been established to protect against deficiency—but unfortunately, none has been set for maintaining health. Major vitamin studies are always newsworthy. In 2001, the Age Related Eye Disease Study (AREDS) confirmed that vitamins actually can protect against vision loss from macular degeneration. All of a sudden, every ophthalmologist who had earlier denied the value of nutritional prevention in eye health changed their minds. Many years earlier, other scientific studies had shown that 6 milligrams of lutein or 4 cups of spinach weekly will provide up to an 80 percent protection against this scourge of old age, macular degeneration.

Why Not Just Eat Right?

In the past, we were told that all we had to do was eat the right foods, properly prepared. Easier said than done. Guidelines are provided and repeatedly revised. We have food groups and pyramids, which are well meaning but of little relevance to the average person. For many, breakfast is a donut or muffin and coffee. Lunch may be a hot dog and cola from the corner street vendor. Dinner may be several beers and pizza, or a trip to the fast-food outlet for a burger, fries, and a soft drink. Most of the foods we are enticed to buy are nutrient-poor and laden with fat. They are heavily processed, which removes vital nutrients, and are loaded with sugar and salt.

In spite of the repeated insistence that diet should serve as our only source of nutrition, surveys repeatedly show that most Americans do not consume a well-balanced diet. About 11 percent of Americans are estimated to be deficient in folic acid, for example. Vitamin-B_6 deficiency is estimated to be present in between 10 to 25 percent of the population of the Western world. Mild vitamin-C deficiency is estimated for 6 percent of the general population. Roughly 6 to 14 percent of healthy adult Western European populations have been reported to be vitamin-D deficient. Another study recently reported that 27 percent of the U.S. population had low blood levels of vitamin E. Less than 10 percent of women in America get adequate calcium, and up to 25 percent of adult women are deficient in magnesium.

A report of the U.S. Senate Committee on Education and Labor stated that "85% of the older population has one or more chronic conditions that have been documented to benefit from nutrition interventions." According to the experts, 55 percent of Americans are overweight. It is said that 49 million Americans are totally sedentary. Diabetes has reached epidemic proportions. We know we have a serious problem and we have to accept the fact that telling people to ignore the advertising promoting unhealthy food and, instead, modify their eating habits to comply with the food pyramid is just not working.

A COMMENT FROM DR. ABEL

The McArthur Twins Study helped answer a very important question about nature versus nurture. People always thought that genes determine our medical future. In actuality, what we eat and our lifestyle may modify our health to a far greater extent. The McArthur Twins Study showed that 70 percent of the diseases that identical twins develop are based on their lifestyle and only 30 percent are determined by heredity.

Easier Said Than Done

Convenience and marketing pressures are not the only factors working against eating right. There are more subtle problems as well. What is right? We were told for quite some time, for example, that butter was unhealthy and margarine was the healthy alternative. A small group of nutritionists and complementary medicine proponents voiced concern about the presence of trans fatty acids in margarine. Only recently has it been acknowledged that these partially hydrogenated oils and spreads (margarine) may be dangerous.

Another example is eggs. Should we or shouldn't we? And what about milk? Is it the "perfect food" or something that should be avoided by humans, especially adults?

Just how healthy is much of the food we buy in the supermarket? Some of it is highly processed, and only a portion of the nutrients removed are replaced. Bread is a good example.

Is Food Really Best?

It may be politically correct to assert that it is always best to get the nutrients we need from food, but in fact, that is not always the case. There are times when nutrients in supplement form are actually more efficiently used by the body than nutrients in food form.

Folic acid is a good example. Folic acid has generated a great deal of attention because of its role in preventing certain types of birth defects and in lowering homocysteine levels. Elevated homocysteine is considered to be a risk marker for heart disease and Alzheimer's disease. It turns out that folic acid, when taken in supplement form and on an empty stomach, is twice as effective as folate in food.

Another problem with food involves processing and contaminants. Quite often, the nutrient content of foods is significantly depleted during processing. The nutrient density is further reduced by the addition of flavoring, processing, and the use of stabilizing agents. Too many foods are no longer what they seem. Instead of drinking fruit juice, we drink concentrate or flavoring in a solution of sugar and coloring. Instead of whole-fruit jam, we use jelly, which is mostly sugar. Instead of cheese, we use cheese spread.

A careful reading of the ingredient listing on food labels reveals an increasing tendency to mislead the consumer about the growing presence of not-so-healthy components. Use of ingredient names such as "dehydrated grape juice" instead of "sugar," for example, is an attempt to mislead the consumer into thinking there is less sugar in the product.

Concern over the increased contamination of foods with pesticide residues, antibiotics, and hormones has resulted in a rapid growth of so-called organic foods.

Whatever the reason, there seems to be an increasing problem with food allergies. For many people, eating a balanced diet has become very difficult because of their inability to tolerate certain foods. The same can be said for people who are frequently on weight loss diets. When reducing caloric intake, the difficulty of maintaining adequate nutrient levels is magnified.

Theoretically Yes, But Practically? No!

Eating right remains a noble goal. But problems with our food supply, lifestyle, and advertising pressures, as well as with reduced intake due to weight loss diets and allergies, make this more difficult than it might seem at first glance.

A COMMENT FROM Dr. ABEL

It is now recognized that many common medications may deplete our cells of necessary vitamins. Ross Pelton, R.Ph., wrote the *Drug Induced, Nutrient Depletion Handbook,* which provides amazing information about drugs that we thought were safe. It appears that artificial estrogens (birth control pills) deplete riboflavin, pyridoxine, folic acid, B_{12}, vitamin C, and zinc. Furthermore, oral contraceptive use results in increased vitamin K, iron, and copper. Vitamin K can increase bleeding, and iron and copper are both prooxidants. Therefore, women taking contraceptive agents should recognize the potential increase of blood coagulation and should maintain the necessary nutrients to counteract this. Drugs, such as the statin family of drugs that reduce cholesterol, also decrease the production of CoQ_{10} and possibly glutathione in the liver. Consumption of sugar-laden soft drinks during the formative teenage years increases urinary calcium excretion and decreases the amount of calcium laid down in bone. People who drink a lot of soft drinks in their teens and twenties are more prone to osteoporosis and fractures in their later years.

It should also be pointed out that we consume fewer calories today than our ancestors did and that our needs for protective nutrients, at the same time, may be greater. We are exposed today to levels of pollution and radiation that place additional burdens on our body's defense systems. We live longer than our ancestors did. Maximizing bone density to prevent osteoporosis may have been less of a concern when the average woman lived only to 50 rather than to 80. To rely only on the myth of a balanced diet to provide us with optimal levels of protective nutrients is impractical given the realities of our environment at this time.

The elderly, as a group, are now considered to be at high nutritional risk. Some have actually gone so far as to propose that what we consider normal signs of aging may actually instead be symptoms of inadequate nutrition.

We have actually reached the point now where even the most conservative nutritionist is acknowledging that there are times when supplements are necessary, even to provide the recommended daily intake of essential nutrients. The National Academy of Sciences, Institute of Medicine, Food and Nutrition Board, has recently increased the recommended daily intake level of vitamin C, for example, to 150 percent of its previous level—90 milligrams daily rather than the previous recommendation of 60 milligrams.

And the recommended intake of calcium has been raised as well, with an admission by the agency that it may be appropriate, or necessary, to use calcium supplements to achieve that level. An acknowledgment of the necessity for using a supplement to satisfy part of the daily nutrient requirement would have been unheard of in years past.

CHAPTER TWO

How to Choose the Right Supplement

Choosing a supplement is not always easy. Which supplements do you need? How do you choose a quality supplement? How should the supplement be taken? Is a capsule better than a tablet? Is there any potential interaction between the supplement and your medications?

There are many choices to be made, some of which are highly individual and related to personal preference. Others require some knowledge of chemistry and physiology, and an ability to differentiate marketing hyperbole from fact. Your personal health problems and needs have to be considered. The information that follows will help you with these decisions.

Choosing the right supplements can be broken down into four steps:

1. Choosing the right type of supplement for you.
2. Choosing supplements tailored to your unique health problems and needs.
3. Choosing the specific brand or product to purchase.
4. Incorporating these choices into a comprehensive program tailored to your needs.

Step One: Choosing the Right Type of Supplement

Tablets and Capsules

Many people think that capsules are superior to tablets because they dissolve better or have fewer additives. This is not correct. A properly manufactured tablet will work just as well as a capsule. The so-called superiority of capsules in this regard is a myth propagated by some companies selling encapsulated supplements.

Theoretically, there may be times when a capsule could contain fewer additives, but this is true only in certain instances. Such a claim must be evaluated on a product-by-product basis and should be verified by full-disclosure labeling. In addition, you should take into account the composition of the capsule itself, which can contain additives as well. Is this really cause for concern? We will answer that question in the next section.

The main factor that should influence this decision is actually ease of swallowing. For many people, it is easier to swallow a capsule. Once it becomes wet, many feel that it slides down more easily. Others prefer tablets. This is purely a personal decision.

One advantage of tablets is that they are usually less expensive than capsules. It costs less to manufacture a tablet than it does a capsule. For those on a tight budget, it usually makes sense to buy tablets. Also, you can squeeze a greater amount of material into a tablet than a capsule. When we discuss multivitamin products later in the book, you will see that the same formula that requires four tablets will require six capsules.

In some cases, an encapsulated product may be more stable than a tablet. If the ingredients are subject to oxidation or are sensitive to moisture, the capsule may offer some additional protection, although tablets can be coated, which also can serve as a protective barrier. This is rarely significant when making your choice. Proper storage is more important. One example, however, where this protective function does come into play is with essential oils such as flaxseed oil. When buying oil, you will notice that it must be kept refrigerated. This is because oil is easily oxidized. But when flaxseed oil is put into soft gelatin capsules, refrigeration is not necessary because the capsule protects the oil from contact with air.

Both tablets and capsules, if manufactured by a responsible company, will be tested for disintegration and dissolution. These are standardized tests, provided for in the United States Pharmacopeia (USP), that show whether or not the product will dissolve and release its active ingredients after being swallowed.

The key here is a responsible company. Theoretically, it is probably easier to make a bad tablet than it is to make a bad capsule. If the tableting process is not done properly and is not carefully monitored, and if the tablet is not formulated properly, a tablet that does not dissolve could be produced. It could be too hard, for example. If the company does not adequately test the tablets, they might not dissolve properly. If you buy products only from reputable companies, this should not be a concern, but if you insist on buying cheap products from questionable sources, you might want to stick with capsules.

Do not be misled by those who tell you to test a tablet by placing it in a glass of water or vinegar. This is not a valid test. The proper testing procedure for disintegration involves much more than this. A tablet may appear to disintegrate in a glass of water or vinegar, but that does not mean the active ingredients have dissolved. This requires a separate test, called the dissolution test, which determines if the ingredients actually dissolve and become available for absorption. And on the other hand, a tablet that does not appear to dissolve in a glass of water may very well dissolve under the proper testing procedures.

Disintegration is actually a measure of how completely a tablet or capsule breaks into small pieces so that its nutrient ingredients can more readily dissolve and be absorbed. A specified apparatus must be used that agitates the tablets or capsules in a measured up-and-down motion in water maintained at a temperature of 37° C.

The dissolution test, on the other hand, is a measure of how fast and completely a vitamin or mineral substance *dissolves*. If the tablet or capsule does not dissolve, its nutrient ingredients cannot be absorbed into the body to do their work. This test involves placing the samples in 0.1 normal hydrochloric acid for one hour, stirring constantly. Six separate samples of the solution are withdrawn during the test period, filtered, and analyzed for vitamin content. To pass, not less than 75 percent of the labeled vitamin content must have dissolved within the one-hour test period.

A vitamin supplement can *disintegrate* quite nicely, then, but still fail the *dissolution* test. In other words, disintegration does not guarantee dissolution or absorption.

In the past, capsules were made primarily of gelatin, an animal product. If you were a vegetarian, or if your religious beliefs forbade the ingestion of animal products, you were pretty much limited to tableted products. While tablets can also contain animal products, it was easier to avoid them when desired. Now, however, vegetarian capsules are available. Kosher and vegetarian supplements can now be obtained in capsules as well as in tablets.

For those who have a problem swallowing any type of solid dosage form, a capsule may offer some advantage. A two-piece hard capsule can be opened and the contents emptied into juice or food. A soft gel capsule can be pricked with a pin and the contents, again, added to food. This may be easier and more convenient than physically crushing a tablet.

THE PHARMACIST SAYS

According to the USP, the disintegration does not imply complete solution of the tablet or capsule, or even of its active constituent. It is defined "as that state in which any residue of the unit, except fragments of insoluble coating or capsule shell, remaining on the screen of the test apparatus is a soft mass having no palpable firm core."

Powders and Liquids

Certain types of supplements lend themselves inherently to the powder or liquid form. Powdered protein and meal-replacement supplements are designed to be mixed with liquids and then administered as a drink. Certain fiber supplements are available as powders, capsules, and tablets. The amount of fiber needed after the initial acclimation period is usually higher than can be conveniently provided by capsules (you would need to take too many capsules), so the powder form is preferred. But for traveling or when eating out, the convenience of capsule fiber supplements may be desirable.

Vitamin supplements are available in powder form as well and a full description of this type of product, along with representative product samples, can be found in Chapter 6.

Theoretically, powdered vitamin supplements should be more economical than tablets or capsules, as one less manufacturing operation is involved in their production.

Liquid vitamin and mineral supplements are available as well, but there are several limitations associated with products of this type. The main problem is stability. In liquid form, the various substances can readily interact with one another. This is why you often find vitamins and minerals in separate products. There is also the problem of taste. To make the product palatable, it is usually necessary to add flavorings and sweeteners to the liquid product. If it is necessary to use a liquid product (for example, for children or for those who cannot swallow tablets or capsules and do not want to be bothered with crushing tablets or emptying capsules), then do so. But read the label carefully. Refer to Chapter 6 for more information.

Hypoallergenic Supplements

Usually, natural supplements are considered preferable over synthetic products. But for those with food allergies or, more often the case, food sensitivities, this may not be the case. Hypoallergenic supplements contain minimal amounts of additives and may utilize synthetic sources of nutrients rather than natural sources. A good example is dl-alpha tocopheryl acetate, which is used rather than the natural d-alpha or mixed tocopherol form of vitamin E.

Hypoallergenic supplements avoid the most common allergens (wheat, dairy, corn, egg, soy). But you cannot rely totally on the term *hypoallergenic*. You must read the ingredient listing.

Allergies

Many people claim they are allergic to certain vitamins or minerals. Hogwash. You cannot be allergic to vitamins or minerals. A vitamin by definition is essential. In other words, you will die without it. If you are alive, you have the various vitamins throughout your body, and you must continue to ingest additional amounts if you want to remain alive.

If you were truly allergic to a vitamin or mineral, therefore, you would be dead.

Rather, you may be allergic, or hypersensitive, to certain components of vitamin supplements. There is a big difference. First, *hypersensitive* is a much broader, more encompassing term than *allergic*. You can be hypersensitive to a B-complex supplement because you cannot tolerate the aftertaste. You can be hypersensitive to vitamin-C supplements because you have a very sensitive stomach. You can be hypersensitive to vitamin-A supplements because belching up fish oil makes you nauseous. That is not an allergy. If you were allergic to fish protein, on the other hand, taking vitamin A from fish oil or cod liver oil could certainly be a problem. If you were allergic to soy oil, taking a vitamin-E softgel could certainly be a problem. But in each case, you are not allergic to the vitamin. You are allergic or hypersensitive to another ingredient that accompanies the vitamin. If you take a form of the vitamin that does not have that other ingredient, you will not have the problem.

Twinlab has a vitamin-A product (Allergy A Caps), for example, that is designed for people who are allergic to fish and fish oil. Allergy Research Group has a hypoallergenic vitamin-E product that contains dl-alpha tocopheryl acetate, the synthetic form of vitamin-E, which is soy-free.

Additives

Tablets and capsules contain various excipients—diluents, binders, flow agents, disintegrants—that facilitate the manufacturing process, enhance disintegration, and increase stability. These are, by law, generally recognized as safe (GRAS) food additives and present in very small quantities.

Think about this: A small capsule will hold about 400 milligrams of powder (depending on the density of the powder). We have a product that consists of 3 milligrams of melatonin. We cannot put only 3 milligrams of powder into a capsule large enough to hold 400 milligrams. Instead, we have to mix the 3 milligrams of melatonin with enough diluent to take up the remaining space in the capsule. This also improves the accuracy of measuring the melatonin, as it is much easier to accurately measure 400 milligrams (of a 0.75-percent dilution) than 3 milligrams. The same holds true for vitamin B_{12}.

The diluent is inert and hypoallergenic. It could be purified microcrystalline cellulose, for example, or dicalcium phosphate. Years ago, lactose was a common diluent, but because of potential problems for those who are lactose intolerant, it is no longer used in the dietary-supplement industry.

So for many products, especially those where the dosage is small, it is impractical, if not impossible, to avoid using some type of diluent. This is a problem for tablets just as it is for capsules. You will not find a capsule small enough to contain 3 milligrams of melatonin and nothing more.

Another commonly used additive is silicon dioxide, which functions as a drying agent or flow agent. To manufacture tablets or capsules, the powder must flow from the storage hopper into the tableting or capsule-filling cavity. If the powder becomes sticky or clumpy, it will not flow smoothly and consistently. Is anything wrong with silicon dioxide? Not at all. Silicon is an essential trace mineral and is often recommended as a supplement, especially for hair, skin, nail, and bone health.

To enhance the flow of the powder, lubricant additives are also commonly used. The best-known tablet lubricant is a combination of stearic acid and magnesium stearate. The only valid complaint against these was the fact that they were derived from animal products. For this reason, vegetable alternatives were developed and are now used almost exclusively in the dietary-supplement industry.

It is important to understand also that these agents are used in very small quantities. And they are used in the dietary-supplement industry only when absolutely necessary. This is not so much because of any real danger, but more because of the public's perception that additives are undesirable.

There is one exception. One question that often comes up is, "What is the difference between drugstore or mass-market vitamin supplements and health-food brands?" There is a difference. In the pharmaceutical industry, little restraint is exercised in the use of additives. Artificial colors will be added, for example, merely to make the tablet look nice. A synthetic vitamin may be used because it is less expensive, with little regard for other factors.

Natural Supplements

Many years ago, the term *natural* was an important part of dietary-supplement and health-food appeal. But today, it is somewhat overrated. Nobody knows what *natural* really signifies when it comes to dietary supplements, and the marketing folks have so overused it that it has become almost meaningless. With few exceptions, there is no legal definition.

There are, however, instances when *natural* is very important. The best example of this is vitamin E. Natural vitamin E may actually be twice as potent, or biologically active, as synthetic vitamin E!

When *Natural* Makes a Difference

Vitamin E is actually not a single entity. From a labeling standpoint, we only look at alpha-tocopherol content when declaring the potency of vitamin E on a dietary-supplement or food label. But there are actually seven other members of the vitamin E family—three more tocopherols and four tocotrienols. All eight of these compounds are present in the natural vitamin E found in food, but only one—the alpha tocopherol—is found in some supplements.

The reason for this is that the Food and Drug Administration (FDA) continues to use outdated nomenclature. Many years ago, the only method available to measure the potency of vitamin E involved its ability to affect the fertility of rats. Using this one measure of vitamin-E activity, the alpha tocopherol form was determined to be the most active of the eight components. The amount of alpha tocopherol was assumed to be most important, therefore, and was used as the measure of its potency, in International Units (IUs). This led to two problems.

First, it turns out that while alpha tocopherol may be most active in preventing reproductive problems in rats, the other components of vitamin E are more active in other areas. The tocotrienols, for example, seem to be more valuable in preventing certain heart-disease problems than the tocopherols. Synthetic vitamin E contains none of the seven other components. The potency on the label (400 IU) refers *only* to the amount of alpha tocopherol. A natural, mixed-tocopherols vitamin-E supplement will provide much more benefit than one that contains only alpha tocopherol, even if the IUs are the same.

Second, the synthetic form of vitamin E, identified on labels as *dl-alpha tocopherol*, is less active than the natural form of vitamin E, identified on labels as *d-alpha tocopherol*. Notice that the difference is the prefix *dl-* or *d-*, with *dl-* indicating synthetic and the *d-* the natural form. Now, it has always been known that synthetic dl-alpha tocopherol is less active than natural *d*-alpha tocopherol. It was thought that the d- form was 36 percent more active than the dl- form, and for this reason, for labeling purposes, the FDA established the following rule: 1 gram of natural vitamin E is equivalent to 1.36 grams of synthetic vitamin E.

What does this mean? It means that if you have 100 milligrams of natural vitamin E (d-alpha tocopherol) in one product and 136 milligrams of synthetic vitamin E (dl-alpha tocopherol) in another product, they would both be labeled as containing 100 IU of vitamin E. And therefore, they would be equal in potency, as both indicate 100 IU of vitamin E (even though they contain different amounts of actual vitamin E).

Or would they? It turns out, based on more sophisticated analytical testing, the 1-to-1.36 equivalency figure is inaccurate. Instead of being 36 percent more active, natural d-alpha tocopherol is double the activity of synthetic dl-alpha tocopherol.

Synthetic vitamin E, therefore, is inferior to natural vitamin E mixed tocopherols for two reasons: dl-alpha tocopherol is less potent than natural, d-alpha tocopherol and synthetic vitamin E does not contain all eight of the naturally occurring components of vitamin E.

When *Natural* Does Not Make a Difference

In most cases, there is no difference between natural and synthetic vitamins. In fact, much to the surprise of many consumers, you could not put natural vitamins into most supplements even if you wanted to. It is just not possible.

Yes, vitamins and minerals occur naturally in food. But the quantities are very small. When taking supplements, we are accustomed to potencies that would be impossible to obtain from natural vitamins in food concentrates. To get 500 milligrams of vitamin C and 10 milligrams of the various B vitamins from natural sources would require a tablet the size of a football.

With a few exceptions—such as vitamin E, natural beta-carotene, and vitamin B_{12}—all of the vitamins used in dietary supplements are synthetic. Regardless of what your local health-food store clerk or multilevel marketing zealot tells you, it's a fact. And it's also a fact that these synthetic vitamins are identical to their natural counterparts. To get high potencies of vitamins and minerals in a dietary supplement, synthetic or highly processed vitamins and minerals must be used.

You cannot have it both ways. High-potency vitamin levels in a product are always the result of added synthetic vitamins. Products without high potencies, on the other hand, are another story. A product that consists of or contains food concentrates will of course contain the natural vitamins native to that food. Many foods contain up to 90 percent moisture, so when dehydrated, their vitamin content can be increased up to tenfold. But this will still not provide the high potencies we have come to expect in our nutritional supplements.

Why not, you might ask, isolate the pure natural vitamin from the food? The answer is that it is totally impractical, prohibitively expensive, and serves no purpose because you would then end up with a pure vitamin that is identical to the synthetic one.

Misleading Claims and False Labeling

Here is one example of the type of intentionally misleading activity that used to be common in the dietary-supplement industry. Companies wanted to capitalize on the appeal of natural vitamins, so they attempted to find a way to make it seem that the vitamins in their product were natural.

For example, companies that manufactured bulk brewer's-type yeast supplied several types of modified yeast. A type that was of interest to the dietary-supplement industry was fortified brewer's-type yeast. This product contained regular brewer's-type yeast with added quantities of B-complex vitamins, giving it a final vitamin concentration that was many times higher than regular brewer's yeast.

The label on the bulk drum of fortified yeast would merely say something like "Fortified Yeast, Type T6361." There would also be a small sticker on the drum with the actual ingredient listing. The listing would read: "Brewer's-type yeast, thiamine hydrochloride, riboflavin, pyridoxine hydrochloride, ascorbic acid." And the specification sheet that accompanied the product would provide the potency of the various B vitamins in the final product.

The dietary-supplement manufacturer would buy this "fortified" yeast and add it to the product. The potencies of the B vitamins would be listed on the label, but the only ingredient included in the ingredient listing would be the brewer's-type yeast. The consumer, when reading the product label, would mistakenly assume that the B vitamins were natural, derived from the yeast, when in fact they were synthetic vitamins that had been added to the fortified-yeast raw material before it was added to the final product.

It is a shame that the consumer can so often be misled by marketing hype embellished with deliberate obscurities and buzzwords. In the case of fortified yeast used to mislead buyers into thinking vitamins are natural, the practice is no longer common—due, perhaps, not so much to a resurgence of moral conscience as to the fact that yeast is no longer viewed as a desirable health food because of its (perhaps undeserved) association with Candida infections.

Instead, variations of the same approach seem to have emerged in the past few years, usually associated with vitamins that are grown or cultured in some way.

How Do You Read a Supplement Label?

Take a good look at the sample label below. It will help you become more familiar with the basic information on a supplement label.

Serving size is the manufacturer's suggested serving expressed in the appropriate unit (tablet, capsule, softgel, packet, teaspoonful).

Amount Per Serving heads the listing of nutrients contained in the supplement, followed by the quantity present in each serving.

International Unit (IU) is a standard unit of measure for fat soluble vitamins (A, D, and E).

Milligram (mg) and microgram (mcg) are units of measurement for water-soluble vitamins (C and B complex) and minerals. A milligram is equal to .001 gram. A microgram is equal to .001 milligram.

The list of all ingredients includes nutrients and other ingredients used to formulate the supplement, in decreasing order by weight.

All supplements should be stored in a cool, dry place in their original containers, out of the reach of children, and should be used before the expiration date to assure full potency.

Supplement Facts
Serving Size 1 tablet

Amount Per Serving	% Daily Value
Vitamin A 5000 IU	
50% as Beta Carotene	100%
Vitamin C 250 mg	417%
Vitamin D 400 IU	100%
Vitamin E 200 IU	667%
Thiamin 5 mg	333%
Riboflavin 5 mg	294%
Niacin 20 mg	100%
Vitamin B_6 5 mg	250%
Folate 0.4 mg	100%
Vitamin B_{12} 6 mcg	100%
Biotin 150 mcg	50%
Pantothenic Acid 10 mg	100%
Calcium 200 mg	20%
Iron 18 mg	100%
Phosphorus 200 mg	20%
Iodine 150 mcg	100%
Selenium 35 mcg	50%
Magnesium 200 mcg	50%
Zinc 15 mg	100%
Copper 2 mg	100%
Boron 150 mcg	*

* Daily Value not established

Ingredients: vitamin A acetate, beta-carotene, vitamin D, dl-alpha tocopherol acetate, ascorbic acid, thiamin mononitrate, riboflavin, niacinamide, pyridoxine hydrochloride, vitamin b-12, biotin, d-calcium pantothenate, potassium chloride, dicalcium phosphate, potassium iodine, ferrous fumarate, magnesium oxide, copperr sulfate, zinc oxide, manganese sulfate, sodium selenate, chromium chloride, sodium molybdate, microcrystalline cellulose, calcium carbonate, sodium carbomethylcellulose.

Storage: Keep tightly closed in dry place; do not expose to excessive heat.

KEEP OUT OF REACH OF CHILDREN

Expiration date: 0 6 / 2 0 0 3
Manufacturer's or distributor's name, address, and zip code

Percent Daily Value (DV) tells what percentage of the recommended daily intake for each nutrient for adults and children ages 4 and up is provided by the supplement.

An asterisk under the "Percent Daily Value" heading indicates that a Daily Value is not established for that nutrient.

The manufacturer's or distributor's name, address, and zip code are required to appear on the label.

Reprinted by permission of the Council for Responsible Nutrition.

Not Necessarily a Bad Thing

Now, there is no question but that taking a vitamin supplement with natural food concentrates and extracts is preferable. And we would have no complaint with a company that made the claim that its natural product was superior because it contained a significant amount of phytonutrient-rich food concentrates. There are many other components in food that are beneficial—the flavonoids, for example, in addition to the vitamins and minerals.

What we object to, however, is the implication that somehow this process has transformed the vitamins themselves into something else, something superior to synthetic vitamins. Just as we cannot turn lead into gold, we cannot change the molecular structure of a vitamin by co-drying it in a slurry of food concentrate or yeast cells.

This is important because such claims can actually get out of hand and cause health threats. Here are two recent examples.

When is 100 milligrams of calcium equivalent to 1,000 milligrams? If you were told that a certain product containing 100 milligrams of calcium in a special food-grown, or cultured, form was equivalent to 1,000 milligrams of calcium in a conventional supplement, would you believe it? Should women be misled into thinking that taking this product would be sufficient to protect them from osteoporosis?

Similarly, think back to the colloidal-mineral boom of a few years ago. There was a lot of hype about how itsy-bitsy, teensy-weensy quantities of minerals in a diluted colloidal suspension were somehow more biologically active and better absorbed than conventional minerals. Who cares? When you got down to the facts, all you had were itsy-bitsy, teensy-weensy (to use the technical terminology) amounts, and even if they were all absorbed, you still had only itsy-bitsy, teensy-weensy amounts! The danger was that people took these products instead of taking proper mineral supplements, thinking they were satisfying their mineral-supplement requirements.

Cheap Products

Much of the advice regarding cheap products is based primarily on common sense. If something seems too good to be true, it most likely is just that—too good to be true. If a product sells for around $10.00 a bottle from all of the well-known companies, should you buy a bottle from a lesser-known company that sells for $2.50?

When demand for a supplement is high, the amount sold to consumers often exceeds the amount manufactured. How can that be?

The answer must be that not every bottle contains what the label says it does.

Assurance of quality is essential. But it costs money. If you decide to buy a product that is suspiciously inexpensive, you may be getting exactly what you pay for.

Kosher and Vegetarian Supplements

What about people who because of religious or moral beliefs seek out products that are labeled as kosher or vegetarian? Such products are available and may be appropriate for those who need them. Some may be seeking out such products for the wrong reason, however, and getting something other than what they think.

A product labeled as vegetarian, or suitable for vegetarians, would be expected to contain no animal products. Does that mean it contains no milk or dairy foods? Does it mean that it contains no ingredients derived from meat, fish, or dairy products? Does it mean that a person who is allergic to milk protein can safely use the product?

A product labeled as kosher would be expected to contain no ingredients derived from those foods that are prohibited in the Bible. For those who are strict in their beliefs, this prohibition is carried to great lengths, and extensive precautions must be taken to ensure that no contamination with nonkosher materials takes place.

For the strictly observant, reading the ingredients on the label is not enough. The product must contain a special seal of approval by one of several rabbinical organizations whose duty it is to inspect and monitor the manufacturing process for total compliance with the kosher guidelines.

Third-party intervention in this instance can be helpful because it is not always easy to tell from the ingredient listing whether or not an item is meat- or dairy-free. Some people might not realize, for example, that gelatin is derived from animal tissue. They might not realize that capsules, unless the label says otherwise, are made with gelatin.

While that may seem obvious, what about stearic acid and magnesium stearate? These are not so obvious. These two ingredients are often used in tablets and capsules in very small amounts as excipients. Stearic acid is usually derived from animal fat.

In each of these instances, non–animal-derived alternatives are available. There are vegetable stearates and nongelatin capsules available. You have to read the label carefully to ascertain which is being used in any given product.

If you have food allergies, you need to exert extra care. The label on a nondairy creamer is a good example. Can anyone be blamed for thinking that *nondairy* would mean the product contains no milk or milk-derived ingredients? The fact is that most nondairy creamers contain as one of their key ingredients sodium caseinate, a milk derivative.

But what about kosher products? Can you assume that a product is free of certain ingredients because it is certified kosher? The answer is no, and this may surprise many people. Shellfish (lobster, oysters, crab) are not kosher. Glucosamine, a popular nutritional supplement, is derived from shellfish. How, then, can a product containing glucosamine be certified as kosher?

Apparently it can be. In an attempt to get an explanation, we contacted one of the kosher certification groups, but were refused an explanation. We found this very disturbing. We can only speculate, then, as to what the reasoning may be, and our best guess is that the ingredient is sufficiently processed such that it, at least from a religious standpoint, no longer shares the properties of the starting material.

THE PHARMACIST SAYS

Another potential pitfall is the reliance on the term *pareve* on kosher foods to indicate "milk-free." If you are allergic to milk, a product labeled *pareve* can satisfy kosher dietary law requirements for "milk-free," but may still contain enough milk protein to cause a problem for milk-allergic individuals.

Step Two: Considering Your Unique Health Requirements

We have explained the role of supplements in preventing overt clinical deficiency diseases (scurvy, pellagra, rickets, beriberi). And we have pointed out that there is a difference between *adequate* and *optimal* when it comes to the amounts needed to ensure good health, vitality, and longevity.

A balanced multivitamin blend, with extra calcium and magnesium, may be all that is needed. In addition, an antioxidant blend would be a good idea. This may be enough to help prevent health problems, fight off disease, and retard the aging process.

But what if you already have a health problem? Or if you are at high risk to various diseases? You may have a family history of heart disease, glaucoma, diabetes, or cancer, for example. Or your lab tests show you have elevated LDL cholesterol. Perhaps your blood pressure is high. Or you are overweight and smoke cigarettes.

There are many situations (pregnancy, illness, stress, old age) that create additional nutritional needs, and there are diseases that can benefit from the therapeutic and healing actions of vitamins, minerals, and herbs. Your supplement program has to be modified to accommodate these additional problems. We will examine some examples in this section and then, in the next section, show you how to incorporate the prophylactic and therapeutic aspects of supplementation into an effective and comprehensive program.

Heart Disease

Cardiovascular disease in the leading cause of death in the United States. If you have a family history of heart disease or if you have elevated cholesterol, elevated LDL cholesterol, high blood pressure, or elevated homocysteine, you should consider using dietary supplements to control the condition or lower your risk.

Folic acid, vitamin B_{12}, and vitamin B_6 have been shown to lower homocysteine levels. Elevated homocysteine is thought to be a specific risk factor for heart disease. Supplementing with extra amounts of these harmless, inexpensive B vitamins may significantly lower your risk of heart disease.

Elevated cholesterol is another risk factor for heart disease. Supplementing with water-soluble fiber supplements (oat bran, psyllium, guar gum, pectin) can lower cholesterol. Many herbs (gum guggul, fenugreek, garlic) can lower cholesterol. Certain plant-derived substances, phytosterols and phytostanols, are very effective. Vitamins such as niacin and pantethine can lower cholesterol. The antioxidant vitamins can prevent the oxidation of LDL cholesterol. A combination of these nutrients and herbs can be as effective as drugs for many people, without the side effects.

Hypertension can sometimes be controlled with supplements. CoQ_{10}, fish oils (EPA, DHA), calcium, garlic, hawthorn, coleus, European mistletoe, and olive leaf extract are some that have been used with success.

Those with cardiac arrhythmia should definitely consider extra magnesium in their supplement program. Those with angina should add additional CoQ_{10} and L-carnitine.

Several studies have found supplementation with 400 to 800 IU of natural vitamin E to be of general benefit to those with heart disease.

Eye and Vision Problems

Cataracts are the result of oxidative damage to the lens of the eye. Those at risk to cataract formation should definitely take additional vitamin B_2 (riboflavin), vitamin C, carotenoids, and other antioxidants.

A COMMENT FROM DR. ABEL

The eye is a bag of water with two lenses: the outer lens is the clear cornea and the inner lens is the crystalline lens of the eye, supported by fibers connected to the circular muscle inside the eye. The inner lens has neither nerves nor blood vessels, and depends on the fluid inside the eye for nourishment. When the proteins in the inner lens break down, opacities form. These are known as cataracts.

What can be done to protect against cataracts?

- *Drink plenty of water.* Try to consume at least six glasses daily.
- *Wear ultraviolet (UV) protective sunglasses.* UV light breaks down the proteins in the lens, accelerating the formation of cataracts.
- *Take supplemental vitamin C.* Vitamin C is a major antioxidant in the lens. Studies show that vitamin C reduces the risk of cataracts by up to 77 percent. Other antioxidant nutrients, such as vitamin E, lutein, glutathione, n-acetyl cysteine (NAC), and alpha-lipoic acid, impart similar benefits.
- *Take supplemental glutathione.* Glutathione, in particular, a cell-membrane antioxidant and enzyme, is extremely important in maintaining the clarity of the lens.
- *Reduce your fat intake.* Dietary fat and obesity are associated with increased risk of cataracts. Therefore, you should make every effort to eat wisely.
- *Increase your intake of the omega-3 fatty acids.* Veterinary

studies have shown that the omega-3 fatty acids, most notably DHA, are in the lens fibers and are important in stabilizing cell membranes.

- *Watch your sugar and alcohol intake.* Elevated blood sugar levels and large amounts of alcohol can damage lens protein. Minimize your risk of diabetes and drink moderately.
- *Don't smoke.* Experts have estimated that as many as 20 percent of cataracts are related to smoking alone.
- *Relax.* Stress stimulates the adrenal gland, releasing steroids and catecholamines, both of which over time are damaging to the metabolism and blood flow.
- *Talk to your pharmacist.* Many medications currently on the market are photosensitizers. In other words, when exposed to sunlight, these drugs increase the susceptibility of the proteins in the lens to potential damage. Those who take systemic steroids or the cholesterol-lowering statin drugs should be especially careful, since these drugs inhibit the production of CoQ_{10} and glutathione in the liver.

Macular degeneration is a leading cause of blindness in older people. Those at risk should make sure that their supplement program includes extra amounts of lutein (carotenoids), zinc, and other antioxidants, such as vitamin C, selenium, and vitamin E.

Migraine Headaches

Studies have shown that people who suffer from migraine headaches can reduce the frequency of attacks by supplementing with magnesium. Other studies have shown that 400 milligrams of vitamin B_2 (riboflavin) per day can reduce the severity and frequency of attacks by two-thirds. Many other supplements have been shown to be helpful, including 5-HTP, omega-3 oils, calcium, vitamin D, SAMe, and the herbs feverfew, butterbur, and ginkgo biloba.

Wouldn't it be foolish for someone suffering from migraine headaches not to avail themselves of one or more of these simple treatments?

Pregnancy

The importance of supplementing with additional folic acid during and before pregnancy is now well recognized. But the importance of optimal nutrition during pregnancy is not so well recognized. Women who get by on the typical American high-sugar, high-fat diet under normal conditions should certainly not do so during pregnancy. Optimal nutrition is related to healthy, higher-birthweight infants. Nutritional needs are greater during this period, and supplementation is most important. Unfortunately, some women are frightened away from supplements by their physicians at a time when it is most important. Vitamin A is a good example. While it is true that too much vitamin A during pregnancy can be harmful, it is also true that too little vitamin A during pregnancy can lead to birth defects.

Benign Prostatic Hyperplasia

Men with benign prostatic hyperplasia have available a number of vitamin, mineral and herbal supplements that can be used to alleviate the condition. Saw palmetto has been shown to be as effective as the most popular prescription drug, without the side effects. Zinc, beta-sitosterol, certain amino acids, and various other supplements should be a part of their supplement regimen.

Osteoarthritis

A person with osteoarthritis has many helpful supplements to choose from. There are the antiinflammatory, healing nutrients such as glucosamine, chondroitin, and MSM. There are natural COX-2 inhibiting herbs, such as ginger and turmeric. SAMe can help, along with antioxidant vitamins. The herb devil's claw has been shown to help.

Diabetes

Alpha-lipoic acid, a powerful antioxidant, has been shown to improve insulin sensitivity and protect against diabetic neuropathy. This agent should be a part of the supplement program of anyone with diabetes. Other nutrients, such as chromium and magnesium, have been found to enhance glucose tolerance in diabetics. Diabetics may benefit from extra vitamin E, GLA-rich oils and/or omega-3 oils, CoQ_{10}, and the B vitamins. Some diabetics benefit from L-carnitine, as it lowers cholesterol and triglycerides and may help alleviate nerve damage. Inositol may help with diabetic nerve damage as well. Fiber supplements can aid in glucose control, and herbs such as gymnema and bitter melon are often recommended.

Menopause

Impressive advances are being made in the use of natural phyto-estrogens (soy isoflavones and herbs such as black cohosh) in the treatment of menopausal symptoms. Calcium and magnesium supplements, along with ipriflavone, can help to ward off bone loss.

Anxiety and Depression

Several herbs are well known as effective in treating mild to moderate anxiety and depression. Kava kava is an excellent antianxiety agent and St. John's wort is an effective treatment for mild depression. But other nutrients should be looked at as well. Extra B vitamins can be helpful. High amounts of inositol can be helpful in treating anxiety. 5-HTP may be helpful in depression.

These are merely some examples of health problems that should be taken into consideration when designing a supplement regimen for each individual. Nutritional requirements differ with age and gender, and this should be reflected in the choice of nutritional supplements as well. Some choices are very transient. Addition of zinc lozenges, extra vitamin C, or elderberry extract at the early signs of a cold, for example, can significantly reduce the duration and severity of the infection. But the zinc should not be taken for more than two or three days. Lysine, vitamin C, and bioflavonoids may be helpful in treating an outbreak of herpes (cold sores, genital herpes), but it might not be desirable to take extra lysine over a long period of time. This will be covered in more detail in Step 4.

Step Three: Choosing Which Brand to Purchase

Now that you have decided what type of supplements you prefer and which specific vitamins, minerals, and herbs fit your unique individual needs, the next problem is to choose the actual products. How do you know which brand is best?

It's not easy. You have to look for clues and use some common sense.

Is Big Better?

In this case of a supplement company, big might indeed be better. The smaller the firm, the less likely they are to have the resources needed to ensure quality, potency, and stability. This does not mean that all large companies use their resources toward this end, but at least they have the ability to do so if they choose. Nor does it mean that a small company is incapable of producing quality products.

To ensure quality, you have to do testing. Total reliance on the supplier of raw materials and on the assurances of the private-label manufacturer (for those companies that do not manufacture their own products) may not be enough. You can send samples to outside laboratories for testing or you can have it done in-house, in your own analytical laboratory. Either way, it costs money.

Raw materials should be quarantined on arrival and not used until tested for purity and potency. Various types of tests must be run during the tableting or encapsulation phase (weight variation, hardness), and every stage of the manufacturing process must be checked and double-checked, from weighing of the ingredients to batch reconciliation after each step (weighing, mixing, tableting, coating, and packaging). The final product has to be tested for potency, disintegration, dissolution, etc. Controls and procedures in place during packaging are designed to prevent product and label mix-ups. And appropriate stability testing, both developmental and ongoing, should be performed.

Again, all of these quality-oriented functions cost money and must be factored into the cost. If a product is too cheap, one has to question whether these steps might not have been taken.

Distributed By or Manufactured For

You can tell if a company manufacturers its own product or has it made by looking at the product label. If it is made by another company, the product will say "distributed by," "manufactured for," or something similar above the company name.

Does the fact that a company manufactures its own product necessarily signify it is of higher quality than products that have been made by a custom manufacturer? Not at all. It is true that for a quality-oriented company, it is easier to monitor all aspects of quality if manufacturing is done in-house. After all, you then have full control over the formulation, manufacturing, and packaging processes. On the other hand, if you are not a quality-oriented company, it might be easier to cut corners, cheat, lie, and deceive if you do not have to involve others in the manufacturing and testing process. So as you see, it is not where the product is made that counts. It is, instead, the integrity of the company that matters.

Custom manufacturers are experts in what they do. Some are honest and some are not. This is true in all industries. For a small or medium-size company, an outside manufacturer may have equipment, expertise, and capacity otherwise unavailable. Smaller companies may be better off spending their money on advertising and marketing, rather than on buying tablet presses and coating pans.

To ensure a quality product from an outside manufacturer, two things are necessary. First, the company for whom the product is being made must want a quality product and must be willing to pay for it. Second, it must be sufficiently knowledgeable to know what to ask for and look for when dealing with the supplier. This is where many problems arise because very often nutritional companies are started up by well-meaning entrepreneurs who know a lot about marketing and sales but little about manufacturing and quality control. They may not have actually inspected the manufacturing facility. Would they know what to look for if they did? They may not have specified shelf-life pa-

THE PHARMACIST SAYS

I (Don) remember once when I was in the private-label powdered-protein manufacturing business. I went calling on a relatively well-known company with a line of powdered protein supplements. I asked for the opportunity to bid on making their product for them. When I returned and sat down with the principles of the company, I gave them my prices, which they acknowledged as being very competitive. But I pointed out that there were a few problems. In one case, the label indicated that the protein source was egg white and there were no coloring agents or other colored ingredients listed. But the product had a yellowish color. So I pointed this out and explained that I could not in good conscience manufacture their product for them with the ingredients listed on their label and have it come out with a yellow color. Initially, they were taken aback, either because they did not themselves know what was in their own product or because they were surprised at my honesty—but then they quickly lost interest and told me that they were happy with their current supplier and didn't want to discuss it anymore.

rameters and inquired as to how the expiration date was determined. Do they know what overages were employed? Have they actually seen the batch formula sheet and checked the calculations? Have they discussed the amount of analytical work required to be performed on each batch of product?

If the appropriate parameters are established by companies of integrity, a "distributed by" or "manufactured for" product can be as high quality as any made in-house.

How Low Can You Go?

There is a point at which a product becomes too cheap. Let's get serious. When you see a bottle of no-name cheapo-supreme CoQ_{10} advertised at a fraction of the price of reputable products and you can buy one and get six free—plus, if you order now, they throw in a 35 millimeter camera for free!—do you seriously think you are getting a quality product?

Certainly, many of us need to pay attention to price. There is no need to pay more than necessary. But if you are careful and patient, you can usually find reputable, well-known brand-name products on sale at discounts up to 30 percent or 40 percent off list price. This is especially true in the major metropolitan areas. Mail order is another alternative, but only if you stick to well-known national brands. There are certain brands that are high quality and priced very competitively.

But if the price is too good to be true, it probably is.

The Bottle in the Window

There are some health food stores that display products on shelves right inside the window. When you are on the street looking into the store, you see the backs of actual products on display. When the sun hits the window, it heats up the bottles. Heat contributes to the deterioration of nutritional supplements.

Do not buy products from stores that may have stored or displayed the items inappropriately. Likewise, if a product is supposed to be refrigerated, it should be on display in a refrigerator, and if the store has a storage area or warehouse, it should have been refrigerated there as well.

The Recommendation

You're in the health food store, looking at the various products on the shelf. Perhaps there is a brand on sale that you have not used before or maybe it is a name you've never heard of. So you ask the clerk, "Is this a good product?"

What you should do is ask yourself, "What are this person's qualifications? Why would he (or she) be capable of evaluating the quality of any given product or brand?" Does he have a scientific background, so that he can separate marketing hyperbole from scientific fact? Has he spoken to anyone from the company other than a sales representative? Has he actually visited the company? Is he getting some type of kickback for selling certain products?

A common tactic in certain stores, especially large health food store chains, is what is called "bait and switch." This can take several forms, but one is very obvious. The store will display the well-known, national brand of a product on one shelf, and right below, it will display the same products under their own house-brand label. You are then pressured to buy the house brand rather than the national brand.

What about a recommendation from your doctor? Most doctors, either directly or indirectly, will admit that they know very little about what distinguishes a high-quality brand from a poor-quality brand. The others will claim they know and perhaps make a recommendation. Doctors are very knowledgeable individuals. They know a great deal about medicine, diagnosis, and treatment. But they don't usually learn about pharmaceutical manufacturing in medical school. They usually learn about products from sales representatives and detail men who, as you might expect, have a tendency to exaggerate. It is very difficult to find a salesman who will not tell you that his products are "the best."

Those doctors who are quick to make recommendations sometimes have ulterior motives. If they sell the products they recommend, their motives may be suspect.

Professional Brands

The good news is that doctors are more supportive of nutritional supplements and herbal remedies than they used to be. Many have come to realize the value of combining conventional and alternative therapies. Some have adopted the term *complementary medicine* to describe this new approach.

The bad news is that a small number of health professionals have taken this a step further and turned it into a business opportunity. They have become supplement retailers. Some involve themselves in multilevel marketing, which we discuss in Chapter 4. Others just stock and sell certain brands of dietary supplements.

THE PHARMACIST SAYS

Some might argue that it is okay for physicians to sell nutritional and herbal supplements from their offices. But the American Medical Association (AMA), in its ethics guidelines, states: "In-office sale of health-related products by physicians presents a financial conflict of interest, risks placing undue pressure on the patient, and threatens to erode patient trust and undermine the primary obligation of physicians to serve the interests of their patients before their own."

The AMA cautions physicians who choose to sell health-related products from their offices to "not sell any health-related products whose claims of benefit lack scientific validity." And they warn that, "because of the risk of patient exploitation and the potential to demean the profession of medicine, physicians who choose to sell health-related products from their offices must take steps to minimize their financial conflicts of interest."

For one thing, as we said above, the AMA suggests that physicians limit sales to products that "serve the immediate and pressing needs of their patients." It suggests that if products are distributed to patients, they should be done so free of charge or at cost. This will avoid the appearance of personal gain and possible "financial conflicts of interest that may interfere, or appear to interfere, with the physician's independent medical judgment."

The AMA goes on to require that physicians disclose fully the nature of their financial arrangement with a manufacturer or supplier. This would include informing patients "about the availability of the product or other equivalent products elsewhere."

What about the so-called professional lines? According to the code of ethics, "physicians should not participate in exclusive distributorships of health-related products which are available only through physicians' offices." The AMA acknowledges that these products may be of established benefit. But it suggests that if this is the case, physicians should encourage the manufacturers to make the products more widely accessible to patients than exclusive physician-distribution mechanisms allow.

Is this a bad thing? According to the ethics guidelines of the American Medical Association, "The relationship between patient and physician is based on trust and gives rise to physicians' ethical obligations to place patients' welfare above their own self-interest and above obligations to other groups, and to advocate for their patients' welfare."

The ethics guidelines say all that needs to be said about the pros and cons of physician retailers. More to the subject of this book is the question of the products being sold. Often, perhaps to justify the fact that they are being sold by the doctor or at a high price, the patient is told that these professional-brand products are superior to those found in retail stores.

This is simply not true. There are high-quality professional lines and there are high-quality retail lines. There is no reason to think that one is higher quality than the other. And it is also highly unlikely that products similar to these cannot be found from other sources.

Are there certain attributes that might distinguish these products from those found in stores? There can be. If the line specializes in hypoallergenic products, for example, the physician may feel more comfortable recommending products from that line if he deals with many patients with allergies. In some cases, these professional lines contain products that are designed for use as part of an integrated therapeutic protocol, and it might not be appropriate for the patient to use the products unless they are under the supervision of the physician. Some of these products are not labeled for retail display. For example, how would a consumer looking at products in a health food store know what Formula XYZ-29B is for?

So, there may indeed be a valid role for supplements that are designed specifically for use under the supervision of physicians, and there may sometimes be justification for physicians making these products available to patients directly from their office.

But is there a valid role for a line of supplements bearing the doctor's label that can be obtained *only* from his office? Is there justification for physicians selling a line of products from their office that cannot be obtained anywhere else, including pharmacies? It's hard to understand how a pharmacy, entrusted with the overseeing and dispensing of the most potent and powerful prescription drugs, cannot be trusted to dispense certain brands of professional vitamin products.

The truth of the matter is that those brands that can be obtained *only* from the doctor are restricted in this manner merely to protect the doctor's financial interest. The company's sales representative goes to the doctor and says, "Hey, Doc, you should carry my line because the patient will not be able to buy it anyplace except from you."

This practice, by the way, is not limited to doctors. The same approach is used by many health food store product lines. Certain companies refuse to sell their products to mass-market stores or pharmacies, and the reason is the same. The sales representative goes into the health food store and says to the proprietor: "Gee, times are tough, aren't they? People are going to the drugstore down the block instead of coming to you to buy their vitamins. Well, they can't get our line over there. We sell only to health food stores."

But let's get back to professional lines and doctors. If the doctor pressures you into buying products from his office, at full price, especially if there are no alternatives, there may be reason for concern. If, on the other hand, he offers products as an accommodation and is open about alternative sources, there may not be a problem. Ask the doctor if you can buy the same product elsewhere. Perhaps you are on a limited budget. Can he recommend some other brand so that you can save a little money?

There is nothing wrong with many of the professional brands. They are quality products and, as we said above, may be specifically formulated for various therapeutic protocols that should indeed be used under the guidance of a health professional. We will be mentioning some of these products in Chapters 6 and 7.

Expiration Dates and Stability

Some consumers have been told not to buy a product that does not have an expiration date on the label. Yes, certain vitamins deteriorate over time and if the bottle has been sitting on the store shelf for a year or so, you might not be getting a product that's up to full potency. But, I'm sorry to tell you, the fact that the bottle has an expiration date on it does not necessarily mean it is any more likely to be up to potency than some similar products without expiration dates.

First, there is not yet any legal requirement that supplements bear expiration dates. This is expected to change and may very soon. But the problem is in how one determines what the appropriate expiration date should be on a given product. This should be a function of the stability, or shelf life, of the product. At the time of manufacture, the supplements should contain at least the full label claim. And at the end of the product's designated shelf life, none of the nutrients should be present in amounts less than 95 percent of the label claim.

How does a reputable supplement manufacturer design a product that will maintain a potency of not less than 95 percent of label claim over a period of two or three years when stored on the shelf of a health food store? And what will be the consequences if it is determined that after two of the three years of designated shelf life, one of the vitamins has dropped to 90 percent of label claim? Does the company recall the product?

If the company takes this seriously, assigning a meaningful expiration date to a product is not something to be taken lightly. What can be done to assure that the product will be stable over that period of time? Care can be taken to select and combine ingredients that will not interact with each other. Sometimes stabilized versions of certain ingredients can be utilized. Overages can be used. If vitamin C, for example, is known to lose about 5 percent of its potency each year and you want a three-year expiration date, you would start off with 115 percent of label claim. This way, at the end of three years, the product will contain more than 95 percent of claim. Each vitamin will require a different overage, based on its stability characteristics. Precautions can be taken during manufacture to ensure minimal loss of potency due to moisture, heat, oxidation, etc. The choice of packaging materials— glass versus plastic—can have a significant effect on stability as well. Vitamins packed in cellophane packets in a cardboard box will not have as long a shelf life as those packaged in glass bottles.

All of these formulating techniques and manufacturing precautions, however, are only the first step in the process. The finished product has to be tested.

The most accurate test would be to take a few cases of the final, packaged product, put them in a storage room maintained at standard conditions of temperature and humidity, and run assays on each ingredient every six months for two or three years. If at the end of the test period, all of the assays were 95 percent of label claim or more, you could then market the product with a meaningful expiration date.

If any changes are made to the formulation or the packaging, of course, the entire testing process would have to be started over again.

Obviously, this is not a very practical approach. Few companies could afford to wait for three years of testing each time they wanted to introduce a new product or modify an existing product. So what you do instead is set up an accelerated stability test. This involves taking quantities of a product and storing them at different temperatures for a shorter period of time, perhaps for three months. Assays are run on each set of products and the results from the higher temperatures are mathematically extrapolated to room-temperature storage. This technique can give an adequate approximation of stability upon which an expiration date can be determined.

> ### THE PHARMACIST SAYS
>
> There is currently some controversy over the use of overages. Some claim that too high an overage is a violation. Historically, however, it has been felt that an excess amount of innocuous substances (such as the B vitamins) can be added in whatever overage is needed to achieve the desired shelf life. Obviously, putting 100-percent overage of vitamin A into a product cannot be tolerated due to potential toxicity issues. In general, overages of more than 5 percent to 10 percent are rarely used.

Reputable companies follow procedures similar to this when placing expiration dates on their supplement products. Some reputable companies have refused to put expiration dates on their products until data of this type can be generated.

Less-reputable companies, however, are not so conscientious. Some companies just pick a date out of thin air and place it on bottles. They have no overages, they do no testing, and they are willing to gamble that no one else will do any testing either.

An expiration date, therefore, is not the assurance of quality you may have thought it was. In fact, in some cases you may be out-and-out deceived. The date means nothing. On the other hand, if a product has an expiration date and that date is near or past, you at least can use that information as an indication that the product is no longer fresh.

How do you know if the expiration date is meaningful or meaningless? Very often, you have no way of knowing for sure. You can ask the company. Ask it what it bases its expiration dates on? Does it have overages in its products? Does it perform ongoing shelf-life testing to verify that the products are still up to potency? What will it do if the tests show that a given product is not up to potency?

If you try to ask these questions, you will most likely find it a very frustrating experience. Instead, you may have to rely on the reputation of the company. Do not buy products from a store that does not move products in volume, regardless of the dates on the bottle. Be aware, once again, that doing the type of testing required is an expensive proposition, and those costs have to be reflected in the product cost. Placing overages in a product adds to the cost as well. In general, a very low priced version of a product is less likely to have had this type of quality built into it.

You can also ask the store personnel. But be aware of the caveats already discussed. Ask the clerk, proprietor, nutritionist, or pharmacist what he or she bases his or her opinion on. Has the person ever spoken to anyone other than the company's sales representative? Has the person seen analytical reports? Has the person visited the manufacturer? Does the person have an educational background sufficient to enable him or her to make a judgment of this type?

Many companies in the health food industry take matters of this type less seriously than they would have you believe. A short time ago, for example, it was revealed that a large health food store chain was knowingly selling expired merchandise. The company, in response to a lawsuit filed by one state's attorney general, agreed to a $1 million dollar settlement. It was accused of selling vitamins that were as much as seven years old.

Remember that, in general, you get what you pay for. This does not necessarily mean that an expensive product is high quality, but it probably does mean that a very cheap product is low quality.

Testing Companies

There has been a confusing mish-mosh of private testing organizations, trade-group certification programs, and proposed semigovernmental analytical programs claiming to provide standards and analytical testing for nutritional supplements. This is both a good thing and a bad thing.

It is good that the importance of nutritional and herbal supplements is now recognized and that meaningful standards and regulations are being established.

Anything that will result in higher standards and product quality is certainly something to be supported by everyone interested in the continued growth and credibility of the dietary-supplement industry. But there are some serious drawbacks to what is available at this time. Currently, for example, when a private laboratory tests a selection of products purchased at random, they report on which products passed their test, but they refuse to divulge which products did not pass. This detracts from the credibility of the entire program. And those companies whose products passed the test cannot use that information unless they pay a fee to the testing company. This further undermines the credibility of the program.

If the testing company is unwilling to withstand the challenges sure to come about from those whose products it claims failed testing, how can we be fully confident in the validity of the results that will not be challenged? Isn't it more important for us to know which products did not pass?

This may be a step in the right direction, but further strides need to be made.

The National Nutritional Foods Association, a leading health food trade organization, has set up a program that awards a Good Manufacturing Practice (GMP) certification to those companies that pass its inspection program. This is a good thing, and we know of a number of companies that upgraded their procedures and facilities to ensure they passed the program. But there is a fee required for a company to participate. This imposes a burden on the smaller companies. And those companies who have their products made for them by several outside suppliers face the need to have multiple facilities inspected and certified.

Also, another source of possible confusion is that the seal, or certification, is not product specific. In other words, it does not mean that a given product has been tested or is certified to be up to potency. The seal merely means that the company follows good manufacturing practice guidelines.

Step Four: Putting It All Together

Now that you have decided which type of supplement is right for you, which supplements accommodate your specific and unique health needs, and which brands or sources you are comfortable with, it is time to put all of this together and set up a regimen tailored to your requirements.

Multivitamin Supplements

The first thing to do is decide on the product or products that constitute the nucleus, or foundation, of your program. This should be a broad-spectrum, balanced multivitamin-multimineral supplement, containing all of the essential vitamins, trace minerals, and perhaps calcium and magnesium. A B-complex formula would not fit this description.

There are four basic types of multivitamin supplements. They differ mainly in two areas: how many times a day will they be taken, and whether or not they contain adequate levels of calcium and magnesium.

The four types are as follows:

- One-per-day multivitamins
- Two-per-day multivitamins
- Complete, or four-to-six-per-day multivitamins
- Specialty multivitamins

One-Per-Day Multivitamins

As the name suggests, this type of multi is designed for a once-per-day dosage. While this may seem convenient to some, the disadvantages of products of this type are very significant:

- *Limited effectiveness.* Most of the nutrients contained in a multivitamin formula are water-soluble. This means that once they are absorbed, they are not stored in the body. Any excess over what is not used at the moment will be excreted. If you assume that most of the content of the one-per-day vitamin will be absorbed in an hour or two and metabolized and excreted in two or three more hours, you will certainly realize that within a half-day, most of what you took will be gone.
- *Lack of calcium and magnesium.* It is easy to fit 10 milligrams of iron or 15 milligrams of zinc into one tablet, along with the vitamins. But for calcium and magnesium, it is a different story. The amounts needed to provide the required level of these two essential nutrients is too great to fit into one, or even two, multivitamin tablets.

All one-per-day multivitamin products suffer from these two serious deficiencies. It does not matter what brand or what source you look at. Because they are taken only once daily, your body gets only limited benefit, and much of what is in the tablet is wasted. And unless you take a separate calcium-magnesium supplement, you are depriving your body of two important nutrients—nutrients certainly no less important than the vitamins.

As we said above, a B-complex is not a daily multivitamin. While such a product may indeed contain plenty of B vitamins, it does not contain many other important nutrients, such as vitamin A, carotenoids, vitamin E, zinc, copper, and selenium.

Even the most potent one-per-day multivitamin products may be poor choices in this regard. People think they are taking a one-a-day multivitamin when they are not. This type of product might be more correctly categorized as a B-complex rather than a multivitamin.

Why is this? Well, a typical one-per-day tablet provides amounts of B vitamins that range from 3,750 percent to 5,000 percent Daily Value, while supplying only 25 percent Daily Value of biotin, 67 percent of zinc, 35 percent of selenium, 21 percent of chromium, and 50 percent of copper. While this type of product does indeed supply some of the fat-soluble vitamins, such as vitamins A and E, it certainly is not a balanced one-per-day type of formula. Perhaps it could best be called a high-potency B-complex one-per-day multivitamin. There may be occasions when a product of this type is appropriate, but not when you are looking for a balanced multivitamin to serve as the cornerstone of your supplement program.

So far, we have had nothing positive to say about the one-per-day type of product. Can we say something positive? Yes—it beats taking nothing!

The fact is that there are some people who adamantly refuse to take more than one tablet or capsule per day in spite of anything they are told. It is just too much trouble. Why worry about osteoporosis, heart disease, diabetes, and cancer now? Many, especially those in their younger years, make the mistake of thinking of these as distant concerns, to be addressed only later in life, in spite of the overwhelming evidence to the contrary. Some people insist that they cannot be bothered with the taking of "pills" more than one time per day.

For these people, I suggest one of the following approaches. Go ahead and take your one-per-day multi, but at the very least, take a separate calcium-magnesium supplement at the same time. If you can swallow only one additional tablet, use the type of calcium-magnesium product that contains around 500 milligrams of calcium and 250 milligrams of magnesium per tablet and take it with a meal.

Even better, especially from a convenience standpoint, would be to take only one or two of the complete, four-to-six-per-day type of product. It could easily be argued that one would derive greater benefit from taking one-half to one-quarter of the daily dose of a four-per-day multivitamin-multimineral than taking one one-per-day multi. The primary reason is that it would be better to get 250 milligrams of calcium and 125 milligrams of magnesium and only 10 to 15 milligrams of each B vitamin than to get 25 to 50 milligrams of each B vitamin and an insignificant amount of calcium and magnesium.

Two-Per-Day Multivitamins

As the name implies, two-per-day multivitamins are designed for a twice-daily dosage. This obviously negates one of the criticisms of the one-a-day product, assuming that one tablet or capsule is taken in the morning and the other in the evening. Taking two at one time would defeat the purpose.

However, the other problem—the lack of meaningful levels of calcium and magnesium—remains and is the major drawback of this sort of product.

But it is certainly better than the one-per-day formula. A product of this type, if taken with a separate calcium-magnesium supplement, can indeed constitute an adequate general-purpose regimen. There are some, however, who resist taking more than one product, and for that group, the next category is ideal.

Complete Multivitamin-Multimineral Supplements

Complete multivitamin-multimineral supplements are the easy way to go for those who do not want to compromise their supplement intake but who want the convenience of a balanced, one-product approach. For those who are looking for the foundation or cornerstone product in a comprehensive supplement program, this type of product is ideal.

With a recommended daily dose of four tablets or six capsules, it is now possible to not only include adequate levels of all the vitamins and trace minerals, but also to include meaningful amounts of calcium and magnesium. Typically, products of this type will contain from 800 to 1,000 milligrams of calcium, along with 400 to 500 milligrams of magnesium.

Such products are comprehensive and balanced, and combine convenience with efficacy. For certain population groups, such as the elderly, the simplicity of combining the necessary nutrients into the fewest products is a big advantage. For those who don't want to be bothered, taking two tablets of one product at breakfast and dinner may seem less intrusive than taking several different products.

Why four or six? A greater quantity of material can be compressed into a tablet than can be filled into a capsule. It typically takes six capsules, for example, to provide the same ingredient quantities as four tablets. Some companies offer the same basic formula in both options. Natrol, for example, offers My Favorite Multi in a tablet form (four per day) or capsule form (six per day). For the advantages and disadvantages of tablets and capsules, see Chapter 1.

Other examples of this type of product are Dualtabs by Twinlab and Willvite by Willner Chemists.

Specialty Multivitamins

This is a category that is somewhat a catch-all for all other types of multivitamin supplements. From a marketing standpoint, it is a popular category, with all sorts of special formulas being promoted—for example, energy formulas, men's and women's formulas, and green formulas.

The problem is that when looking for a product that is to function as the nucleus or foundation of your total supplement program, you have to be careful to not lose sight of what is really important—the essential vitamins or minerals. In other words, remember that your basic, foundation multivitamin-multimineral formula should contain, first and foremost, adequate amounts of *all* the essential vitamins and minerals required for optimal health.

If you want a product that contains additional nutrients, that's fine. Just be careful that these extra ingredients do not take the place of the basic, essential nutrients that must be present in your daily supplement regimen.

Calcium and Magnesium

The next most important components of your program are calcium and magnesium.

THE PHARMACIST SAYS

Here is a recap of the important features to look for in your foundation supplement:

- Whatever you call the product, if the daily dose is only one or two per day, it cannot provide all of the necessary nutrients, especially calcium and magnesium.
- Adding additional cofactors, food concentrates, herbs, and enzymes is fine, as long as they do not take the place of important and essential basic vitamins and minerals. The more room you take up in a tablet with herbs and enzymes, the less room you have for the vitamins and minerals. Always look at the label carefully and look at the amounts of the vitamins and minerals, especially calcium and magnesium.
- Beware of window-dressing. Tossing tiny amounts of numerous accessory food factors (sometimes referred to as *chazzeri*) into a formula to make it look more impressive is nothing but marketing hype. If you really need supplemental CoQ_{10}, for example, the 10 milligrams in a multivitamin are not going to be enough. You will need to purchase a separate, higher-potency CoQ_{10} supplement. Likewise, 10 milligrams of unidentified ginseng, 5 milligrams of papain, or a "base of rose hips" is not going to make any difference.
- Beware of claims that because the vitamin is "derived" from something, or "cultured and grown" in some way, it is more potent than or different from other vitamins. Food concentrates and extracts are great. Taking your vitamins with food, food concentrates, and natural cofactors is definitely desirable. But these types of ingredients do not take the place of the vitamins and minerals themselves.

Supplementing with calcium and magnesium is no less important than supplementing with vitamins. It is not something that should be put off until you get old. It is as important to men as it is to women. As mentioned previously, you have two options. You can choose to use the type of multivitamin supplement that includes 1,000 milligrams of calcium and 400 to 500 milligrams of magnesium in the daily dose of four tablets or six capsules or you can take a separate calcium and magnesium supplement.

There are many types of calcium and magnesium supplements from which you can choose and they are described in Part Two of this book. If you want to minimize the number of tablets or capsules you need, choose the calcium carbonate and magnesium oxide types of products, but be sure to take them with meals. If you cannot be sure of taking them with meals, or if your need for calcium and magnesium is more therapeutic than prophylactic, you should use citrate or chelated forms.

Antioxidant Blends

Now that we have satisfied the basic, foundation requirements for a broad-spectrum multivitamin-multimineral with calcium and magnesium, we can begin to customize your program to meet your unique needs.

What if you have no unique needs? You're just an everyday Joe who lives in our typical toxin-laden environment, who breathes smog and eats the typical sugar- and fat-rich American diet. Here is what we suggest. Add one additional product: an antioxidant blend. Take one in the morning and one in the evening along with your multivitamin, calcium, and magnesium. Check Part Two for suggestions on antioxidant formulas.

The Add-Ons

Most of us, however, will indeed have health problems or health concerns that need to be factored into the program. Maybe our blood pressure is a little high or our cholesterol reading is above normal. Or we're overweight and have diabetes. We are starting to experience the symptoms of arthritis. We feel tired all of the time. We have trouble sleeping. We are worried about Alzheimer's disease, macular degeneration, or the symptoms of menopause.

Not that you have to be old to experience health problems requiring specific supplements. Perhaps you understand, for example, that maintaining optimal bone density in your younger years will lessen your problems with osteoporosis in later years. Maybe you have a family history of heart disease and you don't want to fall victim to the same life-shortening condition experienced by your parents. You hope to become pregnant soon and you know how important preconception nutrition is for increasing your odds of having a healthy baby. Or you exercise regularly and want to maximize your performance and minimize your injury-related downtime.

What you need to do is go to Part Two of this book and check the Therapeutic Cross-Reference. Look at the individual vitamins, herbs, and other nutrients that are beneficial in treating those problems of interest to you. Then check Chapter 6 to find out if there might be a combination product that is appropriate.

These supplements, either individual or combination remedies, should be taken in addition to your basic foundation multivitamin-multimineral, not instead of it.

Chapter THREE

How to Use Supplements

When to Take Supplements

One of the most common questions is, "When should I take my vitamins?" In most cases, this is not as critical a concern as most people seem to think it is, but there are certain situations where it can be very important.

Our bodies are designed to assimilate nutrients from food. This includes the macronutrients such as protein, carbohydrate, and fat, as well as the micronutrients (vitamins and minerals). To accomplish this, we secrete enzymes designed to break down each type of nutrient, and our body adjusts the acidity or alkalinity of each section of the digestive tract to optimize the activity of these enzymes.

With a few exceptions, then, when taking nutritional supplements as sources of nutrients, the best way to take them is to think of them as food. Take them with meals or with food. This will assure that they are broken down and assimilated most efficiently.

What does "with meals" mean? We have seen people almost break out into a sweat in their anxiety over whether "with meals" means before the meal, during the meal, or after the meal. It's not that important. Do whatever makes you comfortable. If you take a large number of supplements, maybe it will be easier if you spread them out, taking some before and some after the meal.

The other advantage of taking your supplements with food is that you will be less likely to experience any gastric discomfort. Some people are very sensitive and find that B-complex vitamins, fish oil supplements, and others can cause a problem if not taken with food.

There are some people who would have you believe that various types of nutrients have to be taken at specific times and that one cannot be taken at the same time as another, and so forth. Pay little attention to this. Remember what we just said about how the body is designed to obtain the nutrients it needs.

One example is calcium. There are some people who advise taking calcium supplements only before bedtime. Bear these facts in mind: First, the body has an elaborate and sensitive mechanism in place to ensure that serum calcium levels remain within a strict and narrow range. As soon as blood calcium levels fall below this range, the body desperately reaches out for any source of calcium it can find to raise calcium back up to the required level. To the body, our bone is a calcium reservoir, a source of calcium when it needs it. When calcium levels in the blood fall, the body pulls calcium out of our bones to correct the deficit. It makes no sense to artificially create a deficit of calcium throughout the day, encouraging bone loss, just to attempt to replenish it at nighttime. Second, it is our nature to obtain calcium from food throughout the day. The optimal way to supplement with calcium is to divide the dosage to two or three times a day.

Another example involves a theory that there is some advantage to eating only one type of nutrient at a time. This makes no sense for many of the same reasons already discussed. Few foods in their natural state consist of only one type of nutrient. A substantial part of the digestive process takes place in the small intestine, under the influence of pancreatic enzymes. The pancreas secretes a mixture of enzymes, composed of proteases, amylase, and lipase (protein-digesting, carbohydrate-digesting and fat-digesting, respectively.) And most vitamins are absorbed through a passive diffusion mechanism.

There are times when supplements should not be taken with food. This usually is when the item is being used as a therapeutic agent rather than as a nutrient.

One example would be the amino acids. If you are using amino acids, especially in a mixture, as a source of efficient protein supplementation, you could take the supplement at any time. But if you are taking an individual amino acid for its therapeutic activity, you should take it between meals, when there is no other protein present to compete with its absorption.

Another example would be proteolytic-enzyme supplements designed to be used as anti-inflammatory agents rather than as digestive enzymes. When taking an enzyme supplement containing proteolytic enzymes (trypsin, chymotrypsin, papain, bromelain) for the purpose of enhancing the digestion of dietary protein, the obvious time to take the product is with meals. But if the intention is for these enzymes to be absorbed and exert a systemic anti-inflammatory action, you do not want to take them with meals, where they would be partially deactivated by interacting with food. Instead, take them between meals, so that more will be absorbed into the bloodstream.

Usually, if a supplement is intended to be taken at times other than with meals, the directions on the container will state that. As a general rule, you can assume that unless stated otherwise, a supplement should be taken with food. If in doubt, ask a qualified health professional, such as a nutritionally trained pharmacist or physician.

How Often to Take Supplements

To obtain maximum benefit, it is usually best to divide your supplements in two or three doses per day. Many nutrients are water-soluble. They will be absorbed in an hour or two, reach maximum blood levels, and then begin to be eliminated from the body. Within a half-day, much of the dose is gone. When you take several doses (at least two) throughout the day, you maintain blood levels over a much longer time. This is why we have suggested that a two-a-day multivitamin is much superior to a one-a-day multivitamin.

For fat-soluble nutrients (such as vitamin A, vitamin D, and CoQ_{10}), this is less of a problem, as they are stored for a much longer period in the body. To maximize the utilization of these nutrients, take them with food, especially food that contains some fat or oil. CoQ_{10} is now available suspended or emulsified in oil in soft gel capsules.

Storing Supplements

The best way to store supplements is in a cool, dry place, away from direct sunlight. Cool does not necessarily mean cold, and storing vitamins in a refrigerator is not generally recommended. The reason for this is that the opening and closing of bottles stored in a refrigerator may cause moisture condensation, and moisture is no less a cause of deterioration than heat or oxygen. In fact, moisture may be the biggest culprit. Keep the bottle tightly closed. If you do not have a cool place to store your supplements in the summer, do not purchase large bottles.

Vitamins will gradually deteriorate on storage. Heat and moisture will accelerate that deterioration. As a vitamin supplement deteriorates, it loses potency. It does not turn into something toxic or dangerous. Instead of having a tablet that contains 500 milligrams of vitamin C, it may now contain only 400 milligrams of vitamin C.

You can often tell if a vitamin supplement is old. Vitamin C starts to turn brownish in color. So what may have been a white tablet when first purchased is now off-white or lightly brown. In a multivitamin, you might start to see dark brown spots throughout the tablet, and you will notice a strong vitamin smell.

Minerals are very stable, and you seldom have to worry about the age of a mineral supplement. Herbs, if kept dry, will remain stable for long periods as well.

Storing Oils and Probiotic Supplements

Some types of supplements are inherently unstable. Certain oils, for example, may easily be oxidized and must be stored in glass bottles and refrigerated. Flaxseed oil is a good example.

Probiotic (acidophilus) products are another good example. Many of the cultures used in probiotic supplements are very vulnerable to the effects of heat. You want to have as high a content as possible of live, viable organisms. Pasteurization of yogurt kills the beneficial microorganisms. In supplements, theoretically, freeze-dried cultures should be reasonably stable, but in the race to see who can claim the highest potencies, refrigeration is necessary to preserve the extremely high levels now being marketed.

Once again, this does not mean you have to carry a battery-operated portable refrigeration unit with you on the bus so that you can protect your probiotic supplement from deterioration on the way home from your neighborhood health food store. Instead, what you should do is enhance its potency and shelf life by making sure it is refrigerated in the store and keeping it refrigerated once you get it home. Short periods of exposure to ambient temperatures should not significantly impact the integrity of the product. If instead of containing 2.5 billion trillion organisms per quarter-teaspoon, it contained only 2.4 billion trillion organisms per quarter-teaspoon, the world will not come to an end. Luckily, however, new, stabilized probiotic supplements are now being introduced that do not require refrigeration. One example is a new product from Jarrow Formulas, Jarro-Dophilus EPS.

Side Effects, Interactions, and Toxicity

Some people would have you believe that just because something is natural, it cannot be harmful. This is obviously not true. Many of history's most popular poisons are natural substances.

On the other hand, time-tested therapeutic herbs have not been used continuously for 2,000 or more years because they kill half the people who take them! Nor does an herbal remedy continue to be used for hundreds of years if it has no beneficial action. To the contrary, trial and error has led us to herbs and nutrients that have been shown to be helpful in treating various disorders without causing side effects and toxic reactions. It is a mistake to ignore evidence based on traditional experience and history of use.

Most of the cautions associated with dietary supplements are commonsense cautions. In other words, you don't take a supplement that lowers blood pressure if you have low blood pressure. If you are taking antidepressant medication, you don't start taking a bunch of antidepressant herbs at the same time.

There are those in conventional medicine, however, who resent the implication that anything other than drugs is effective in treating or preventing disease. Others, including many dietitians, jealously guard against any suggestion that food alone is not sufficient and that supplements might be an appropriate adjunct to improved health and vitality. They embrace anything negative about dietary supplements that they can find. The problem is that they cannot find very much.

So they resort to harping on marginally appropriate concerns to the point of absurdity.

"Don't take vitamin E because it may cause thinning of the blood." "Don't take fish oil, ginkgo biloba, garlic, or feverfew if you are taking blood-thinning medication." People are walking around scared to death that if they get a paper cut, they will bleed to death, merely because they took 400 IU of vitamin E that morning.

Goodness gracious. If these concerns were at all valid, you would expect to see people lying about in pools of blood . . . a scene reminiscent of *Night of the Living Dead*. Zombie-like folks, holding bottles of vitamins, staggering about with a squishing sound as blood oozes from their skin and pools in their shoes. All because they took fish oil supplements and vitamin E.

THE PHARMACIST SAYS

The antisupplement contingent would have you believe that dietary supplements are unproven, unregulated and potentially dangerous. Dietary supplements are in fact regulated by the FDA and the Federal Trade Commission, albeit not entirely the same way that drugs are regulated. They are proven to varying degrees, and while anything can be dangerous, they are certainly considerably less dangerous than drugs. They imply that all drugs are reliable, proven effective, and safe. Yet the news is filled with one prescription drug after another that has been found to cause dangerous side effects and problems *after* approval and a period of use. According to a study published in the *Journal of the American Medical Association,* new research shows that approximately 20 percent of recently approved prescription drugs have serious and even life-threatening side effects. One recent example is the cholesterol-lowering drug Baycol, from Bayer, which has been found to have caused more than 100 deaths before being voluntarily recalled. And there is an ongoing investigation as to how much medical research and how many published studies are tainted because of the financial ties between researchers and the companies whose products are involved in the studies. This is not to say that there is not a lot to respect and appreciation about modern medicine and the wonderful pharmaceutical agents now available to us. But let's not throw stones from the window of our glass house.

It is hard to find an herb, vitamin, food, or human activity that does not cause some degree of thinning of the blood. This is usually a good thing. We want the blood to clot only when it is absolutely necessary (such as when we cut our finger and do not want to bleed to death). We do not want blood to clot in our blood vessels, block flow, etc. This is especially true if we have health problems that heighten this danger. That is why doctors prescribe blood-thinning drugs such as Coumadin. This is why they urge daily use of low-dose aspirin. Supplements (such as fish oil, ginkgo, and feverfew) also have a slight blood thinning action. Obviously, if you are taking Coumadin, a powerful blood-thinning agent, you need to be aware of the other things that have this since they will all work to increase the total effect. As Grandma used to say, too much is not always good.

If these various supplements have so significant an effect on blood clotting, then why not use them rather than Coumadin? They have other beneficial actions as well, so wouldn't it be better to use them as anticlotting agents if indeed they exert this action? Or why shouldn't the doctor adjust the dose of Coumadin to accommodate the anticlotting activity of vitamins and herbs rather than the other way around?

Exercise reduces blood-clotting time. Why are we not being cautioned to cut back on exercise as well if we take blood-thinning medication?

Subtle Misinformation

Bias creeps into the information presented on side effects, toxicity, and safety of supplements. A good example is the supposed toxicity of vitamin B_6.

In a column, "Q & A: Be Careful With B's," which appeared in the January 22, 2002, edition of *The New York Times,* the following question was asked: "I heard dietary supplements may contain harmful amounts of B vitamins. Which ones?"

The response indicated that niacin and vitamin B_6 were potentially harmful. The comment on vitamin B_6 was as follows: "The R.D.A. for vitamin B_6 is two milligrams. Neurologic problems that can alter balance and sensations are associated with more than 100 milligrams a day."

The author goes on to provide a reference: "For more information, *The PDR for Nutritional Supplements,* edited by Dr. Sheldon Saul Hendler and David Rorvik, summarizes many studies of dietary supplements." There is also a reference to the FDA's website, where you can find recent reports of adverse reactions to dietary supplements. The implication, clearly, is that these references support the information presented by the author of the column.

Unfortunately, this is not at all the case. In fact, the book by Dr.

Hendler does not support the author's warning about vitamin B_6 at all. Dr. Hendler actually concludes:

"The Food and Nutrition Board of the Institute of Medicine of the U.S. National Academy of Sciences has concluded that reports and studies showing sensory neuropathy at doses of pyridoxine less than 200 mg/day are weak and inconsistent, with the weight of evidence indicating that sensory neuropathy is unlikely to occur in adults taking pyridoxine at doses less than 500 mg/day."

Back in 1983, there was a report of sensory neuropathy in seven patients who had been taking between 2,000 milligrams to 6,000 milligrams per day of vitamin B_6 for two to forty months. There were other reports, again during the 1980s, of neuropathy resulting from doses ranging from 1,000 milligrams to 4,000 milligrams per day.

In addition, at about that same time, there were reports of toxicity from lower doses. These reports were evaluated and dismissed for various reasons (such as methodological flaws) as being unreliable. A detailed explanation is readily available.[1]

All of this took place back in the mid-1980s. In more than twenty years, no additional evidence of vitamin B_6 toxicity has been published. Certainly, no evidence in support of a contention that doses of vitamin B_6 in the 100-milligrams, 200-milligrams, or even 500-milligrams-per-day level is harmful.

In fact, the Food and Nutrition Board has set the Lowest-Observed-Adverse-Effect Level (LOAEL) for vitamin B_6 at 500 milligrams per day and the No-Observed-Adverse-Effect Level (NOAEL) at 200 milligrams per day.

Now, this information was also presented in Dr. Hendler's book, the very same one quoted as a reference in *The New York Times* column. Yet the author made the statement implying that a dose of 100 milligrams per day of vitamin B_6 may be harmful.

Why then did the author say this? As we said earlier, those who have an antisupplement bias are hard-pressed to justify their sentiments. This is the best they can do.

---

[1] "Dietary Reference Intakes for Thiamine, Riboflavin, Niacin, Vitamin B_6, Folate, Vitamin B_{12}, Pantothenic Acid, Biotin, and Choline." A Report of the Standing Committee on the Scientific Evaluation of Dietary Reference Intakes and Its Panel on Folate, Other B Vitamins, and Choline and Subcommittee on Upper Reference Levels of Nutrients, Food and Nutrition Board, Institute of Medicine, National Academy of Sciences, 1998. National Academy Press, Washington, D.C. (pp. 184–86).

A Comment from Dr. Abel

Remember to look at the benefits versus risks of different therapies. Doctors may tell patients that certain natural therapies cause bleeding, kidney stones, or emotional problems. If one looks quite carefully at the literature, we find that there are very few examples of overdoses of vitamin A or vitamin D; only fat-soluble vitamins can accumulate. Few of us dine regularly on polar-bear liver, a rich source of vitamin A. Vitamin C rarely causes kidney stones. The calcium-oxalate kidney stones are more often caused by our modern diet. Therefore, it is more important to look carefully at the risks of any therapy. Certainly prescription drugs, whether approved by the FDA or under study, always seem to have the potential for adverse reaction. The risk of a natural therapy in a recommended dose is extremely unusual. A frequent risk of many bioflavonoid compounds and vitamin E (tocopherol) is thinning of the blood. These natural elements decrease platelet adhesiveness, which interferes with the effect of Coumadin and other blood-thinning agents. Because you can measure bleeding time, the Coumadin dose can be adjusted. I personally recommend to my patients that they take E or ginkgo biloba to thin their blood unless their cardiologist insists on aspirin. Stopping aspirin will not normalize blood clotting for seven to ten days, whereas stopping ginkgo or another supplement two days before surgery will normalize blood clotting. I have an interesting story to share. A friend's father was undergoing a transurethral prostate operation for his benign prostate hypertrophy. During the operation, he bled profusely and received 4 pints of blood. His urologist had not obtained a history that he had been on daily aspirin. If the bleeding hadn't been stopped, the simple aspirin-a-day therapy could have cost him his life. It is always important to remember to look to your medications and ask your doctor, especially before surgery, which ones you should or should not be taking. I think it is a mistake to worry so much about supplements while not considering the potential risks of your prescription medications.

When Not to Take Supplements

If you are trying to become pregnant, if you are pregnant, or if you are nursing, avoid using any herbal supplements, amino acids, or high-dose vitamins and minerals without first consulting your physician. A good, balanced multivitamin-multimineral, with at least 800 micrograms of folic acid, on the other hand, should be taken during this period.

If you are allergic to a supplement or any of the ingredients associated with the supplement, do not take it.

Use common sense. If the supplement raises blood pressure, don't take it if you have high blood pressure. If it lowers blood pressure, don't take it if you have low blood pressure. If the supplement stimulates the mind (or central nervous system), don't take it if you are nervous or cannot sleep. If it makes you drowsy, don't take it if you do not want to go to sleep.

If you take medication, consult with a nutritional pharmacist or knowledgeable doctor to make sure there are no contraindications or interactions. Make sure, however, that the doctor knows enough about the supplement to offer a meaningful response. Sometimes, if a doctor does not know anything about a particular nutritional or herbal supplement, he will take the path of least resistance, telling you not to use it (rather than going to the trouble of finding out what it actually is).

CHAPTER FOUR

Too Good to Be True?

We have already given you some examples of things to watch out for when shopping for nutritional supplements in the section on choosing which brand to purchase. Here are some additional pointers.

What a Deal! Or Is It?

Watch out for discounts that are not as impressive as they seem. For example, "Buy one and get another at half price" is not as impressive a deal as it might sound at first. If the cost is based upon list price, then this deal translates to 25 percent off list. That does not sound nearly as impressive as it did at first, does it? Especially when the store down the street has the same or similar products on sale at 30 percent off list price. And you have to buy only one bottle, not two.

Another common ploy is to put a big poster in the window touting a large discount, perhaps "40 percent off." Only when you read the fine print or go into the store do you discover that this discount applies only to selected items or only to the store's house brand.

Watch out for deals that cost. A chain of health food stores makes you an offer. You can purchase a special membership card that will enable you to purchase supplements at a 20 percent discount one day a month. The card costs twenty-five dollars, but you will certainly recoup that after just the first month or two. What a deal.

Or is it? The other health food stores in the area carry similar products, if not a wider selection, at everyday discounts of 20 percent off list price. And they frequently run specials, with discounts of 30 percent to 40 percent off list price. And you do not need to buy a card to obtain these larger discounts. We still cannot figure out why people are so willing to pay for the privilege of getting less.

Something to Hide?

Watch out for product labels that contain proprietary blends of ingredients. As far as we are concerned, there should be no such thing. During a time when efforts are being made to bring increased accountability and credibility to the nutritional-supplement industry, there is no excuse for not listing the actual composition, both quantitatively and qualitatively, on the product label.

For example, there is a line of herbal supplements with formulas designed for a wide variety of disorders that bear ingredient statements in this format:

Amount Per Serving:
Proprietary Blend:
　　St. John's Wort Extract 0.3% (leaves/stems), L-tyrosine, Kava Kava
　　Extract 30% (root), Ginkgo Biloba Extract 24% (leaves), Royal Jelly
　　Extract 3x, Siberian Ginseng Powder (root).

We do not approve of products that do not list the quantity of active ingredients on the label.

Multilevel Marketing or Pyramid Schemes

Watch out for claims made by those involved in multilevel marketing. Why? Because the claims are almost always exaggerated and unfounded.

There is an inherent thread of deception that runs through most multilevel-marketing programs. Deception is necessary for several reasons. The products being promoted are by necessity substantially more expensive than similar products being sold through normal retail channels. This is because there is the need to support so many additional levels of discounts and commissions. To justify these higher prices, exorbitant claims of uniqueness, efficacy, and superiority are made by people who have no responsibility for what they say. They are independent contractors. If you have ever tried to obtain substantiation for any of the claims being made by these representatives from the actual company, you know what we are talking about.

In fact, whenever you are presented with testimonial after testimonial in support of a product, you should be very suspicious. And this is primarily what you get with multilevel marketing. You are also typically told about the team of Nobel Prize scientists who developed the product, the billions of dollars the company made last month (after all, how can there be any doubt of the integrity of the product or the program when so much money is being made?), reminded about Mom and apple pie, and bombarded with buzzwords such as *natural, environment,* and *organic.* You, of course, are also told about the great amount of money you can make if you buy into the program.

And this leads to the second reason why deception is involved. The fact is, you are not really buying products when you get involved with multilevel marketing. Instead, you are buying into the business plan, the opportunity to get rich quick at other people's expense. The organizers or recruiters sit you down and delude you into thinking that it is easy to recruit people into level after level of distributors, each of whom is paying you a portion of their sales proceeds. It rarely works out that way.

THE PHARMACIST SAYS

What is multilevel marketing? Some would have you believe it is merely a way for people to pursue the American dream, empowering the average person to sell directly to others, bypassing the evil, wicked, bad, and nasty conventional retail sales infrastructure. But that is not the case. You can do that without getting involved in multilevel marketing. What differentiates this from other sales methods, including direct sales, is that you are buying into an opportunity to participate in a modified pyramid scheme. In its pure sense, pyramid schemes, or Ponzi schemes, are now illegal. Here is how it works: Participants buy into the program. The money from new participants is distributed to the previous participants, or those higher up in the ever-expanding pyramid. The more people you recruit, the more money you make. And the new recruits go out and recruit new people, who buy in, and they in turn recruit more people . . . until you start to run out of new recruits. At that time, the pyramid collapses. Those who were lucky enough to have risen to the upper part of the pyramid laugh on their way to the bank and those at the bottom of the pyramid suddenly wonder where their money went.

To avoid the illegality of a Ponzi scheme, the recruits have to obtain something tangible in return for their initial investment, something other than an opportunity to participate in the pyramid. So they do. They get a starter kit, for example, or a business plan. All they have to do now is go out and pitch the product and entice the prospective recruit with the lure of easy wealth. It's so easy. Talk to ten people. Three of them will buy into the program. You get a commission on their sales. For every ten people with whom each of those three talk, three more will buy into the program. You also get a commission on their sales. That's twelve people now downline from you. And for every ten people with whom each of these folks talk, three will sign on. You, of course, get a commission on their sales as well. That adds an additional twenty-seven downline people feeding you commissions, for a total of thirty-nine. And it just keeps on going. There can be as many as five levels of commissions involved. What are you going to do with all that money? You will have to buy a bigger home, so that you can have a larger garage to accommodate your new cars. One for each day of the week.

Of course, it rarely works out that way, does it? There is nothing wrong with the American dream. And there is nothing wrong with direct sales, door to door, over the Internet, or whatever. But when it involves false and misleading claims, deceptive promises and the lure of easy money, that's another story. Selling product is fine, but selling an opportunity to participate in a modified pyramid scheme is not our idea of the American dream.

It's not as bad as it used to be. At least the products sold by many of the larger multilevel marketing companies are decent products with honest labels. If you read the label, dismiss the false and misleading information being provided by the distributor, and don't mind paying more than you have to for a product, go ahead and do so.

Radio Infomercials

Watch out for advertising in disguise. In magazines, they put a heading at the top of the page warning you that it is an advertisement. On the radio or television, the disclaimer is often not that obvious.

If you read the biographical information on the cover of this book, you will see that two of the authors, Don Goldberg and Arnie Gitomer, host a two-hour radio program every Sunday afternoon in New York. When we hear some of the infomercials that air on the radio, we are embarrassed to be associated with this industry. It is a shame that such blatant misinformation is allowed to be broadcast.

What is an infomercial? It is a block of radio time, usually thirty minutes, purchased by people who have a product to sell. They, apparently, can say anything they want to. And they say it well. If you don't listen carefully, and if you are not knowledgeable about the subject matter, it is easy to be impressed with their pitch.

But the facts are rarely as they make them out to be. For example, does the fact that a couple of scientists received the Nobel Prize for discovering the effect of nitrous oxide on blood vessels really mean that those same scientists are endorsing an herbal impotency cure?

It all boils down to what we have said over and over again. If something sounds too good to be true, assume it is too good to be true!

If we told you that peppermint schnapps cured impotency, baldness, cancer, halitosis, Alzheimer's disease, and athlete's foot, would you believe us? Would you pick up the phone and order a bottle? Well, people do it. And they must do it in large numbers because these ads and infomercials go on and on.

Do you really believe that Maud, who couldn't get out of bed because of her severe case of "arther-itis," rubbed this miracle cream on her back and the very next morning was able to jump out of bed and start training for the New York marathon? And she was so impressed, she gave some to her husband, Howie, who had been confined to a wheelchair for the past three years. And, you guessed it, the next day Howie threw away his cane and rejoined the bowling team. Is this wonderful or what?

How many of you noticed the comment "results may vary" at the end of the commercial?

Do you want to lose weight? Just take a few spoonfuls of this miracle liquid (no mention is made during the commercial as to what it contains, by the way) before bedtime and when you wake up in the morning, "You are well on your way to losing weight!"

What does that mean, "well on you way to losing weight"? Does that mean that this miracle liquid causes you to lose weight overnight while you were sleeping? Or does it mean that if you follow the rest of the program—reduced calorie intake, increased exercise, etc.—you will maybe then lose weight?

What about the "second-grade schoolteacher" who invented the cure for the common cold? We have the highest respect for second-grade schoolteachers, but why would we believe that a second-grade schoolteacher was successful in inventing a cure for the common cold when the leading pharmaceutical scientists throughout the world have yet to do so?

Grow Your Vitamins?

Watch out for people who can turn lead into gold. There are some companies that sell products containing vitamins that are supposed to be different from others. These vitamins have been somehow grown or cultured with food or yeast, and incorporated into these organic plant cells. And as a result of this, the vitamins are supposedly changed, altered in some way such that they are no longer the same as "regular" vitamins. They are better, more potent, better assimilated, more politically correct.

In Chapter 2, we explained the ploy used to "fortify" brewer's-type yeast. B vitamins would be dumped into a yeast culture and the resultant mixture of yeast and B vitamins would be co-dried. The product would be called fortified brewer's-type yeast and have very high potencies of the various B vitamins. The high potency, of course, was due to the added vitamins. Companies would put this "yeast" into their vitamin products and mention only "yeast" on the label's ingredient panel. But they would list the high potencies of the B vitamins. The consumer would be misled into thinking that the vitamins came from the yeast, rather than from the regular, synthetic vitamins that were added to the yeast.

The "food-base," "cultured," or "grown" vitamin supplements are variations of this same approach. That's okay up to a point. We firmly support the inclusion of as much natural food concentrate and food isolates as possible into a supplement program. Foods, especially fruits and vegetables, are rich sources of beneficial phytonutrients—flavonoids, polyphenols, etc.—and the more the better.

But that is all these products are—mixtures of regular vitamins and minerals with yeast or other food concentrates. The vitamins have not been altered in any way.

This culturing process does not change the vitamins. The vitamins are not incorporated into the yeast or food cells and somehow made more potent. A mixture of food concentrate and vitamins is formed, dried, and incorporated into the supplement. That's all. And as long as we accept that for what it is, no harm is done—except remember that there is only so much space in a tablet or capsule. The more of that space that is taken up by the food concentrate, the less the space that is available for the actual vitamins and minerals. It is difficult, if not impossible, then, to have a high-potency vitamin or mineral supplement of this type.

There is an exception to this situation. Certain trace minerals can indeed be assimilated by plant cells in higher than normal levels. Perhaps the best example of this is selenium. A selenium-enriched yeast culture has indeed been developed and commercially produced. This is an exception, as plants usually are genetically limited in how much of a given nutrient they can utilize.

Our main concern regarding these types of products is that there is a tendency to mislead consumers into thinking they are getting more than they really are. Overspending is one thing, but if a woman takes one of these "food-grown supplements" with only 75 milligrams of calcium, for example, thinking that this will have the same effect as 1,000 milligrams of regular calcium, there is a serious problem. As we said before, food concentrates are fine. But they should be taken as an adjunct to an appropriate nutrient supplement, not as a replacement for it.

THE PHARMACIST SAYS

There is a Cal Mag Whole Food Complex Dietary Supplement that supplies 75 milligrams of calcium as a "Bio Grown Food-Cultured Nutrient." Do not be misled into thinking that 75 milligrams is anything other than 75 milligrams. Seventy-five milligrams of calcium, whether "food-cultured" or brewed in a witch's cauldron, is not equivalent to 1,000 milligrams of calcium.

What's That Smell?

Watch out for what's not there. A few year's ago, there was a very popular powdered protein supplement being sold in health food stores and advertised on the radio. It was originally packaged in a large plastic bottle and later in a fiber can. The front of the label said it was soy protein with papain and bromelain (enzymes). There was no mention of any type of flavoring. On the back side of the label, the ingredient listing showed only the following: "Soy Protein Isolate, Papain, Bromelain." Again, there was no mention of any flavoring agents.

But there was a distinct vanilla odor associated with the product. Without even opening the bottle, you could smell the vanilla. Where was that vanilla odor coming from?

Well, in spite of the fact that there was no mention of it on the label, the product contained vanilla flavoring. You did not have to be a brain surgeon to realize that something was not right. The product was mislabeled.

Why did the manufacturer mislabel the product? There is no way for us to know, of course, except the fact that the source of the odor was vanillin, or artificial vanilla, rather than natural vanilla flavoring might have had something to do with it.

We discussed the problem of identifying quality brands back in Chapter 2. This is a good case in point. You have to look for clues, and very often the clues are easy to spot. You pick up a product from the store shelf and it smells of vanilla. You see no mention of vanilla on the label. *Voilà*, the product is mislabeled and you have reason to wonder about the general integrity and competency of that particular brand.

Why Does It Fizz?

Here is another example. If you look at the label on a jar of one particular brand of buffered ascorbate powder currently on store shelves, you might notice several things. You will notice a lot of space devoted to statements explaining what is not in the product. You will also notice that it bears a full disclosure label, indicating no hidden or inactive ingredients. The ingredient listing is provided as follows:

Vitamin C (triple recrystallized) 1,584 mg
Potassium (as ascorbate) 99 mg
Calcium (as ascorbate) 40 mg
Magnesium (as ascorbate) 16 mg
Zinc (as ascorbate) 600 mcg

Everything sounds good so far, but under the directions, you are told to mix one rounded half-teaspoon with 4 ounces of liquid.

Now, you notice one more thing. You are instructed to wait for effervescence to stop before drinking.

What effervescence? Mixing various mineral ascorbates with water will not result in effervescence. Instead, you need to have some type of bicarbonate present. There was no mention of ingredients on that "full disclosure label" that would lead to effervescence. Does it contain potassium (as ascorbate), as the label claims, or does it instead contain potassium bicarbonate? Is this true as well for calcium bicarbonate, magnesium bicarbonate, and zinc bicarbonate? Does it contain citric acid? Should I have to guess? Or should it be clearly stated on a full disclosure label?

Now, this particular label may or may not be legal in the strictest sense. That's not the point. Perhaps the implication is that after the reaction is completed (the chemical reaction between the bicarbonate and the acid when stirred into water), all that you have left is vitamin C and mineral ascorbates. But full disclosure labeling should be just that.

This is especially true when there are competing products on the market that contain fully reacted ascorbates. These other buffered vitamin C products do not rely on the acidic vitamin C reacting with the mineral ascorbate after being stirred into water. They provide the vitamin C in an already-reacted, fully buffered form, as a true mineral ascorbate.

For more information on buffered vitamin C products, refer to Chapter 5.

Just the Facts, Please

Country Life has a product that tells you everything except what you need to know—at least, not directly.

The product is labeled as follows:

Triple Strength Bromelain
500 mg
2,000 G.D.U. per gram
The highest potency proteolytic . . .
Serving Size: 1 tablet
Amount per Serving
Bromelain Powder (2,000 G.D.U./g) . . . 500 mg

Okay, now what you really want to know is what is the bromelain potency in one tablet? The answer is 1,000 G.D.U., but you would have a hard time figuring that out without a calculator, wouldn't you? To explain, the label is saying that the bromelain powder in the product contains 2,000 G.D.U. per gram, but only 500 milligrams of that powder is used in one tablet. Since 500 milligrams is .5 gram, one tablet contains only 1,000 G.D.U. of bromelain activity. When comparing products, you have to read the label very carefully. See Chapter 5 for more information on this.

THE PHARMACIST SAYS

G.D.U. stands for Gelatin Digesting Units, which is a commonly accepted measure of the potency of proteolytic (protein-digesting) enzymes. Another unit that you may see on labels is M.C.U., which stands for Milk Clotting Units. The advantage of labeling activity in units is that it is easy to compare the potencies of products.

Fluff

Watch out for fluff. What do we mean by fluff? Here are examples:

"Biochemically formulated"
"Fully bioactive"
"100% vegetable, energized formula"
"Hand-crafted in small batches in an exclusive alchemic process . . . "
"Our own unique super-oxygenated, energized, structured distilled living water"
"These powerful tinctures are electromagnetically infused with color frequencies known to heal the organ or system."
"Nutrients that are hydroponically farmed (grown on nutrient activated in water)"

"The inherent benefits of Vital Food Factors not found in ordinary vitamins and minerals"

Fluff sounds impressive but means nothing. The more fluff we see on a label, the more suspicious we should get.

Unregulated Dietary Supplements and Hidden Ingredients

There is a big difference between the claim that nutritional supplements are unregulated and the claim that they are poorly regulated.

There is a persistent tendency among those in the news media, and especially those with a bias against supplements, to talk about unregulated nutritional supplements.

In a recent example, there was an article in the January 30, 2002, *New York Times* titled "U.S. Athletes Must Guess on Supplements." In this story, the various Olympic organizations were criticized for sending "mixed messages" to Olympic-caliber athletes. On the one hand, the Olympic organizers accept endorsement money from various companies that manufacture and sell nutritional supplements. On the other hand, they tell athletes, according to *The New York Times*, "Do not take a vitamin and put it in your mouth, period."

Why so harsh an admonition? Why advise the most highly trained athletes in the world to not avail themselves of the health benefits of optimal nutrition? The reason, according to various Olympic officials and news reporters, is that supplements are unregulated, and may contain hormones, steroids, and their precursors. They claim that these substances are not listed on the product labels and, therefore, the athlete may inadvertently end up with blood levels of prohibited substances sufficient to disqualify him or her from competition.

The *Times* article quoted Frank Shorter, who is now chief of the United States Anti-Doping Agency, as saying, "The people who are manufacturing this stuff have no reason not to lace it." It also quotes The American Bobsled Federation as saying it "does not believe that the athletes should bear the burden of an unregulated supplement industry that can not guarantee all ingredients are identified on its labels."

As if there still might be any question as to whether or not the problem is due to a lack of regulations, the *Times* also stated the following:

"F.D.A. approval is not required to market supplements, which are considered foods and not drugs, under the Dietary Supplement Health and Education Act of 1994."

The implication is obvious. Supplement manufacturers can include undeclared ingredients in products with impunity because the products are unregulated, or not subject to FDA approval.

This is not true. Supplements are regulated, just as foods are regulated. All ingredients must be declared on the label. Unapproved food ingredients cannot be included in the product, let alone not declared on the label. Drugs cannot be hidden in foods or nutritional supplements. Doing so is illegal, and the FDA has full authority to prevent and prosecute those who break the law.

The regulatory status of dietary supplements is clearly set forth in the law, and the authority of the Food and Drug Administration as the enforcers of the regulations is clearly defined. Why, then, does the media persist in stating otherwise? In another story published in *The New York Times*, "Drug Testing in U.S. Comes Under Fire from Olympic Officials,"published on September 26, 2000, the following statement is included:

"The supplements are classified as food, and as such, are not regulated by the Food and Drug Administration. Steroids can be sold in the supplements legally, even when not labeled, as long as no medical claim is made, said Dr. Don Catlin, who operates the Olympic drug testing lab at U.C.L.A. and is a member of the I.O.C.'s doping commission."

How absurd! "Foods are not regulated by the Food and Drug Administration"? Perhaps the name of the agency should be changed to the Drug Administration?

"Steroids can be sold in supplements legally"? This is news to us, and we're sure that it comes as a great surprise to the FDA. Why are we so worried about the high cost of prescription drugs? All we need to do, it seems, is stop by our local health food store and get our steroid medications there.

This type of misinformation is not limited to news organizations such as *The New York Times*. According to an article published in the *Journal of the American Medical Association*,[1] nutritional supplements

---

[1]"Recent Patterns of Medication Use in the Ambulatory Adult Population of the United States," *Journal of the American Medical Association,* January 16, 2002.

are "by law not subject to FDA regulation." Again, this is just plain false.

As explained by the Council for Responsible Nutrition in its report "The Truth Must Be Told About Dietary Supplement Regulation" (www.crnusa.org):

> In media coverage, it is often falsely claimed that dietary supplements are "unregulated" since passage of the Dietary Supplement Health and Education Act of 1994 (DSHEA). In fact, the 1994 law reaffirmed that dietary supplements are regulated like foods. They have been regulated as a category of foods since the current Food, Drug, and Cosmetic Act was enacted in 1938. They are not drugs and have never been regulated as drugs. Like foods, dietary supplements are required to be safe. There is a procedure requiring notification of the FDA before new ingredients are introduced into dietary supplements, and the agency has disapproved numerous ingredients on safety grounds. The FDA has authority to remove products from the market that are unsafe. In recent years, the FDA has in fact taken action against a number of dietary supplements.
>
> Like foods, dietary supplements are required to provide full information to consumers through product labeling. This includes information such as nutrition labeling and ingredient labeling. The extensive labeling regulations are codified in Title 21 of the Code of Federal Regulations. The law requires that all labeling for dietary supplements be truthful and not misleading, and the FDA has authority to take action against any false statements made in labeling. The DSHEA imposed some additional requirements on dietary supplements, requiring companies to notify the FDA when claims are made about beneficial effects on the structure or function of the body ("structure/function claims").

Are there mislabeled dietary supplements being sold? Certainly. There are unscrupulous people in every business. But it should be kept in mind, however, that people often get what they ask for. This is true for the athlete who buys a miracle supplement, advertised in the back of a muscle magazine, containing herbs from Uganda mixed with Argentinian bull-testicle extract and guaranteed to build muscle, burn fat, increase endurance, improve sexual performance, and increase

SAT exam scores by 500 points—to provide the benefits of anabolic steroids without the risks associated with taking anabolic steroids! It's true for the college basketball player who blithely accepts unidentified capsules from some other player on the team bus. It's true for the consumer who sends in money for miraculous arthritis cures advertised on the radio.

This tendency to issue blanket condemnations of the dietary-supplement industry because a small number of supplements may be mislabeled is irresponsible. The statement that dietary supplements are unregulated is blatantly false. Instead, what the Olympic officials and *The New York Times* writers probably want to say is that dietary supplements are poorly regulated.

The regulations are in place, and they are adequate to address the problems encountered by the Olympic officials. Perhaps the FDA does not enforce the regulations to their satisfaction. That may be the case, but that does not mean the products are unregulated. It may mean the regulations are poorly enforced. Do athletes really have to "guess on supplements"? No, they do not. Do they have to use a little common sense and resist the temptation to ingest products claimed to provide the benefits of anabolic steroids without affecting test results? Yes, they do. Should they err on the side of caution? Yes, they should.

Does this mean dietary supplements are unregulated? Of course not. Where was *The New York Times* and the various Olympic officials when the FDA removed tryptophan supplements from the market? What about the numerous instances of contaminated Chinese herbal imports that were seized and removed from the market? What about comfrey and chaparral, which may contain an ingredient that might be harmful to the liver? Or red yeast rice, which has been virtually removed from the market because the FDA considers it a drug rather than a food supplement due to the claims being made. When the FDA feels it is necessary, it has no problem enforcing the laws that are on the books.

PART TWO

A Supplement Encyclopedia

Cautions: If you are pregnant or nursing, do not take any supplements without first consulting your obstetrician. If you are taking a medication, do not take any supplements without first discussing the possible interactions with your health-care provider. Do not take a supplement if you are hypersensitive to any of the ingredients it contains.

CHAPTER FIVE

Individual Nutrients and Herbs

In this chapter, we will provide information on individual nutrients and herbs. Each listing will provide the following information:

- *Related Items.* Other nutrients of similar or related composition.
- *Description.* A general description of the nutrient or herb.
- *Uses.* A discussion of the item's function and properties.
- *Indications.* A listing of health conditions for which the nutrient or herb may be useful.
- *Dosage.* How much and how often to use the nutrient.
- *Cautions.* Cautions or contraindications specific to the nutrient.
- *Products.* Representative examples of retail products. The company, product name, potency, and size are provided. Links to more detailed product information will be available on the web site www.bestsupplementsforyourhealth.com.

If you want information about a particular nutrient, look it up alphabetically in the chapter. If you have a specific health concern and want to find out which nutrients might be indicated, look in the therapeutic cross reference on page 297. Then check the appropriate listings in the chapter.

5-HTP

Related Item: Tryptophan.

Description: 5-hydroxytryptophan (5-HTP) is a neurotransmitter used by the body to make serotonin and melatonin. In supplements, 5-HTP is extracted from the seed of the plant *Griffonia simplicifolia.*

Uses: As a precursor to serotonin, 5-HTP may induce sleep, as well as influence mood. It has been recommended for mild depression and as an appetite suppressant. Increasing serotonin results in increased melatonin, the natural hormone that regulates the body's sleep cycle.

Indications: Anxiety, depression, fibromyalgia, migraine headaches, seasonal affective disorder, weight loss, obesity, insomnia, headaches.

Dosage: Generally, 300 milligrams per day is recommended. For sleep, as little as 100 milligrams before bedtime may be sufficient. For weight loss, up to 600 milligrams or more daily may be required.

Cautions: Use caution if you are already taking antidepressant medication.

Products:

Jarrow: 5-HTP, 100 mg, 60 capsules.
Doctor's Best: 5-HTP Best, 100 mg, 60 capsules.
Allergy Research: 5-HTP, 50 mg, 100 capsules.
Natrol: 5-HTP, 50 mg, 30 capsules.
Country Life: 5-HTP Tryptophan, 50 mg, 50 capsules.
Jarrow: 5-HTP, 50 mg, 90 capsules.

5-Hydroxytryptophan

See 5-HTP.

7-Keto DHEA

Related Item: DHEA.

Description: 7-keto DHEA is a metabolite of the hormone dehydroepiandrosterone (DHEA). Its chemical name is 3-acetyl-7-oxo-dehydroepiandrosterone.

Uses: DHEA is one of the primary adrenal steroid hormones, serving as, among other things, a precursor to estrogen and testosterone. 7-keto is not converted to these sex hormones.

Indications: Anti-aging, obesity, weight loss, energy, low immune system, sexual performance, stress.

For those who feel they would benefit from DHEA but fear the possible side effects of increased estrogen or testosterone production, 7-keto is offered as a substitute.

As we age, the production of DHEA and related hormones by the adrenal glands drops. It is thought that supplementing with those hormones may retard the aging process, boost the immune system, boost thermogenesis, and generally enhance the quality of life.

Dosage: For weight loss, the suggested dose is 100 milligrams, twice daily. For anti-aging purposes, from 25 to 100 milligrams daily is a general recommendation.

Cautions: 7-keto is chemically related to steroid hormones and long-term usage has not been studied for safety. Also, 7-keto may affect thyroid function, increasing T_3 levels, so those with thyroid disorders should exert caution before using 7-keto or DHEA.

Products:

Enzymatic Therapy: 7-Keto Naturalean, 100 mg, 30 capsules.
Enzymatic Therapy: 7-Keto DHEA, 25 mg, 60 capsules.
Twinlab: 7-Keto Maxilife, 25 mg, 60 capsules.
Twinlab: 7-Keto Fuel, 50 mg, 30 capsules.

Acerola Vitamin C

Related Item: Vitamin C.

Description: Acerola is the fruit of the small shrub *Malphighia glabra*. The fruit contains a very high concentration of vitamin C.

Uses: A concentrate or extract of acerola can be used in supplements as a source of natural vitamin C. Although natural vitamin C is no different from synthetic vitamin C, there are other substances in acerola (flavonoids, other vitamins, minerals) that offer additional benefit.

Just as it is desirable to take vitamin C with bioflavonoids rather than vitamin C alone, it may be of some benefit to take vitamin C either from acerola or with acerola concentrate.

What is important is to be careful not to be misled about what is actually in the product. If it is a high-potency vitamin C supplement, it is unlikely to provide vitamin C only from acerola. Instead, it is more likely a mixture of acerola-derived vitamin C and synthetic vitamin C. Read the label carefully.

Products:

Pure Encapsulations: Acerola Plus, 233 mg of vitamin C total, from 25.5 mg acerola extract, 6 mg ascorbyl palmitate, 200 mg ascorbic acid, with 150 mg hesperidin methylchalcone and 150 mg naringin, 120 vegicaps.

Acetyl-L-Carnitine

Related Item: Carnitine.

Description: Acetyl-L-carnitine is the acetyl ester of L-carnitine, commonly referred to as carnitine. As a supplement, it functions as a source of L-carnitine and acetyl groups.

For the cardioprotective action of carnitine, use a carnitine supplement rather than acetyl-L-carnitine. (See Carnitine for more information.) As a contributor of acetyl groups, however, acetyl-L-carnitine offers benefits not found with carnitine alone.

Uses: The acetyl component of acetyl-L-carnitine functions as a precursor for the formation of acetylcholine, one of the neurotransmitters in the brain thought to be involved in age-related dementias, including Alzheimer's disease.

Indications: Anti-aging, infertility, Alzheimer's disease, cardiovascular disease, neuropathies, Down syndrome.

Dosage: Generally, 500 to 1,000 milligrams two or three times daily is recommended.

Products:

Jarrow: Acetyl-L-Carnitine, 500 mg, 60 capsules.
Twinlab: Acetyl-L-Carnitine, 500 mg, 30 capsules.
Solgar: Acetyl-L-Carnitine, 250 mg, 30 vegicaps.
Allergy Research: Acetyl-L-Carnitine, 500 mg, 100 capsules.

Acidophillus

See Probiotics.

ALA

See Lipoic Acid.

Alkylglycerol

Related Items: Shark liver oil, squalene.

Description: Alkylglycerols are fat-soluble substances found naturally in the spleen, liver, bone marrow, and breast milk. In dietary supplements, they are concentrated from shark liver oil.

Uses: Alkylglycerols from shark liver oil are often included in cancer treatment protocols. They may help reduce the side effects of conventional cancer therapy. They are also thought to enhance immune system function, raise white blood cell counts, and exert some anti-inflammatory action.

Indications: Cancer, immune system, arthritis, psoriasis, HIV.

Dosage: A general dose is about 500 milligrams of shark liver oil or 100 milligrams of concentrated alkylglycerols. For serious infections, cancer, or human immunodeficiency virus (HIV), complementary physicians sometimes use up to 1,500 milligrams daily.

Products:

Amino Acid & Botanic Supply: Shark Liver Oil, 1,000 mg=200 mg, alkylglycerols, 60 softgels.
Lane Labs: Immunofin, 250 mg shark liver oil, 20% G-E lipids, 60 softgels.
Lane Labs: Immunofin, 250 mg shark liver oil, 20% G-E lipids, 120 softgels.
Scandinavian Natural: Alkyrol, 250 mg=50 mg alkylglycerols per cap, 60 softgels.
Scandinavian Natural: Alkyrol, 250 mg=50 mg alkylglycerols per cap, 120 softgels.
Scandinavian Natural: Alkyrol, 500 mg =100 mg alkylglycerols per cap, 120 softgels.
Solgar: Shark Liver Oil Complex, 500 mg=50 mg alkylglycerols per cap, 60 softgels.

Aloe

Description: Aloe (*Aloe vera*) is one of the oldest medicinal plants known to man. Different parts of the plant yield compounds with widely differing therapeutic actions.

Uses: There are two major parts of the aloe plant. A bitter latex is found in a layer of cells just under the outer rind of the leaves. The dried latex that is derived from this part of the leaf is a strong laxative.

It contains anthraquinones (bar-baloin, or aloin A & B, and aloe-emodin) that can exert a potent cathartic action. The aloe vera gel is derived from the inner, central part of the leaf. This mucilage-nous liquid is the part used topi-

> *Indications:* Aloe vera gel, topical: Burns, wound healing, psoriasis. Aloe vera gel juice: Diabetes, gastrointestinal disorders. Aloe vera bitter latex: Constipation.

cally and internally for its healing, antimicrobial, and anti-inflammatory activity.

Unfortunately, there are several problems associated with aloe products. First, there is a paucity of studies supporting the many claims made for aloe, especially those associated with oral use. Second, there is still some question as to what the active ingredients are in aloe. In turn, this leads to a problem with standardization and potency of the various commercial products on the market. There is considerable variation in product composition from one brand to another. This makes it very difficult to distinguish between good products and bad. And third, the nomenclature and labeling of many aloe products is very confusing. It is often difficult to discern what is actually in the container by reading the label.

For example, contrary to some claims, there is no difference between the gel and the juice, except for the addition of thickening agents. When first taken from the plant, aloe gel is naturally viscous, or gel-like. But the enzymes naturally present in the gel cause it to become watery in a short time. So any product, regardless of whether it is labeled as a gel or juice, will contain thickeners (such as gums or starches).

Theoretically, a product labeled "aloe vera gel" should refer to the natural, undiluted gel obtained from the inner portion of the leaf. Without additives (preservatives), it would be difficult to package or store this material. An aloe vera concentrate should theoretically consist of the natural gel with the water removed. Neither of the two above-mentioned products would be appropriate for internal use. Aloe vera juice, which should be the gel diluted with water (usually up to 50 percent), would be the form appropriate for ingestion.

The most universally accepted use of aloe gel involves its external healing and soothing action on various skin disorders, including burns, wounds, and minor skin aliments. The discovery that aloe gel may contain prostaglandin precursor fatty acids such as gamma-linolenic acid (GLA) may explain why it appears to exert anti-inflammatory activity. This may explain, for example, why it proved helpful in treating psoriasis in one study.

Aloe gel juice is used internally for other types of problems, ranging from gastrointestinal upset to diabetes and ulcers. But again, there is currently little research to support this.

Further complicating matters is that some research indicates that the anthraquinones emodin and aloe-emodin may be effective against *Helicobacter pylori*, which is thought to cause gastric ulcer. But these substances, as already mentioned, are not supposed to be present in the aloe gel except in very small quantities. They are found in the latex, and at the appropriate dosage have powerful laxative action.

Some aloe products are labeled as "whole leaf." What does that mean? Does it mean that it contains the bitter latex as well as the gel? Until some standardization of terminology and content is adopted, it remains difficult to make meaningful product recommendations. Some investigators have analyzed commercial aloe products and found that some contain no aloe (just maltodextrin), some contain a mixture of maltodextrin and aloe, and some are pure aloe.

Cautions: There are two types of aloe products. The type that contains the bitter latex is a potent laxative. The aloe gel or juice products should not contain the laxative components of aloe. Do not confuse the two.

Aloe is a stimulant laxative and should be used with caution. It should not be used for a prolonged period of time, as this may cause dependence and impaired bowel function.

Products:

Nature's Herbs: Aloe Vera Inner Gel, 250 mg aloe vera inner gel, 100 capsules. Note: This product is labeled as a "mild stimulant laxative," with the appropriate warnings and cautions.
Nature's Herbs: Aloe Vera Gel, 50 mg aloe vera gel, 200:1 extract, 50 softgels.
Lily of the Desert: Aloe Vera Juice (aloin and aloe emodin removed), quart.
R Pur Aloe: Super Gelly (contains aloe vera gel), 4-oz gel.

Alpha-Lipoic Acid

See Lipoic Acid.

American Ginseng

Related Items: Ginseng, Siberian ginseng.

Description: There are several types of ginseng—different species of the same genus. According to Chinese medicine, American ginseng (*Panax quinquefolis*) is less stimulating, or less "yang," than Asian ginseng (*Panax ginseng*). The main active ingredient are the ginsenosides.

Uses: Chinese medicine considers American ginseng to have different uses than Asian ginseng. Western medicine does not. If you are following a protocol of diagnosis and treatment based upon traditional Chinese medical philosophy, choose the type of ginseng dictated by that philosophy. For others—that is, for most of us—our suggestion is to consider the two as almost interchangeable. Historically, ginseng has retained a reputation as one of the premier general tonic herbs for more than 5,000 years. It is used as a tonic to revitalize and replenish vital energy. This does not mean you should expect the type of energy jolt you get from a dose of caffeine. The effect is more subtle, especially with American ginseng. It is a tonic that revitalizes the function of the organism as a whole, building resistance, reducing susceptibility to illness, and promoting health and longevity.

> *Indications:* Immune system, athletic performance, energy low, anti-aging, cold & flu, erectile dysfunction, fertility (male), chronic fatigue syndrome, cancer, diabetes.

Dosage: For standardized extracts, the dose is 200 to 500 milligrams per day. For non-standardized concentrates, the dose is higher. For liquid tinctures, follow the directions on the label or use 2 to 3 milliliters three times a day.

Cautions: American Ginseng may be contraindicated for persons with hypertension.

Products:

Root to Health: American Ginseng, 500 mg *Panax quinquefolius* per capsule, 100 capsules.
Solgar: American Ginseng Extract, 100 mg Panax quinquefolius root extract (10% ginsenosides), 200 mg *Panax quinquefolius* powder (5% ginsenosides), 15 mg ginsenosides total, 60 vegicaps.

Androstenedione

Related Item: DHEA.

Description: Androstenedione is a steroid hormone, naturally found in the adrenal glands. It is derived from DHEA and converted in the body to testosterone, estrone, and estradiol.

Use: It is used by bodybuilders and athletes in the belief that it increases blood levels of testosterone, which in turn leads to increased muscle. Whether or not it really exerts this action remains controversial.

Cautions: Prudence dictates that androstenedione supplementation is best undertaken only on the advice and guidance of a physician. Higher dosage levels should definitely not be used without medical supervision. The long-term effects of androstenedione supplementation are unknown. Those who are at risk for prostate, breast, uterine, or ovarian cancer should not take androstenedione. The most common adverse reactions seem to be androgenic effects, such as acne, and increased facial hair.

Products:

Olympian Labs: Androstene Power, androstenedione, 50 mg, 90 capsules.

Antioxidants

Related Items: Vitamin E, vitamin C, selenium.

Description: Antioxidants, in general, are substances that can neutralize unstable molecules that can cause damage. In biological systems, we are concerned about damage to DNA, cell membranes, etc. These unstable molecules are sometimes referred to as "free radicals."

One type of instability involves oxidation. Free radicals can do damage by acting as runaway oxidizing agents. Antioxidant nutrients can neutralize this potential hazard. They sacrifice themselves to protect other cells in the body from oxidative damage.

There are many, many antioxidant substances found in foods and supplements. In addition to the well-known vitamins and minerals (vitamin C, vitamin E, beta-carotene, and selenium), there are phytochemicals such as flavonoids. Lycopene, lutein, quercetin, catechins, polyphenols, OPCs, PCOs, anthocyanins—these are now being recognized as perhaps even more powerful antioxidants than vitamins C and E.

Equally important is the realization that the antioxidants usually function most effectively when used in combination. This may be why some studies show better results with antioxidant-rich foods than with isolated, or supplemental nutrients.

Arginine

Description: Arginine is a semi-essential amino acid. In addition to the usual functions of amino acids in general, i.e. protein formation, arginine is involved specifically as a precursor to nitric oxide (NO), and the amino acids ornithine and proline.

Uses: Most of the reasons for using supplemental arginine relate to its role as a precursor to nitric oxide (NO). Nitric oxide is produced throughout the body, and plays an important role in

> *Indications:* Cardiovascular disease, wound healing, athletic performance, erectile dysfunction, fertility (male), immune system.

cardiovascular system, immune system, and nervous system function.

Nitric oxide has been shown to reduce platelet stickiness and mononuclear cell adhesion, dilate blood vessels, and inhibit free radical production. It is, therefore, useful to those with atherosclerosis, elevated cholesterol levels, and other types of cardiovascular disease.

Because of the vasodilating action of nitric oxide, there is some interest in the use of arginine in treating erectile dysfunction. Research has also shown that arginine may be helpful in treating male infertility, improving sperm count and motility.

Arginine is also thought to be beneficial for improving wound healing, burns, and other types of trauma, as well as enhancing immune system function. There is ongoing interest in the use of arginine by those with various types of cancer, AIDS, and HIV infection.

High doses of arginine have been shown to increase levels of human growth hormone. It has been used by bodybuilders to increase muscle, reduce fat, and improve energy levels. Studies in this area have yielded mixed results. It is sometimes taken along with another amino acid, ornithine.

Dosage: It should be noted that most of the research on arginine utilizes doses in excess of 5 to 10 grams daily. In treating cardiovascular and fertility problems, up to 20 grams a day may be recommended.

Doses of up to 15 grams daily seem to be well tolerated.

Cautions: The herpes simplex virus protein contains high levels of arginine. Some are concerned that supplemental arginine might in some way enhance or encourage the growth of the herpes simplex virus. They caution against taking arginine supplements if you have recurrent oral herpes outbreaks. This concern is more speculative than factual, but bears mentioning nevertheless.

Products:

Solgar: Arginine, 500 mg, vegetarian and kosher, 250 vegicaps.
Jarrow: Arginine, 1,000 mg, 100 tablets.

Artichoke Leaf

Description: Artichoke leaf (*Cynara scolymus*) is an herb or herbal extract derived from the leaves of the globe artichoke. This is not the part normally eaten as a vegetable, which is the unopened flower head, or bud, and bracts. The leaves are found below the flower head, and are very bitter in taste.

Uses: The official use is for the treatment of dyspeptic problems, or indigestion. But most of the current interest in artichoke leaf

> *Indications:* Cholesterol problems, indigestion, irritable bowel syndrome, liver disorders.

involves its ability to stimulate bile production (choleretic), lower cholesterol, and protect the liver from damage by toxins and free radicals.

These actions are supported by clinical evidence. In the past, it was thought that the active ingredient in artichoke leaf was cynarin, but now it is felt that a combination of ingredients are responsible, including cynaroside and luteolin.

Standardized extracts, in capsule form, are available, as are liquid tinctures. Artichoke leaf is not usually prepared as a tea (infusion).

Cautions: Caution should be exercised if you have gallstones or bile duct blockage.

Products:

Nature's Herbs: Artichoke Power, 100 mg, Std 15% caffeoylquinic acids; 375 mg artichoke pwd., 60 capsules.
Enzymatic Therapy: Artichoke Extract, 160 mg, Std 13-18% caffeoylquinic acids as cholerogenic acid, 90 capsules.
Nature's Way: Artichoke Extract Standardized, 300 mg, Std 5% (15 mg) caffeoylquinic acids, plus 150 mg milk thistle, 60 capsules.
Flora: Cynarol, 500 mg, 11:1 concentrate, 40 softgels.

Ascorbic Acid

See Vitamin C.

Ascorbyl Palmitate

Related Items: Vitamin C, ascorbic acid.

Description: Vitamin C is a water-soluble vitamin and antioxidant. To convert vitamin C from a water-soluble substance to a fat-soluble substance, it can be chemically modified by reacting it with the long-chain saturated fatty acid palmitic acid. This results in an ester, ascorbyl palmitate, which is now fat-soluble.

Why is this important? If you want to incorporate vitamin C as an antioxidant in a fat-based food product, or oil, you need a form of vitamin C that will dissolve in oil. Ascorbyl palmitate, being fat-soluble, can be used in products of that type. It can also be used in topical skin creams and ointments, intended for cosmetic and therapeutic purposes.

Uses: In addition to its fat-solubility-related uses as an additive in foods and cosmetics, ascorbyl palmitate is thought to

Indications: Skin conditions (topical), cholesterol problems.

possibly offer some advantage as a nutritional supplement. If ascorbyl palmitate is absorbed intact, it may be more active in the lipid-rich parts of the body, such as the cell membranes, helping to lower LDL cholesterol, etc. It may be more effective in regenerating vitamin E than vitamin C.

While interesting, these possible advantages of ascorbyl palmitate over regular vitamin C have yet to be proven.

Dosage: The recommended daily allowance for vitamin C is 75 to 90 milligrams for nonsmokers and 110 to 125 milligrams for smokers. The amounts typically found in supplements provide 500 and 1,000 milligrams daily, although some claim that 200 milligrams are enough to ensure maximum tissue levels. Many take much higher amounts. Some, for example, take 4 to 5 grams daily to ameliorate the symptoms of a cold. Some research studies have used doses in the 5-gram-daily range. Daily intakes of up to 2 or 3 grams a day are generally considered benign. Too high a dose will result in diarrhea.

Products:

Pure Encapsulations: Ascorbyl Palmitate, 214 mg ascorbic acid from 500 mg ascorbyl palmitate, 90 capsules.

Ashwagandha

Description: Ashwagandha (*Withania somniferum*) is a plant that is popular in Indian or Ayurvedic medicine. It belongs to the pepper family. The roots are used medicinally.

Uses: Many of the constituents of ashwagandha resemble those in Asian ginseng, and in fact, it seems to function as an adapto-

> *Indications:* Immune system, stress, arthritis.

gen, a nonspecific tonic that strengthens the body's ability to handle stress of all types.

Ashwagandha is used for most problems affecting the immune system, as well as an anti-inflammatory for treatment of arthritis.

Products:

Nature's Answer: Ashwagandha Root Alcohol Free, 2,000 mg ashwagandha fluid ext (1:1) per 2 ml, 2 fl oz.
America's Finest: Ashwagandha Root Extract, 300 mg, 1.5% withanolides, 4.5 mg, 60 capsules.
Nature's Herbs: Ashwagandha, 300 mg, 1.5% withanolides, 4.5 mg, 50 tablets.
Solgar: Ashwagandha Root Extract, 300 mg, 1.5% withanolides, 5 mg, plus 100 mg ashwagandha rt pwd., 60 vegicaps.
Solaray: Ashwagandha, 470 mg, 1.5% withanolides, 7 mg, 60 capsules.
Herb Pharm: Ashwagandha Whole Root, organically grown; (1:4) dry herb/menstrum, 1 fl oz.

Astragalus

Description: Astragalus (*Astragalus membranaceus*) is a plant native to northern China. The portion of the plant used medicinally is the 4–7-year-old dried root.

Uses: Astragalus is one of the premier immune-enhancing, adaptogenic herbs known to Chinese medicine. It is thought to be espe-

> *Indications:* Cancer, immune system, liver disorders, stress, cold and flu, hepatitis.

cially valuable as a preventive agent, and for its ability to renew vitality and energy after an illness has passed.

It is perhaps the herb of choice, according to some, for treating serious illness, including cancer. Most of the research on astragalus is in

Chinese, but it is currently under investigation as a cancer treatment and has been shown to also be especially beneficial in protecting the liver.

Dosage: Available in capsule and tincture form, the recommended dosage is often high, typically 400 to 500 mg, eight times daily.

Products:

Nature's Answer: Astragalus Root Alcohol Free, 2,000 mg astragalus root fluid Ext (1:1) per 2 ml, 1 fl oz.
Nature's Herbs: Astragalus Power, 200 mg, 7% polysaccharides, plus 250 mg astragalus root, 60 capsules.
Solgar: Astragalus Root Extract, 225 mg, 0.5% triterpene glycosides (1 mg), plus 250 mg astragalus root, 60 vegicaps.
Nature's Answer: Astragalus Root Extract, 250 mg, 0.3% astragalosides, plus 250 mg astragalus root, 60 vegicaps.
Nature's Way: Astragalus Root, 470 mg astragalus root, 100 capsules. Note: This is a concentrate, not an extract.

Barberry

Description: Barberry (*Berberis vulgaris*) is an herb found in Europe and North America. The root and stem bark are used medicinally. It contains berberine, a compound also found in goldenseal and Oregon grape.

Uses: Thought to exert antimicrobial action, barberry has been recommended for chronic candidiasis, parasites, and other infections, but this is not supported by current research.

> *Indications:* Immune system, psoriasis, candidiasis, ventricular arrhythmias, urinary tract infections.

There is some interesting speculation that it may be of value in treating ventricular arrhythmias and psoriasis, but again, strong supporting evidence is not yet available.

Products:

Nature's Answer: Barberry Root, 2,000 mg barberry fluid extract (1:1) per 2 ml, 1 fl oz.

Barley Grass

Related Items: Spirulina, green foods, wheat grass, chlorella, chlorophyll, blue green algae.

Description: Dried barley grass concentrates, like all green food supplements, are relatively rich in protein, chlorophyll, and carotenoids.

Uses: Green food concentrates of this type are claimed to have anticancer activity, modulate immune system function, lower cholesterol, treat gastrointestinal problems, and function, generally, as detoxification agents.

While convincing proof of all of these actions may be lacking, there is certainly no reason not to include one of the green food concentrates in a comprehensive supplement program. They are all rich in phytonutrients, antioxidants, and varying amounts of trace nutrients. The problem with these supplements is that exaggerated marketing claims often accompany the products, and consumers may overestimate their value. As a general rule, they should be considered adjuncts to other supplements, not replacements or alternatives to them.

Cautions: Green food supplements may be rich in vitamin K, so caution should be exercised if you are taking anticoagulant medication.

Products:

Nature's Answer: Barley Grass, 900 mg organic barley grass per 3 vegicaps, 90 vegicaps.
Kyolic: Kyo Green Drink Powder, combination of young barley and wheat grasses with chlorella, brown rice, and kelp, 5.3 oz powder.
Green Kamut: Just Barley, dried juice from organic barley leaves, 80 g powder.
Green Foods: Green Magma Original Powder, dried juice from young barley leaves, 5.3 oz powder.

Bee Pollen

Related Item: Flower pollen.
Description: Bee pollen is plant pollen, the male germ seeds of plants, collected by worker bees. The bees combine the pollen with plant nectar and bee saliva. This material is then used as food for drone bees.
Uses: In spite of the fact that bee pollen has been a popular health food supplement for many years, there is little justification for its use. There is even some question as to whether it has any value as a food for humans as the pollen grains may not be digestible. There is no support to early claims by athletes that it increased stamina and performance.

We suggest using flower pollen, rather than bee pollen.

Cautions: Bee pollen should be avoided by anyone who is allergic or hypersensitive to bee venom.

Products:

Nature's Way: Bee Pollen Blend, 580 mg bee pollen from China and Europe, 100 capsules.
Nature's Answer: Bee pollen, 1,000 mg high desert bee pollen per ml, 1 oz liquid.

Beta-1,3-Glucan

Description: Beta-glucan is a complex polysaccharide derived from the cell wall of certain yeasts, mushrooms, oat fiber, barley fiber, and seaweed. Depending on the source, it consists of a mixture of varying proportions of beta-1,3-glucan, beta-1,6-glucan, and/or beta-1, 4-glucan.

Uses: The primary use of this material is as an immune system modulator, and a cholesterol-lowering agent.

Indications: Cancer, immune system, cholesterol problems.

Numerous studies show that the beta-glucans are effective in activating certain white blood cells. These white cells are essential for optimal immune system function, and are even involved in battling tumor cells.

Some research indicates that beta-glucans modulate immune function without causing it to be overactive. This is valuable in treating autoimmune disorders such as rheumatoid arthritis.

Beta-glucans may be the component of soluble fibers such as oat bran responsible for lowering cholesterol levels.

Cautions: Persons with food allergies should be aware of the source of the beta-glucans in the supplement being used.

Products: We have provided a selection of products, but you will notice that the "potency" varies over a wide range, from 20 to 500 milligrams. What does that mean? We don't know. In our opinion, there seems to be a lack of standardized terminology in this product category, making it very difficult to compare one product to another.

Natrol: Beta Glucans 20 mg, "Beta Precise," beta 1,3 & 1,6 glucans, 20 mg, 30 capsules.
Nutrition Supply Corp: NSC 100 (Immunition), dSM beta 1,3/1,6 glucan 10 mg, micronized from Saccharomyces cerevisiae, 60 capsules.

Source Naturals: Beta Glucan, Purified beta 1,3 glucan, 7.5 mg, 60 capsules.
America's Finest: Beta 1,3 Glucan, 500 mg, 100 capsules.

Beta-Carotene

Related Items: Carotenoids, lutein, lycopene, zeaxanthin, alpha-carotene, canthaxanthin, vitamin A.

Description: Beta-carotene is a yellow-orange plant pigment, which may be converted in the body to vitamin A. Beta-carotene is one of many carotenoids found in green vegetables and fruits, but is the one that is most readily converted to vitamin A.

Not all ingested beta-carotene is converted to vitamin A. The body uses only the amount needed, and the rest is stored. For this reason, beta-carotene is not as toxic as vitamin A, and larger amounts can be consumed with no harm to health.

Uses: Beta-carotene has two important functions. First, it can be converted to vitamin A by the body, as needed. Second, beta-carotene is a powerful antioxidant.

> *Indications:* Cancer, cardiovascular disease, HIV, immune system, leukoplakia, night blindness, asthma, cataracts, macular degeneration, HIV.

Numerous studies, over many years, indicated that people with the lowest intake of beta-carotene had the highest incidence of cancer. In the mid-1990s, much to everyone's surprise, studies were published showing that beta-carotene, in certain instances (among smokers), actually made cancer worse. The best explanation for this, so far, is that synthetic beta-carotene, the type used in those studies, does not function the same as natural beta-carotene, or perhaps even more to the point, natural mixed carotenoids.

On a supplement label, the synthetic form is identified only as "beta-carotene," while the natural form is usually accompanied by "...from *D. salina*," "...from algae," or "...from palm," etc.

Beta-carotene remains a powerful protective agent, effective against various types of cancer, heart disease, infections, and immune system problems. Some clinicians feel that beta-carotene is an essential component in the treatment for people with acquired immune deficiency syndrome (AIDS).

Cautions: Large doses of beta-carotene, or other carotenoids, can produce a harmless, and reversible, yellowing of the skin. Smokers should avoid supplements containing synthetic beta-carotene, and high levels of isolated beta-carotene.

Products:

Jarrow: Marine Beta Carotene, 25,000 IU, natural beta-carotene (*D. Salina*), 100 softgels.
Solgar: Beta Carotene, 10,000 IU, natural beta-carotene, dry, vegetarian, 250 tablets.
Solgar: Beta Carotene, 11,000 IU, natural beta-carotene from carrot oil 100 softgels.
Twinlab: Carotene Caps, 25,000 IU, synthetic beta-carotene, dry, water dispersed, 120 capsules.

Beta-Hydroxy Beta-MethylButyrate

See HMB.

Betaine

Related Items: Choline, trimethylglycine, betaine hydrochloride.

Description: A substance closely related to choline. It functions, biochemically, as a methyl donor. It is also involved in the synthesis of the essential amino acid methionine from homocysteine.

Choline has four methyl groups. When choline reacts chemically, and donates one of those methyl groups to another molecule, it forms betaine (trimethylglycine). When betaine donates one of its methyl groups, it forms DMG (dimethylglycine).

Uses: In enhancing the conversion of homocysteine to methionine, which requires folic acid, vitamin B_6, and vitamin B_{12}, betaine may lower the risk of heart disease. Betaine and choline may be in-

Indications: Cholesterol problems, liver disorders, cardiovascular disease.

volved in prevention of fatty liver, neurotransmitter function, and the metabolism of fat. Agents that facilitate the liver's ability to process fats are called lipotropic agents.

The body manufactures choline from methionine, with the aid of folic acid and vitamin B_{12} as coenzymes.

Another form of betaine often seen in supplement form is betaine hydrochloride. This form is usually used as a source of hydrochloric acid, for appropriate digestive problems, rather than as a source of betaine.

Products:

Jarrow: TMG-500, anhydrous betaine, 120 tablets.
Jarrow: TMG Crystals, anhydrous betaine, 1 teaspoon equals 2.6 g, 50 g.
Source Naturals: TMG 750 mg, 120 tablets.

Betaine Hydrochloride

Related Items: Betaine, trimethylglycine.

Description: A form of betaine that contains hydrochloric acid, intended for use as a digestive aid.

Uses: Betaine hydrochloride is intended for those with insufficient levels of stomach acid. Hydrochloric acid is normally secreted in the stomach, and is necessary for proper digestion of food. Betaine hydrochloride often comes in combination with pepsin, the proteolytic enzyme found in the stomach.

Some feel that certain health problems, such as food allergies, asthma, and candidiasis, are related to incomplete or inefficient digestion of protein.

A dose of 650 milligrams of betaine hydrochloride, or 10 grains, should be sufficient. Higher doses should be used only under the guidance of a physician.

Cautions: Discontinue use if a burning sensation (heartburn) is experienced unless advised otherwise by your physician.

Products:

Solgar: Beta Pepsin, betaine HCl, 325 mg; pepsin (1:10,000) 59 mg, 250 tablets. Caution: Do not take in cases of stomach or duodenal pain or history of ulcers.
Advanced Medical Nutrition: Betaine Hydrochloride, betaine HCl, 648 mg, 90 capsules. Does not contain pepsin. Do not use if gastric hyperacidity or peptic ulcers are present.
Twinlab: Betaine HCl, betaine HCl, 648 mg, pepsin (1:10,000) 130 mg, 100 capsules. Warning: Do not take on an empty stomach.

Beta-Sitosterol

Related Items: Phytosterols, phytostanols.

Description: Beta-sitosterol is a phytosterol, a compound found in plants that is chemically similar in structure to cholesterol, which is found only in animals. Beta-sitosterol is the most common type of phytosterol found in the diet. High levels of beta-sitosterol are also found in saw palmetto, pumpkin seed, and pygeum.

Uses: Beta-sitosterol most likely has cholesterol-lowering activity similar to that of the phytosterols and phytostanols in

> *Indications:* Benign prostatic hypertrophy, cholesterol problems.

general. But the interest in beta-sitosterol is related more to its apparent role as a treatment of benign prostatic hyperplasia (BPH).

Numerous studies have shown that beta-sitosterol and products containing beta-sitosterol are effective in improving the symptoms associated with BPH.

Dosage: The amount varies with the nature of the product. In Europe, products containing between 20 to 130 milligrams of beta-sitosterol, three times daily, with meals, have been used. For maintenance, about one-half that amount is used. Substantially higher doses are used for cholesterol reduction.

Cautions: There is a possibility that beta-sitosterol interferes with the absorption of carotenoids, vitamin E, and lycopene.

Products:

Natrol: Beta Sitosterol, 120 mg beta sitosterol, 60 mg campesterol, 40 mg stigmasterol, 60 tablets.

Bilberry

Related Item: Bioflavonoids.

Description: Bilberry (*Vaccinium myrtillus*) is used as an herbal supplement because it is rich in anthocyanosides and other flavonoids, which are powerful antioxidants. Bilberry is closely related to the American blueberry. Today, the berries are used in the preparation of supplements, although the leaf was also used historically.

Uses: The anthocyanodin flavonoids in bilberry protect and maintain the tone of small blood vessels, thus enhancing the flow of oxygen-rich blood to areas such as the retina of the eye.

> *Indications:* Diabetes, retinopathy, cataracts, macular degeneration, night blindness, cardiovascular disease, diarrhea, hemorrhoids, varicose veins.

Because of this ability to enhance microcirculation, and protect against oxidative damage, bilberry appears to be valuable in preventing and treating many of the vision problems associated with aging, including cataracts and retinopathies (including diabetic retinopathy), along with, possibly, glaucoma and poor night vision.

There is also some evidence that bilberry anthocyanosides enhance the regeneration of rhodopsin, or visual purple, found in the rods of the eye. This might explain its effect on night vision.

All flavonoid-rich substances like bilberry have a tonifying effect on the circulatory system. It is used for easy bruising, hemorrhoids, varicose veins, spider veins, and before surgery to minimize bruising and excessive bleeding.

Wild bilberry produces small, astringent berries. Cultivated bilberry, however, produces a larger, sweeter berry that is almost identical to the North American blueberry (*Vaccinium angustifolium*). It might seem that blueberries and bilberries could be used interchangeably, then, and for many purposes, that might be correct. On the other hand, certain of the traditional uses, such as treating diarrhea with the dried berries, might be dependent to a degree on the wild berries' astringent properties. Cultivated bilberry, or blueberry, would not be expected to be as effective.

A COMMENT FROM DR. ABEL

Bilberry is a bioflavonoid found in the berries of a small shrub, *Vaccinium myrtillus*. The berries are loaded with anthocyanins. The bilberry, or huckleberry, is a relative of the grape and blueberry. The anthocyanins contribute to the production of rhodopsin, and improve vision at night. In fact, there is a story from World War II that cites bilberry jam as the reason British pilots could see so well at night. Many references cite bilberry as having preventive and therapeutic value in a host of diseases including cataract, glaucoma, macular degeneration, and diabetes. The fact remains that it is a minor player, even in diabetes, where it helps support blood vessel function. There are other bioflavonoids such as quercetin, which is a natural antihistamine and prevents oozing from blood vessels. Bilberry as a supplement may be helpful for night driving; those who are not diabetic can gain an equivalent effect from blueberries.

Dosage: A dose of between 160 and 320 milligrams daily, in divided doses, is usually recommended, although higher doses can be taken if necessary. A standardized (25% anthocyanosides) form is now most often used, in capsule form. Liquid extracts are also available.

Cautions: As is the case for most phytotherapeutic supplements of this type, bilberry has a slight blood-thinning effect. This is generally a beneficial property, but use caution if taking blood-thinning medications.

Products:

Solaray: Bilberry One Daily, 160 mg bilberry extract providing 36% anthocyanosides, 30 capsules.

Solgar: Bilberry Vegicaps, 60 mg bilberry extract providing 25% anthocyanosides, 100 mg bilberry powder, and 322 mg ginkgo leaf powder, 50 vegicaps.

Scandinavian Natural: Strix, 80 mg bilberry extract providing 25% anthocyanosides, 60 tablets.

Jarrow: Bilberry Grapeskin, 80 mg bilberry extract providing 25% anthocyanosides, and 200 mg grapeskin providing 30% polyphenols, 120 capsules. Note: this is actually a combination product, containing both bilberry and grapeskin, which we feel is complementary to the action of bilberry.

Biotin

Description: Biotin, also known as vitamin H, is a water-soluble B vitamin involved in the metabolism of protein, fat, and carbohydrates.

Uses: Biotin is thought to be useful in high doses for preventing brittle nails and hair loss. It may be useful in diabetes, enhanc-

> *Indications:* Skin disorders, hair, skin, and nails, diabetes.

ing glucose metabolism and preventing diabetic neuropathy.

Dosage: The recommended daily value for biotin is 300 micrograms.

Cautions: There are no known toxic effects.

Products:

Allergy Research: Biotin 5000, 5 mg (5,000 mcg) biotin, 60 capsules.

Country Life: Biotin, 5 mg (5,000 mcg) biotin, 60 capsules.

Ecological Formulas: MegaBiotin 7500, contains 7.5 mg (7,500 mcg) biotin, 50 capsules.

Black Cohosh

Description: Black cohosh (*Cimicifuga racemosa*) is native to North America, and has been widely used by Native Americans, early settlers, and herbal doctors. Black cohosh was a main ingredient in Lydia Pinkham's "Vegetable Compound." Supplements of black cohosh consist of the fresh or dried rhizome with the attached roots.

Uses: Black cohosh influences the hormonal regulatory systems, greatly alleviating the symptoms of menopause. A considerable number of clinical studies have

> *Indications:* Menopause, menstrual irregularities, premenstrual syndrome, osteoporosis.

been published on a product Remifemin, in Germany, supporting the usefulness of black cohosh for premenstrual and menopausal conditions. Black cohosh may be the best documented herbal preparation for these types of problems.

Dosage: Follow instructions on bottle.

Products:

Nature's Herbs: Black Cohosh Extract, 80 mg black cohosh root ext (2.5% terpene gylcosides), and 380 mg black cohosh root powder, 60 capsules.

Nature's Answer: Black Cohosh, 1,000 mg black cohosh root in 28 drops, 1 oz liquid.

Smithkline Beecham: Remifemin Menopause, 20 mg black cohosh root and rhizome from black cohosh root and rhizome extract, 60 tablets.

Black Currant Seed Oil

Description: Black currant seed oil is derived from the seed of the plant *Ribes nigrum.* It is a rich source of gamma-linolenic acid (GLA), 15 to 20 percent, as well as alpha-linolenic acid (ALA), 12 to 14 percent, and stearidonic acid (SDA), 2 to 4 percent.

Other oils rich in GLA are borage oil and evening primrose oil, but black currant oil is unique in the fact that it contains ALA along with the GLA. Alpha-linolenic acid is present in high amounts in flaxseed oil.

Uses: GLA is an omega-6 oil. Not all omega-6 oils are undesirable. The predominant omega-6 oils in the diet—linoleic, linolenic, and arachidonic—can be both detrimental and beneficial. Linoleic acid is essential to life. In the body, these oils are converted into powerful, hormone-like substances called prostaglandins. The omega-6 oils can form two types. One type, the 2 series, is usually detrimental,

> **Indications:** Cardiovascular disease, arthritis (rheumatoid), cancer, ulcerative colitis, diabetic neuropathy, skin disorders, eczema.

causing inflammation, etc. The other type, the 1 series, is beneficial, reducing inflammation. The GLA type of omega-6 oil leads to the beneficial, series 1 type of prostaglandin. The beneficial actions of series 1 prostaglandins are similar to those of the series 3 prostaglandins derived from omega-3 oils, ALA (flaxseed oil), and EPA (fish oil). Thus, GLA, from borage, black currant, and evening primrose oil, provides much the same benefit as the omega-3 oils from fish and flaxseed.

Some nutritionists prefer recommending the omega-3 oils, and others recommend the GLA-containing oils. But black currant seed oil may offer the best of both, as it contains GLA, which is metabolized to series 1 prostaglandins, and ALA, which is metabolized to EPA, the precursor to series 3 prostaglandins. Stearidonic acid is also metabolized to EPA.

Dosage: The dose can vary widely, with an average ranging from three to six capsules daily.

Cautions: This item has a slight "thinning" effect on the blood. This, generally, is a good thing. But if you are taking "blood-thinning" medications, check with your doctor.

Products:

Health from the Sun: Black Currant Oil, 1000 mg, 60 softgels.
Natrol: Black Currant Oil, 500 mg, 90 softgels.

Blue Green Algae

Related Items: Spirulina, green foods, wheat grass, barley grass, chlorophyll, chlorella.

Description: All green-food supplements are relatively rich in protein, chlorophyll, and carotenoids. Marketing claims to the contrary, there is little documented therapeutic difference among them.

Uses: Green-food concentrates of this type are claimed to have anticancer activity, modulate immune system function, lower cholesterol, treat gastrointestinal problems, and function, generally, as detoxification agents.

While convincing proof of all of these actions may be lacking, there is certainly no reason not to include one of the green-food concentrates in a comprehensive supplement program. They are all rich in phytonutrients, antioxidants, and varying amounts of trace nutrients. The problem with these supplements is that exaggerated marketing claims often accompany the products, and consumers may overestimate their value. As a general rule, they should be considered adjuncts to other supplements, not replacements or alternatives to them.

Cautions: Green-food supplements may be rich in vitamin K, so caution should be exercised if you are taking anticoagulant medication.

Products:

Klamath: Blue Green Algae, 500 mg blue green algae, with 2% plant enzymes, 130 vegicaps.

Bone Meal

Related Item: Calcium.

Description: Bone meal is used in supplements as a source of calcium. It is made from the ground bones of cattle.

Uses: Bone meal can contain over 20 percent calcium. Theoretically, it might seem that ground bones would represent an ideal source of nutrition for the bone. Unfortunately, it may contain undesirable substances as well, such as lead. It is also an animal product, which some people find undesirable. With the plethora of other sources of calcium that are available, there seems little reason to use bone meal.

Products:

Solgar: Bone Meal Powder, 1,000 mg calcium, 600 mg phosphorus, 25 mcg vitamin B_{12}, and 20 mg bone marrow per teaspoon, 12 oz powder.

Borage Oil

Related Items: Black currant oil, evening primrose oil.

Description: Borage oil is derived from the seeds of the borage plant, *Borago officinalis*. The oil contains the highest concentration of gamma-linolenic acid (GLA). GLA is a precursor to the inflammation-suppressing series 1 prostaglandins.

Uses: The therapeutic value of borage oil supplements results from its high concentration of GLA, an omega-6 oil. Not all

> *Indications:* Arthritis (rheumatoid), skin disorders, eczema.

omega-6 oils are undesirable. The predominant omega-6 oils in the diet—linoleic, linolenic, and arachidonic—can be both detrimental and beneficial. Linoleic acid is essential to life. In the body, these oils are converted into powerful, hormone-like substances called prostaglandins. The omega-6 oils can form two types. One type, the 2 series, is usually detrimental, causing inflammation, etc. The other type, the 1 series, is beneficial, reducing inflammation. The GLA type of omega-6 oil leads to the beneficial, series 1 type of prostaglandin. The beneficial actions of series 1 prostaglandins are similar to those of the series 3 prostaglandins derived from omega-3 oils, ALA (flaxseed oil) and EPA (fish oil). Thus, GLA, from borage, black currant, and evening primrose oil, provides much the same benefit as the omega-3 oils from fish and flaxseed.

Borage oil has been shown to be effective in treating rheumatoid arthritis, Sjogren's syndrome, and ulcerative colitis. It is also thought to have possible benefit in treating osteoporosis, diabetic neuropathy, hypertension, and elevated triglycerides.

Dosage: The usual dose is 360 to 480 milligrams of GLA daily, but the amount can vary over a wide range.

Cautions: The presence of pyrrolizidine alkaloids in certain parts of the borage plant has caused some to worry about using borage oil. Pyrrolizidine alkaloids (also found in comfrey, for example) can be hepatotoxic and carcinogenic. So far, these substances have not been found in the oil, and would not be expected to be. Those using high doses of borage oil, over a long period of time, however, should exert caution.

This item has a slight "thinning" effect on the blood. This, generally, is a good thing. But if you are taking "blood-thinning" medications, check with your doctor.

Products:

Solgar: Super GLA 300, 300 mg GLA from 1300 mg cold-pressed borage oil, 60 softgels.
Health from the Sun: Borage Liquid Gold, 280 mg GLA from borage oil, 4 oz liquid.

Boron

Description: Boron is a trace mineral. It has been known to be essential for plants, but its essentiality to humans has only been recently determined.

Uses: Boron seems to be important in helping to maintain healthy bone and joints. Although the actual mechanism is still

> *Indications:* osteoporosis, arthritis.

under investigation, studies have shown that boron, perhaps through involvement with calcium and vitamin D, enhances bone formation. This leads to the recommendation that it may be one of the nutrients important in preventing osteoporosis.

Boron has also been shown to be helpful in treating arthritis, both rheumatoid and osteoarthritis.

Other claims for boron, including its purported ability to increase muscle, mental function, etc., have yet to be substantiated.

Dosage: The actual quantity of boron required by humans is not yet determined, but the safe level of intake seems high. For osteoporosis prevention, 1 to 3 milligrams are usually used. For those with osteoporosis, at risk for osteoporosis, or suffering from arthritis, the usual dose is 3 to 9 milligrams daily.

Boron is available in supplements is several different forms, often in combination, but the form may not be too important. Regardless of the form, it seems to be readily converted to boric acid, and distributed throughout the body in that form.

Cautions: Some have voiced a concern that boron may raise estrogen levels. Boron may enhance or mimic the action of estrogen on calcium metabolism in postmenopausal women. This is good. Osteoporosis is bad, and a boron deficiency may be a significant factor leading to the high incidence of osteoporosis and other menopausal symptoms.

Products: A good osteoporosis formula, containing boron in addition to all of the other nutrients directly involved in bone health, is Twinlab's Tri-Boron Plus. It provides, in four capsules, a full supply of boron, calcium, magnesium, vitamin D, zinc, manganese, copper, and betaine hydrochloride to enhance absorption.

Vitaline: Boron, 6 mg, 6 mg boron from boron citrate and boron aspartate, 90 tablets. One-half tablet can be used, if desired.
Twinlab: Tri Boron, 3 mg boron from boron citrate, glycinate, and aspartate, 100 capsules.

Boswellia

Description: The resin from a tree found in India, boswellia (*Boswellia serrata*) is an important Ayurvedic remedy. It is closely related to frankincense.

Uses: Modern interest in boswellia is related to its ability to reduce inflammation and pain. The active ingredient seems to be the boswellic acids. It has been shown in many studies to be an effective

Indications: arthritis, irritable bowel syndrome, Crohn's disease, ulcerative colitis, sports injuries, asthma.

treatment of both rheumatoid and osteoarthritis, possibly with significant advantages over nonsteroidal anti-inflammatory drugs. It reduces pain and joint stiffness. There is some evidence that boswellia may be helpful in treating leukemia, but this is very preliminary.

It is thought that boswellic acid blocks leukotriene synthesis. Leukotrienes are the prostaglandins responsible for inflammation and pain.

Dosage: The dose varies, depending on the standardization of the product. For a product standardized to 60 to 65 percent boswellic acid, such as those listed below, the usual dose is three tablets or capsules daily. This will provide a total of approximately 600 milligrams of boswellic acid.

For products standardized to a lower potency, higher doses may be required.

Products:

Nature's Herbs: Boswellin, 60%X250mg=150mg per tab, 50 tablets.
Nature's Way: Boswellia Extract, Standardized, 65% boswellic acids 65%X307mg=200mg per tab, 60 tablets.
Solgar: Boswellia Resin Extract, 65%X350mg=228mg per cap, 60 vegicaps.

Bovine Cartilage

Related Items: Bovine cartilage, shark cartilage, glucosamine, chondroitin, green-lipped mussel extract, sea cucumber.

Description: Cartilage is the gristle or connective tissue attached to the ends of bones. It is a component of joints, and helps cushion and support the bones.

In general terms, cartilage is composed of collagen and proteoglycans, which in turn contain glycosaminoglycans (GAGs) or mucopolysaccharides, which in turn contain chondroitin sulfate, which in turn contains glucosamine. There is considerable argument and debate in the nutritional supplement industry over which of the forms of cartilage—shark cartilage, bovine cartilage, glucosamine sulfate, chondroitin sulfate, or other mucopolysaccharide-rich substances such as green-lipped mussel extract or sea cucumber—are most effective. There is no clear answer, as there is some degree of support for each argument, and there is clinical evidence supporting the efficacy for each supplement.

Uses: The primary use for this supplement is to rebuild damaged connective tissue and joints, re-

Indications: Cancer, arthritis

duce inflammation, and relieve the pain associated with osteoarthritis and sports injuries. Cartilage supplements, however, have historically been used for a different purpose—as a treatment for certain forms of cancer. The basis for the use of cartilage in treating cancer is that it was thought to inhibit the formation of new blood vessels (angiogenesis). In spite of early enthusiasm in this area, followup research has not been forthcoming.

It is difficult to assign a specific use for shark or bovine cartilage supplements today. Rich in the minerals and protein building blocks of bone and connective tissue, they certainly could be part of any supplement regimen involving arthritis or osteoporosis. But as a primary treatment for a condition such as arthritis, glucosamine sulfate and/or chondroitin sulfate should perhaps be given precedence. For cancer, the advice of a qualified health professional should be sought out, to determine whether or not cartilage treatment is appropriate.

Dosage: For cancer, extremely large doses were utilized. For arthritis and in support of other supplements, up to 2 grams a day is sufficient.

Products:

Vita Carte: Bovine Cartilage, bovine tracheal cartilage, 750 mg.

Broccoli Extract

Related Items: Cruciferous vegetables, indole-3-carbinol.
Description: Broccoli is a member of the cabbage family.

It contains substances such as indole-3-carbinol, sulforaphane, and diindolylmethane that have been reported to have anticancer activity. It is also a good food source of carotenoids, flavonoids, vitamin K, and vitamin C.

Indole-3-carbinol and sulforaphane are sulfur-containing compounds that may prevent certain cancers by stimulating some of the natural detoxification systems of the body.

Broccoli extracts rich in these substances may be especially helpful in preventing breast and cervical cancer due to its effect on estrogen metabolism.

More research is needed to determine just how effective this material may be.

Uses: While additional corroborative research is desirable, a person who is considered at risk

> **Indications: Cancer**

for breast cancer would seemingly be well advised to utilize a product of this type as part of her supplement regimen.

Products:

Solgar: Broccoli Cruciferous Extract, 500 mg, 2% (10 mg) glucosinolates, 50 vegicaps.
Nature's Herbs: Broccoli Power, 250 mg cruciferous blend providing 2% glucosinolates, including sulforaphane, 60 capsules.

Bromelain

Description: Bromelain is the protein-digesting enzyme (cysteine protease, or proteolytic enzyme) found in pineapple. It has a long history of medicinal as well as food use. It is a principal active ingredient in meat tenderizer, for example.

Uses: Its primary uses as a dietary supplement fall into two categories. First, because of its protein-digesting qualities, it is often included in digestive en-

> **Indications: Indigestion, sports injuries, arthritis, diarrhea, asthma, wound healing, sinusitis, digestive aid.**

zyme formulas, to assist in the breakdown of food proteins. Second, it seems to exert an anti-inflammatory action, making it valuable in treating sports injuries, sprains, strains, tendinitis, sinusitis, prostatitis, and possibly rheumatoid arthritis.

There is some question as to whether or not it needs to be absorbed from the intestine to exert some of these actions, and the exact mechanisms are unknown. For this reason, some bromelain-containing products that are designed to exploit its anti-inflammatory actions are enteric-coated, and the product is to be taken between meals. Obviously, when taken as a digestive aid, it should be taken with meals.

Dosage: The most important thing about bromelain dosage is to be sure it is labeled in units of potency. Milligrams, alone, is not sufficient. Bromelain is available in up to twelve different potencies as a raw material, and a product that is labeled only in milligrams is totally meaningless, and should not be purchased. The two most common units of potency that should appear on a label are GDU (gelatin-digesting units) or MCU (milk-clotting units). One GDU is equal to about 1.5 MCU. The usual dose can vary from 500 to 2,000 GDU, one to three times daily. If taken as a digestive aid, take the product with meals. If taken for its anti-inflammatory and healing activity, take it between meals.

Caution: There are some products on the market that contain bromelain (and papain, another protein-digesting enzyme) in "chewable" wafers. If you have ever experienced the sore mouth and tongue that sometimes results from eating raw pineapple, you should wonder how you could chew a wafer that contained any appreciable amount of bromelain or papain without experiencing the same phenomenon. Thus, it is likely that a chewable product would be of fairly low potency.

Cautions: Bromelain may have a slight blood-thinning action, so caution should be exerted if you are taking anticoagulant medication.

Products:

Solgar: Bromelain, 500 mg, 1,000 GDU bromelain per tablet, vegetarian, 60 tablets.
Twinlab: Mega Bromelain, 600 GDU bromelain per capsule, 90 capsules.
Country Life: Bromelain, 500 mg (2,000 GDU), 1,000 GDU bromelain per tablet, vegetarian and kosher, 60 tablets. Here is a product that could be labeled in a less-confusing way. See Chapter 4, "Just the Facts, Please," for more information.

Buffered Vitamin C

Related Items: Vitamin C, effervescent C.
Description: Buffered vitamin C refers to a product that consists of

a mineral ascorbate of vitamin C designed to reduce the acidity associated with regular ascorbic acid.

Uses: Some people find that regular vitamin C, ascorbic acid, is too acid. By converting all or some of the vitamin C to mineral ascorbates, the acidity is reduced, and the supplement may be more tolerable, especially in high doses. The minerals commonly used are calcium, magnesium, potassium, and zinc. Sodium also works but is rarely used because some individuals are on low-sodium diets. When all of the vitamin C in the product is converted to mineral ascorbate, the resulting pH is close to neutral.

Some "buffered C" products contain mixtures of mineral bicarbonates and vitamin C, and when mixed with water, the bicarbonate reacts with the vitamin C, releasing carbon dioxide (the "fizz") and forming mineral ascorbates (calcium ascorbate) which is less acid than free vitamin C. Some products add a little extra citric acid, etc., to enhance the "fizz factor." Some are flavored, and some are not.

A Comment from Dr. Abel

A four-year British study evaluating nearly 20,000 people between the ages of 45 and 79 found an inverse relationship between vitamin C levels in the blood and mortality. The 20 percent group with the highest vitamin C blood level experienced approximately a 20 percent reduction in all causes of mortality. Sounds good to me. (*Lancet*, March 31, 2001; 357: 657–63)

Other "buffered C" products consist of "fully reacted" mineral ascorbates (calcium ascorbate), rather than a mixture of free vitamin C and mineral carbonate/bicarbonate (vitamin C and calcium carbonate). These products would not be expected to "fizz" when stirred into water. But there is also no question as to how completely the acidic vitamin C has been neutralized.

If you are taking a buffered vitamin C powder because you find an effervescent liquid more palatable, then the bicarbonate form is what you want. If you are taking buffered vitamin C powder because you are very sensitive to the acidic nature of vitamin C, then those products containing the fully reacted ascorbates might be the better choice.

Remember, however, as we explained in Chapter 4, if it fizzes, it is not "fully reacted" no matter what the ingredient statement on the label might imply.

Products:

Allergy Research: Buffered Vitamin C Powder, 900 mg vitamin C as calcium, magnesium, and potassium ascorbates per ½ teaspoon, 240 g. This product contains vitamin C and mineral carbonates, which react when added to water. It is hypoallergenic, and produces a moderate "fizz." This same formulation is also available in capsule form.

Alacer: Emergen-C, 1,000 mg vitamin C as mineral ascorbates, and all the B vitamins, per packet, 36 packets. This product is a mixture of bicarbonates, vitamin C, citric acid, etc., resulting in a pronounced fizz. It comes in numerous flavors, etc.

Twinlab: Super Ascorbate C Powder, 2,000 mg vitamin C, from calcium, magnesium, zinc, and manganese ascorbates, with bioflavonoids, rose hip, acerola, etc., 8 oz. This product is an example of one that contains "fully reacted" mineral ascorbates. It does not fizz.

Alacer: Super Gram II, 1,000 mg timed-release vitamin C as 7 fully reacted mineral ascorbates, 260 tablets.

Butcher's Broom

Description: Butcher's broom (*Ruscus aculeatus*) is an evergreen shrub native to Mediterranean Europe and parts of Africa. The dried rhizome and root are used medicinally, and contain the steroid saponins ruscin and ruscoside.

Uses: Historically, butcher's broom was used as a laxative and diuretic agent. Now, especially in Europe, it is used for problems involving the circulatory system, including venous fragility, varicose veins, and hemorrhoids.

Indications: Varicose veins, hemorrhoids, leg cramps, chronic venous insufficiency.

The German Commission E has approved butcher's broom for the treatment of "chronic venus insufficiency." What is this? It is a term used to describe what happens when veins become chronically swollen and inflamed. It results in an aching, tired feeling in the legs. There may be pain, itching, leg ulcers, and changes in skin pigmentation. It is commonly associated with varicose veins. The standard treatment for chronic venous insufficiency is compression using bandages or support stockings, drugs, or surgery.

Dosage: Generally, use an amount of extract equivalent to about 10 mg total ruscogenin.

Products:

Solgar: Butcher's Broom, 50 mg butcher's broom root extract (5:1), 283 mg butcher's broom root powder, 100 vegicaps.
Nature's Herbs: Butcher's Broom Root, 470 mg, 100 capsules.

Calcium

Related Items: Calcium carbonate, oyster shell calcium, calcium citrate, bone meal, dolomite, MCHC, calcium lactate, calcium gluconate, calcium phosphate, chelated calcium.

Description: Calcium is an essential mineral. Its best-known role is as a major constituent of bones and teeth, but calcium plays numerous other important roles in the body, including muscle contraction, nerve transmission, blood coagulation, heart contractions, energy, and immune function. Calcium makes up 1 to 2 percent of total body weight, and about 99 percent of the body's calcium is found in the bone and teeth.

Uses: Calcium is necessary for proper bone growth. Up to age 35, calcium along with other minerals is needed to build up maximum bone density. After that age, bone density starts to decline and calcium is needed to retard that decline. More than half of the young people today fail to get the required amount of calcium. Most women only get 60 percent of the recommended level of calcium, and 95 percent of women get less than 800 milligrams daily. Twenty-five percent of men fail to get enough calcium. When calcium intake is too low, and bone density decreases, osteoporosis results.

In addition to preventing and treating osteoporosis, calcium may also reduce the risk of colon cancer and may help lower blood pressure in those with hypertension.

In recognition of the importance of adequate calcium supplementation, the recommended intake levels have recently been increased. The "adequate intake" for teenagers is now 1,300 milligrams per day. The adequate intake for men and women below 50 years of age is 1,000 milligrams per day, and 1,200 milligrams per day for those over 50.

It is almost impossible to achieve adequate calcium intake without taking a calcium supplement. Unfortunately, choosing the proper calcium supplement can be difficult.

Because the daily requirement is so high (1,000 to 1,200 milligrams or more), it is difficult to obtain the necessary amount in only one or two tablets. It is impossible to obtain it in a "one-a-day" multivitamin supplement.

Calcium comes in many different forms, and each form provides different amounts of calcium. This means that depending on the form, you may need anywhere from two to twelve tablets to get the same 1,000 milligrams of calcium. Why is that?

Calcium is always present in combination with another component. It never occurs by itself. Here is a list of some of the commonly used calcium compounds in nutritional supplements:

Calcium carbonate, 40 percent calcium
Calcium phosphate tribasic, 35 percent calcium
Microcrystalline hydroxyapatite, 25 percent calcium
Calcium phosphate dibasic, 23 percent calcium
Calcium citrate, 21 percent calcium
Calcium lactate, 13 percent calcium
Calcium gluconate, 9 percent calcium

What this means is that it is necessary to use 2,500 milligrams of calcium carbonate to get 1,000 milligrams of "elemental" calcium. Likewise, it is necessary to use 4,750 milligrams of calcium citrate, and 11,100 milligrams of calcium gluconate to get the same 1,000 milligrams of elemental calcium. You can understand, then, why you may need to take only two tablets of calcium from calcium carbonate, but you may need four tablets of calcium from calcium citrate to get that same 1,000 milligrams of elemental calcium. It gets worse, as you would need 18 tablets of calcium from calcium gluconate to get 1,000 milligrams.

Let's look at it another way. Here is a selection of calcium products from one manufacturer, Solgar, and the number of tablets needed to obtain at least 1,000 milligrams of elemental calcium:

Calcium 600—2 tablets (1,200 milligrams calcium)
Calcium citrate—4 tablets (1,000 milligrams calcium)
Calcium gluconate—18 tablets (1,080 milligrams calcium)
Calcium lactate—12 tablets (1,013 milligrams calcium)
Chelated calcium—6 tablets (1,000 milligrams calcium)

So now you are probably wondering, "Why would anyone take eighteen tablets to get 1,000 milligrams of calcium when they could take two?"

Unfortunately, there is a reason. And that reason is related to
the fact that these different forms
of calcium are not absorbed

> Indications: Osteoporosis, cancer (colon), hypertension.

equally well. The calcium carbonate form, for example, may work fine if you have plenty of hydrochloric acid in your stomach and/or always take it with food, while the calcium citrate form is well absorbed regardless of the level of gastric acid that might be present. People tolerate certain forms better than others. For more information on the pros and cons of each form, look up the individual listings.

There are other considerations as well. For optimal efficacy, magnesium should be taken along with calcium, either separately, or as a combination in the same product. This further increases the tablet size. And for many people with concerns about osteoporosis, additional vitamin D may be appropriate as well, and some calcium supplements include vitamin D along with the calcium.

In general, for optimal absorption, calcium supplements should be taken two or three times a day, with meals. If blood levels of calcium fall below a certain point, the body compensates by pulling calcium out of the bone. To the body, maintaining the required calcium level in the blood is more important than maintaining bone density, so it treats bone as a backup calcium storage depot. This is why you should supplement with calcium throughout the day, rather than at night.

It is important to emphasize, relative to osteoporosis and bone growth, that calcium will not do the job alone. The other minerals, magnesium and trace minerals, are necessary as well. It is a mistake for doctors to recommend calcium supplements without also recommending the other minerals as well.

Cautions: Depending on the type of kidney stone, calcium, when taken with meals, may actually prevent kidney stone formation. Talk to your doctor.

There are certain conditions that result in hypercalcemia (hyperparathyroidism, hypervitaminosis D, sarcoidosis, cancer). Do not take supplemental calcium if you already have too much.

Certain drugs interact with calcium supplementation; check with your pharmacist. Certain nutritional supplements may do so as well. Inositol hexaphosphate (phytic acid) may bind calcium and block its absorption, while supplementation with FOS may increase its absorption.

Products: See individual forms of calcium for product recommendations.

Calcium Carbonate

Related Item: Calcium.

Description: Calcium carbonate is used in supplements as a source of calcium. It can be derived from several sources, including oyster shell and limestone. *See* Calcium for more information.

Uses: Calcium carbonate provides the highest concentration of calcium for use in nutritional supplements. It contains 40 percent calcium, and to obtain 1,000 milligrams of elemental calcium, you would need about 2,500 milligrams of calcium carbonate. This means you can get a full day's calcium requirement in only two tablets.

There is a downside, however. Calcium carbonate is "inorganic" calcium. For optimal absorption by the body, it needs to be ionized. Normally, gastric acid will achieve this. But if stomach acid levels are low, it may not be well absorbed. Low stomach acid is not uncommon in older people. Other forms of calcium, the organic chelated forms such as the citrate, lactate, and glycinate, are not as dependent on gastric acid for absorption.

If fewer number of tablets is more important than optimal absorption, take calcium carbonate supplements, but be sure to take them in divided doses—for example, one tablet with breakfast and one tablet with dinner—and be sure to take it with meals. On the other hand, if you are at high risk of osteoporosis and may not have optimal gastric function, you should consider getting at least part of your calcium supplementation from more easily absorbed forms.

Calcium carbonate from natural sources, such as oyster shell, contain small amounts of lead. This is of little concern as long as the amounts are below accepted standards. Avoid buying a cheap oyster shell calcium supplement. It is a relatively inexpensive product, and you should buy only well-known, reputable brands.

Cautions: For optimal bone health, all of the minerals are needed. Magnesium is required, usually at levels equal to half of what is recommended for calcium. Taking a calcium supplement alone may not be helping you as much as you think. It is not difficult to get the microminerals (zinc, copper, etc.) in your daily multivitamin, but to get the proper amount of magnesium, you will need to take it separately, or in combination with calcium. Vitamin D is also required for optimal absorption of calcium.

Products:

Twinlab: Cal 1000 with Vit D, 1,000 mg calcium from carbonate and citrate, 400 IU vitamin D, 120 tablets.
Solgar: Cal 600, 600 mg calcium from carbonate (oyster shell), 300 IU vitamin D, 120 tablets.
NOW Foods: Calcium Crave Chewy Chocolate, 500 mg calcium (400 mg as carbonate, 100 mg as citrate), 100 IU vitamin D per chew, 60 chews. This is an excellent alternative to tablets and capsules, containing a mixture of carbonate and citrate, in a tasty chewy "candy."

Calcium Citrate

Related Item: Calcium.

Description: Calcium citrate is used in supplements as a source of calcium.

Uses: Calcium citrate is an excellent source of calcium because it is well absorbed, and contains about 21 percent elemental calcium. It is more expensive than calcium carbonate, and you will need four tablets rather than two to get 1,000 milligrams of elemental calcium. But it is well tolerated and well absorbed even if stomach acid levels are low.

If your need for calcium supplementation is critical, it is best to use a supplement such as calcium citrate rather than calcium carbonate.

If you are taking acid-blocking drugs, you will need to use calcium citrate, or other chelated forms of calcium, rather than calcium carbonate.

Cautions: For optimal bone health, all of the minerals are needed. Magnesium is required, usually at levels equal to half of what is recommended for calcium. Taking a calcium supplement alone may not be helping you as much as you think. It is not difficult to get the microminerals (zinc, copper, etc.) in your daily multivitamin, but to get the proper amount of magnesium, you will need to take it separately, or in combination with calcium. Vitamin D is also required for optimal absorption of calcium.

Products:

Solgar: Cal Citrate with Vit D, 250 mg calcium from citrate, 150 IU vitamin D, kosher and vegetarian, 240 tablets.

NOW Foods: Calcium Citrate Powder, 700 mg calcium in 1 teaspoon (3 g) of calcium citrate, 8 oz.
Allergy Research: Calcium Citrate, 150 mg, 180 capsules.

Calcium Gluconate

Related Item: Calcium.
Description: Calcium gluconate is used in supplements as a source of calcium.
Uses: This form of calcium is well absorbed and well tolerated, but provides only 9 percent elemental calcium. There seems little reason to use this form rather than calcium citrate.
Products:

Solgar: Calcium Gluconate, 650 mg, 60 mg calcium from gluconate, 250 tablets.
Willner Calcium Gluconate, 500 mg, 46 mg calcium from gluconate, 250 capsules. Elemental calcium not stated on the label.

Calcium Lactate

Related Item: Calcium.
Description: Calcium lactate is used in supplements as a source of calcium.
Uses: Calcium lactate contains about 13 percent calcium, and is well absorbed and well tolerated. It provides less calcium per unit weight than calcium citrate, however, and more tablets are required to achieve the same intake of elemental calcium.

Contrary to what some believe, calcium lactate does not contain lactose, and is quite suitable for those with lactose intolerance or milk allergies.
Products:

Twinlab: Calcium Lactate, 100 mg calcium from 740 mg calcium lactate, 250 capsules.
Solgar: Calcium Lactate, 650 mg, 250 tablets.

Calcium Pantothenate

See Pantothenic Acid.

Calcium Phosphate

Related Item: Calcium.

Description: There are several forms of calcium phosphate used in nutritional supplements. Dibasic calcium phosphate and tribasic calcium phosphate are two examples.

Uses: These forms of calcium are used in various nutritional formulations, sometimes as fillers. Theoretically they can serve as a source of calcium. The dibasic form contains about 23 percent calcium and the tribasic form contains about 35 percent calcium. But this is inorganic calcium and, perhaps most important, has a high phosphorous content. This may actually interfere with the bone-building action of calcium.

Phosphate forms of calcium are generally not recommended.

Canthaxanthin

Related Items: Carotenoids, beta-carotene.

Description: Canthaxanthin is a carotenoid but, unlike beta-carotene, cannot be converted to vitamin A.

Uses: Some research shows that canthaxanthin might be effective in lowering risk of cancer.

Caprylic Acid

Description: Caprylic acid is a medium-chain (8-carbon) saturated fatty acid. It is found naturally, in the form of triacylglycerols, in palm oil, coconut oil, and butterfat.

Uses: Caprylic acid has been used as a natural antifungal agent, especially for the treatment

Indications: Candidiasis.

of chronic candidiasis. It has remained a popular treatment for this condition, but some feel that its effectiveness has not been convincingly demonstrated.

Products:

Solgar: Caprylic Acid, 365 mg caprylic acid as calcium, magnesium, zinc, and potassium caprylates, 250 tablets.
TE Neesby: Mycopril 680, 680 mg caprylic acid as calcium magnesium caprylate, 250 capsules.

Carnitine

Related Item: Acetyl-L-carnitine.

Description: L-carnitine, also known as just carnitine, is an amino acid derivative that facilitates the transport of long-chain fatty acids across the cell membrane into the mitochondria, where they are metabolized (oxidized) to produce energy (in the form of ATP, or adenosine triphosphate).

Uses: Carnitine's primary value lies in its ability to alleviate various problems associated with cardiovascular disease. This includes heart attack, angina, elevated triglyceride levels, conges-

> *Indications:* Cardiovascular disease, diabetes, weight loss, cholesterol problems, energy (low), triglycerides (High), athletic performance.

tive heart failure, and intermittent claudication. It has been called a "cardioprotective" agent. It lowers triglyceride levels and increases levels of HDL cholesterol.

A COMMENT FROM DR. ABEL

Carnitine is an essential nutrient because it is the only chemical in the body that transports fat across cell membranes into the mitochondria, where the fat can be metabolized. It can be synthesized from the amino acids lysine and methionine, requiring the presence of vitamin C, niacin, pyridoxine, and iron. Deficiency of carnitine means a deficiency of fat, which results in decreased energy and memory. As you might expect, the production of carnitine decreased with age. This phenomena could be one of the contributors of memory loss and Alzheimer's disease. I have personally found that the combination of acetyl-L-carnitine, vitamin E, magnesium, and CoQ$_{10}$ have improved cognitive thinking in several people with senile depression and age-related memory loss. People do not need to wait until they have severe depression and memory loss before benefiting from supplementation of 500 to 1,000 milligrams twice daily, with meals.

There are other possible benefits from carnitine supplementation, but they are not as well documented. These other uses revolve around its role in energy production, and include chronic fatigue syndrome, athletic performance, diabetes, and weight loss.

Acetyl-L-carnitine is a related compound, but is not utilized for the same purpose. Acetyl-L-carnitine has a neuroprotective action, and is used for age-related cholinergic-deficit problems such as Alzheimer's disease.

Dosage: From 500 to 2,000 milligrams daily, in divided doses, with or without food.

Products:

Twinlab: CarniFuel Liquid, 1,000 mg of carnitine per tablespoon, 8 oz.

Phytotherapy: Carnitine Fumarate, 250 mg carnitine from 450 mg carnitine fumarate, 60 capsules. Highly stable and absorbable.

Jarrow: Carnitine, 500 mg, 500 mg carnitine from 750 mg carnitine tartrate, 100 capsules.

Carnosine

Description: Carnosine is a compound made up of the two amino acids histidine and alanine. It is found in muscle tissue and the brain. It appears to be a strong water-soluble antioxidant. It might possibly function as a neurotransmitter substance.

Uses: There is speculation that carnosine may play a role in immune function, wound healing, heavy metal chelation, and cancer

Indications: Ulcer (peptic), anti-aging.

treatment, but the research supporting these uses is still preliminary. There is evidence that carnosine, as a zinc salt, may be of value in treating peptic ulcers, and may actually kill *Helicobacter pylori.*

Current interest in carnosine seems centered around its possible anti-aging action. It is thought to retard glycosylation, or biochemical cross-linking between proteins and certain sugars.

Dosage: The suggested dose for treating ulcers is 150 milligrams, twice a day.

Products:

Jarrow: Carnosine 500, 90 capsules, 500 mg L-carnosine (alanyl-histidine) per capsule.

Carotenoids

Related Items: Beta-carotene, lycopene, lutein, cryptoxanthin, and xeaxanthin.

Description: Carotenoids, or carotenes, are the red, orange, and yellow plant pigments that protect against oxidative damage during photosynthesis. There are over 600 carotenoids in nature.

Uses: Carotenoids, in general, serve two main functions: as antioxidants and as precursors to vitamin A.

Only a small number of carotenoids can actually be converted to vitamin A in the body (beta-carotene, alpha-carotene). Others, such as lycopene and lutein, function as powerful antioxidants.

It should be noted that there is more evidence that a deficiency of dietary carotenoids, or beta-carotene, is a cause of increased cancer, heart disease, cataracts, and immune system problems than there is evidence that supplemental beta-carotene reduces those disorders. This leads to the conclusion that for maximum value, natural mixed carotenoids, in moderate dosage, is superior to synthetic beta-carotene, in high doses, and that it is important that carotenes be administered along with the other antioxidant nutrients.

A COMMENT FROM DR. ABEL

The colored compounds are very helpful in vision. The carotenoids and bioflavonoids, in particular. Bioflavonoids in grapes, bilberry, and other berries and the orange fruits and vegetables provide the necessary ingredients for vitamin A and rhodopsin. Rhodopsin is the important chemical that allows for night vision. Carotenoids, most notably lutein and zeaxanthin, protect the photoreceptors responsible for daytime vision. Not only does it ward off the toxic short wavelengths, UV, and blue light, but also serves as an antioxidant and binds components of cell membranes together. These colorful compounds are nature's way of protecting plants against light and toxins. They also are nature's way of protecting our bodies and our vision.

Dosage: There is a very wide range of bioavailability among the various individual carotenoids. Bioavailability is also influenced by other foods, such as fiber, which lowers it, and fat, which improves it.

Various carotenoids interfere with each other as well, and the amount absorbed decreases as the amount ingested increases.

On labels, carotenoids are usually labeled as an equivalent to vitamin A, but this value has been the subject of much debate and disagreement, even between government agencies. For reference purposes, 15 milligrams of beta-carotene is equivalent to 25,000 IU of vitamin A or 5,000 Retinal Equivalent. The DV (Daily Value) for vitamin A is 5,000 IU (or 1,000 RE).

Supplements generally provide up to the equivalent of 25,000 IU of vitamin A (up to 15 mg of beta-carotene). There is little reason to have more than 4,000 to 5,000 IU of preformed vitamin A in a general multivitamin supplement; the balance should be from natural beta-carotene.

For those of you who think 25,000 IU of vitamin A from beta-carotene is a lot, we should point out that one raw carrot contains over 20,000 IU of vitamin A (from beta-carotene).

Cautions: During pregnancy, it is advisable to avoid more than 8,000 IU of supplemental preformed vitamin A. Because of this, some physicians think the same limit should apply to carotenoids. This is incorrect. Supplemental carotenoids should be perfectly safe during pregnancy. Orally ingested carotenoids, such as beta-carotene, show no detectable toxicity, even at very large doses.

On the other hand, prudence and caution should rule during pregnancy. Unless there is a compelling reason to take exceptionally high doses of carotene during pregnancy, it would seem best not to do so. The levels usually present in balanced multivitamin supplements should not be of concern. Too much caution can be a problem as well. Studies have shown that plasma carotene levels during pregnancy, in mothers who smoke, was directly related to birthweight.

The only condition associated with high doses of beta-carotene is a yellowing of the skin. When the dose is reduced, the discoloration disappears.

Products:

Twinlab: Maxilife Multi Carotene, 20,000 IU vitamin A as beta-carotene, 6 mg lutein, 5 mg lycopene, and 4 mg carrot oil (9.5% carotenoids), 60 capsules.

Solgar: Advanced Carotenoid Complex, 25,000 IU vitamin A as beta-carotene, plus alpha-carotene, gamma-carotene, lutein, lycopene, and capsanthin, 60 softgels.

Nature's Way: Multi Carotene, 40,000 IU vitamin A as beta-carotene and alpha-carotene, plus gamma-carotene and lycopene, 60 softgels.

Cartilage

Related Items: Bovine cartilage, shark cartilage, glucosamine, chondroitin, green-lipped mussel, sea cucumber.

Description: Cartilage is the gristle or connective tissue attached to the ends of bones. It is a component of joints, and helps cushion and support the bones.

In general terms, cartilage is composed of collagen and proteoglycans, which, in turn, contain glycosaminoglycans (GAGs) or mucopolysaccharides, which, in turn, contain chondroitin sulfate, which, in turn, contains glucosamine.

There is considerable argument and debate in the nutritional supplement industry over which of the above—shark cartilage, bovine cartilage, glucosamine sulfate, chondroitin sulfate, or other mucopolysaccharide-rich substances, such as green-lipped mussel and sea cucumber—are most effective. There is no clear answer, as there is some degree of support for each argument, and there is clinical evidence supporting the efficacy for each supplement.

One persuasive argument for the use of glucosamine sulfate is that it is the smallest entity of the group and, thus, may be the form most readily absorbed. The same argument may hold for the use of chondroitin sulfate over the various cartilage extracts.

There is also some evidence that the sulfate component is important as well, and that the sulfate forms are more effective than other forms.

Uses: The primary use for these supplements, in general, is to rebuild damaged connective

Indications: Arthritis, cancer.

tissue and joints, reduce inflammation, and relieve the pain associated with osteoarthritis, sports injuries, etc.

Cartilage supplements, however, have historically been used for a different purpose—as a treatment for certain forms of cancer. In spite of early enthusiasm in this area, follow-up research in support of this use has not been forthcoming. The basis for the use of cartilage in treating cancer was that it was thought to inhibit the formation of new blood vessels (angiogenesis).

It is difficult to assign a specific use for shark and bovine cartilage supplements today. Rich in the minerals and protein building blocks of bone and connective tissue, they certainly could be part of any supplement regimen involving arthritis and osteoporosis. But as a primary treatment for a condition such as arthritis, one would have to wonder if glucosamine sulfate and/or chondroitin sulfate should take precedence. For cancer, likewise, the advice of a qualified health professional should be sought out, to determine whether or not cartilage or other treatments are most appropriate.

Dosage: For cancer, extremely large doses were utilized. For arthritis, in support of other supplements, up to 2 grams a day are sufficient.

Products:

Vita Carte: Bovine Cartilage, 750 mg, 375 capsules. Contains bovine tracheal cartilage.
Seagate: Shark Cartilage, 650 mg, 100 capsules.
Lane Labs: Benefin Caplets, 750 mg shark cartilage per caplet, 270 caplets.

Cat's Claw

Description: The type of cat's claw used commercially is either *Uncaria tomentosa* (popular in the United States) or *Uncaria guianensis* (popular in Europe). It is common in the Amazonian rain forest, and the source of most commercial herb is either Peru or Brazil. The Spanish common name is *una de gato.*

Uses: Interest in cat's claw skyrocketed a few years ago. Rumors about its use as a South American folk remedy against cancer provided fodder for entrepreneurs,

Indications: Arthritis, cancer, HIV, immune system Crohn's disease, irritable bowel syndrome.

who began touting its value as a treatment not only for cancer, but also for HIV, arthritis, and intestinal disorders.

Unfortunately, almost all of the evidence for this was anecdotal. Cat's claw may turn out to enhance immune system, help prevent or treat cancer, and reduce the pain and inflammation associated with arthritis. But firm evidence is still lacking.

Products:

Jarrow: Cat's Claw 6:1, 500 mg of a 6:1 extract of the inner bark, 100 capsules.
Nature's Herbs: Cat's Claw, 500 mg cat's claw bark, 250 capsules.
Nature's Answer: Cat's Claw Alcohol Free, 14 drops contain 500 mg of a 4:1 extract of cat's claw inner bark, 2 oz liquid.

CDP-Choline

Related Items: Choline, phosphatidylcholine, lecithin.

Description: Cytidine 5'diphosphocholine (CDP-choline) is a naturally occurring substance that is a precursor to the biosynthesis of phosphatidylcholine.

Uses: CDP-choline is thought to be especially useful for mental function and cell-membrane integrity. As an essential intermediate for the synthesis of phosphatidylcholine, some feel that CDP choline is more active in brain biochemistry.

> *Indications:* Cardiovascular disease, mental function, Alzheimer's disease, tardive dyskinesia, Parkinson's disease, brain injury, stroke.

Dosage: 500 to 2,000 milligrams daily. CDP-choline contains about 21% choline.

Products:

Jarrow: CDP Choline, 250 mg, 60 capsules.

Cetyl Myristoleate

Description: Cetyl myristoleate (CMO) is a waxy, lipid substance, an ester, that is composed of cetyl alcohol and myristoleic acid.

Uses: Cetyl myristoleate is thought to be of value in alleviating the discomfort of arthritis, both osteo and rheumatoid. This

> *Indications:* Arthritis, fibromyalgia.

is based upon a small number of animal studies, patent filings, and one human study that was published in a non–peer-review journal—all by the same researcher.

This lack of convincing evidence of its effectiveness does not mean, of course, that cetyl myristoleate will not be shown to function as a joint "lubricant" and anti-inflammatory agent, as has been claimed. But until then, other anti-inflammatory supplements should be tried before turning to cetyl myristoleate. If other substances have been used, with only partial success, cetyl myristoleate is certainly worth trying.

Dosage: 400 to 500 milligrams daily, for at least 30 days.

Products:

Natrol: Cetylpure, 550 mg cetyl myristoleate, 120 capsules.

Chaste Tree Berry

Description: Chaste tree (*Vitex agnus castus*) is originally native to the Mediterranean area. The ripe, dried fruits are the source of medicinal components.

Uses: Chaste tree fruit has been used for at least two thousand years. It is now officially approved by Commission E for irregularities of the menstrual

> *Indications:* Premenstrual syndrome, fibrocystic breast disease, infertility, menopause, menstrual irregularities.

cycle, premenstrual complaints, and mastodynia (breast tenderness).

Chaste tree fruit itself does not contain hormones, but it has an effect on the pituitary gland, and seems to cause an increase in the release of progesterone during the second phase of the menstrual cycle. It may also lower prolactin levels.

It is used for many female problems, including PMS, heavy or frequent menstrual cycles, infertility, menopausal symptoms, uterine fibroids, and it is used to increase the flow of breast milk.

Dosage: Tinctures, follow instructions on bottle. Capsules, one capsule, up to three times a day.

Products:

Nature's Answer: Vitex Chaste Berry Drops, 2,000 mg vitex berry fluid extract in 56 drops (2 ml), 1 oz liquid.
Nature's Answer: Vitex Agnus Castus, 40 mg chaste tree berry, 90 capsules.

THE PHARMACIST SAYS

What is the Commission E? In Germany, herbal products are widely used, and the government has taken measures to guarantee that the public is assured of their safety and efficacy. In 1978, the *Bundesgesundheitsamt* (Federal Health Agency) established an expert committee on herbal remedies charged with evaluating the safety and efficacy of phytomedicines. This organization of experts is called the Commission E. When the Commission evaluates an herbal remedy, it publishes its findings in monograph form. Some of the findings are positive, and others are negative. These collected monographs have been translated into English by the American Botanical Council and published as, *The Complete German Commission E Monographs: Therapeutic Guide to Herbal Medicines,* edited by Mark Blumenthal (American Botanical Council, Integrative Medicine Communications, 1998). A more informative, expanded version was later published by the same organization under the name *Herbal Medicine: Expanded Commission E Monographs* (2000).

Chelated Calcium

Related Item: Calcium.

Description: Chelated calcium is a form of calcium supplement utilizing calcium that is bound to another substance, usually an amino acid.

Uses: Properly defined, a chelate would indicate a certain type of cyclic compound formed between an organic molecule and a metallic ion. In this case, calcium is the metallic ion, and the organic compounds used are generally amino acids. Perhaps the best-known "chelating agent" is EDTA. A good example of a chelated calcium compound would be one in which the calcium is bound by, or chelated to, the amino acid glycine. The compound calcium bisglycinate, for example, is a true calcium chelate. Other forms of chelated calcium are identified as amino acid chelates, or protein chelates.

Not all products labeled as "chelated minerals" are true chelates, however. In the past, unscrupulous manufacturers would merely dump some inorganic mineral into a slurry of soy protein, stir it up, spread it onto trays, and dry it. *Voilà.* Instant "chelated mineral"! Obviously, this does not yield a true mineral chelate.

Another use of the term *chelated mineral* is a looser definition, referring to what more correctly would be organic calcium compounds rather than inorganic compounds. Examples would be calcium gluconate, lactate, and citrate. While the nature of the chemical bond in these compounds may not fit the true definition of a chelate, the end result is pretty much the same—enhanced absorption and tolerance, and less dependence on the ionizing action of gastric acid. Unfortunately, chelates contain relatively low amounts of calcium, necessitating a greater number of large tablets.

Products:

Solgar: Chelated Calcium, 1,000 mg calcium from calcium glycinate in 6 tablets, 250 tablets.

Chelated Magnesium

See Magnesium Glycinate.

Chitosan

Description: Chitosan is a type of fiber derived from chitin. The chitin used as a source of chitosan is usually the shells of shrimps, crabs, and so forth.

Uses: Chitosan, when taken orally, binds with dietary fat in the stomach. This prevents the fat from being absorbed into the body. It may exert this action by complexing with lipids because of its opposite electronic charge, and/or by functioning as a bile acid sequestrant, similar to cholestryamine drugs (Questran, Cholestid).

Indications: Cholesterol problems, weight loss.

Theoretically, chitosan should be useful as a cholesterol-lowering agent and as a weight loss agent. Its effectiveness in weight loss, however, has yet to be convincingly demonstrated. There is some preliminary research that shows a possible role for chitosan in preventing atherosclerosis, as well as wound healing, diabetes, and liver disease.

Dosage: For cholesterol lowering, 1,000 milligrams, twice a day, with meals, with water.

Cautions: Chitosan can interfere with the absorption of nutrients and medications, and should not be taken at the same time. If taking chitosan, it is very important to take a full-spectrum multivitamin-multimineral supplement at different times of the day.

Products:

Natrol: Chitosan, 120 capsules. Fat-soluble vitamins (A,D,E, and K) should be taken 4 hours before or after chitosan.

Chlorella

Related Items: Spirulina, blue green algae, chlorophyll.

Description: All green-food supplements are relatively rich in protein, chlorophyll, and carotenoids. Marketing claims to the contrary, there is little documented therapeutic difference among them.

Uses: Green-food concentrates of this type are claimed to have anti-cancer activity, modulate immune system function, lower cholesterol, treat gastrointestinal problems, and function, generally, as detoxification agents.

While convincing proof of all of these actions may be lacking, there is certainly no reason not to include one of the green-food concentrates in a comprehensive supplement program. They are all rich in phytonutrients, antioxidants, and varying amounts of nutrients. The problem with these supplements is that they are often accompanied by exaggerated marketing claims, and consumers may overestimate their value. As a general rule, they should be considered adjuncts to other supplements, not replacements or alternatives to them.

Cautions: Green-food supplements may be rich in vitamin K, so caution should be exercised if you are taking an anticoagulant medication.

Products:

Natrol: China Chlorella, 500 mg, 120 tablets. Cell walls "cracked" for easier assimilation.

Sun: Chlorella Granules, 3 g of chlorella per pack, 20 packs. "Broken cell walls" for easier assimilation.

Jarrow: Yaeyama Chlorella, 400 mg chlorella, providing "chlorella growth factor," 150 capsules.

Chlorophyll

Related Items: Spirulina, green foods, wheat grass, barley grass, chlorella, blue green algae.

Description: Chlorophyll is the green pigment found in plants, including algae. It is involved in photosynthesis, the process in which a plant converts light and carbon dioxide to carbohydrates and oxygen.

Chlorophyll is similar in chemical structure to hemoglobin (the heme group); among the differences is that chlorophyll contains magnesium while heme contains iron.

There are different types of chlorophyll, but this may not be of significance in nutritional supplements.

All green food supplements are relatively rich in protein, chlorophyll, and carotenoids.

Uses: Chlorophyll-rich green food concentrates are thought to have anticancer activity, modulate immune system function, lower cholesterol, treat gastrointestinal problems, and function, generally, as detoxification and protective agents.

Indications: Detoxification, immune system, cancer, odor, kidney stones.

The basis for most of these functions of chlorophyll lie in animal testing only, although its use in reducing body odor, fecal odor, gas, and constipation has been verified in a small number of human studies.

Some preliminary work indicates that chlorophyll may be of some value in preventing calcium oxalate kidney stones.

Cautions: Green food supplements may be rich in vitamin K, so caution should be exercised if you are taking anticoagulant medication.

Products:

Nature's Way: Chlorofresh, 50 mg copper chlorophyllin complex from alfalfa, 90 softgels.
Nature's Way: Chlorofresh Liquid Mint Flavor, 1 tablespoon equals 50 mg copper chlorophyllin complex from alfalfa, 16 oz.

Choline

Related Items: Lecithin, phosphatidylcholine, CDP-choline.

Description: Choline is now recognized as an essential nutrient. It is used in the body to make phosphatidylcholine and sphingomyelin, the structural components of biological membranes, as well as other crucial intercellular compounds. It is also a precursor for acetylcholine biosynthesis, essential to proper brain function, and functions as a methyl donor.

Uses: Choline is important for the formation and maintenance of normal cellular membranes, brain function, cardiovascular function, and liver function.

Indications: Alzheimer's disease, cholesterol problems, liver disorders, hepatitis, manic depression, mental function, Parkinson's disease, tardive dyskinesia.

Acetylcholine, one of the major neurotransmitters, requires choline for its synthesis. There is some evidence that inadequate levels of acetylcholine in the brain may lead to certain types of dementia, including Alzheimer's disease.

Choline is converted in the body to betaine, which is involved in preventing elevated homocysteine levels, a risk factor for cardiovascular disease.

In Europe, choline in the form of phosphatidylcholine is widely used for various liver disorders, including fatty liver, hepatitis, cirrhosis, etc.

Choline is available alone or as choline bitartrate, choline citrate, or choline chloride. While these forms provide the highest level of choline per dose, they are not as well tolerated as other forms.

Dosage: The amount taken as a supplement can vary over a wide range. The new "dietary reference intake" is 550 milligrams daily and the suggested "upper limit" is 3,500 milligrams daily.

To achieve the level of 550 milligrams daily, you would have to use approximately 770 milligrams of choline chloride, and 1,339 milligrams of choline bitartrate.

Cautions: At high dosage levels, over 3 or 4 grams daily, choline can cause a fishy body odor and gastrointestinal discomfort.

Products:

Solgar: Choline, 267 mg choline from 650 mg choline bitartrate, kosher and vegetarian, 100 tablets.
Twinlab: Choline, 350 mg, 350 mg choline from choline bitartrate 100 capsules.

Chondroitin

Related Items: Cartilage, glucosamine.

Description: Chondroitin sulfate is a glycosaminoglycan (GAG), or mucopolysaccharide material that helps to lubricate the joints by drawing water into the area, as well as helping to regenerate collagen and connective tissue.

Uses: Chondroitin has been shown to be useful in treating osteoarthritis and injuries by reducing inflammation, enhancing the regrowth of connective tissue, and cushioning the area within the joint.

Indications: **Arthritis, sports injuries.**

It is often used in conjunction with glucosamine sulfate; there is no convincing evidence that taking chondroitin sulfate along with glucosamine sulfate is more effective than taking either one by itself. Combination products seem to work better, but this may be because the total amount of chondroitin and glucosamine is greater than the amount usually taken individually.

Dosage: 400 to 500 milligrams, three times a day.

Products:

Twinlab: CSA, 250 mg, 100% chondroitin sulfate A from bovine trachea, 120 capsules.
Solgar: Chondroitin sulfate, 600 mg, 60 tablets.

Chromium

Related Item: Chromium picolinate.

Description: Chromium is an essential trace mineral, thought to be necessary for normal carbohydrate metabolism.

Chromium is found in nature in several chemical forms. The most common are the trivalent and hexavalent forms. In food, the trivalent form is predominant, and is often referred to as "GTF chromium." GTF stands for "glucose tolerance factor." The other form of chromium, the hexavalent form, is toxic and potentially carcinogenic.

The use of "GTF" in the labeling of chromium dietary supplements is redundant, as all forms of chromium approved for use in foods and supplements are, by definition, GTF-chromium.

Uses: Chromium works with insulin to control blood sugar levels, and seems to be a valuable supplement for those with diabetes and hypoglycemia. It also seems to help in lowering elevated cholesterol levels.

Indications: Diabetes, cholesterol problems, weight loss, triglycerides (high), hypoglycemia.

There is also some interest in chromium supplementation for athletes, to enhance muscle formation and facilitate weight loss. Support for this use remains problematic, as some studies are positive, and others are negative.

Dosage: Normal dosage is 200 micrograms daily. For those with problems managing glucose levels, and those with blood lipid problems, doses up to 400 micrograms daily may be appropriate. Higher levels are sometimes prescribed by health professionals, but caution should be observed at high doses, over 800 micrograms, especially with the well-absorbed forms such as picolinate.

Chromium is available as a high-chromium brewer's-type yeast, chromium picolinate, chromium polynicotinate, and chromium chloride. The absorption of the chloride form may be less efficient than the others.

Products:

Solgar: GTF Chromium, yeast derived, vegetarian and kosher, 250 tablets. *See* individual product listings for other chromium products.

Chromium Picolinate

Related Items: Chromium, chromium polynicotinate.

Description: Chromium is an essential trace mineral, thought to be necessary for normal carbohydrate metabolism. It potentiates the action of insulin, and may affect lipid balance.

Chromium is available as an organic complex for enhanced absorption and bioavailability. The three most popular forms are high-chromium brewer's-type yeast, chromium picolinate, and chromium polynicotinate. Chromium picolinate is a complex formed by reacting picolinic acid, a natural metabolite found in breast milk, related to the B-vitamin niacin, with chromium.

Marketing claims to the contrary, all three forms are well utilized, and there is little evidence that one is substantially better than the other.

Uses: Chromium works with insulin to control blood sugar levels and seems to be a valuable supplement for those with diabetes and hypoglycemia. It also seems to help in lowering elevated cholesterol levels.

Indications: Diabetes, cholesterol problems, weight loss, triglycerides (high), hypoglycemia.

There is also some interest in chromium supplementation for athletes, to enhance muscle formation and facilitate weight loss. Support for this use remains problematic, as some studies are positive and others are negative.

Dosage: Normal dosage is 200 micrograms daily. For those with problems managing glucose levels, and those with blood lipid problems, doses up to 400 micrograms daily may be appropriate. Higher levels are sometimes prescribed by health professionals, but caution should be observed at high doses, over 800 micrograms, even though some research has shown high levels to be beneficial and safe.

Products:

Twinlab: Chromic Fuel, 200 mcg yeast-free chromium, 200 capsules.
Solgar: Chromium Picolinate, 500 mcg, 500 mcg yeast-free chromium, 120 vegicaps.

Chromium Polynicotinate

Related Items: Chromium, chromium picolinate.

Description: Chromium is an essential trace mineral, thought to be necessary for normal carbohydrate metabolism. It potentiates the action of insulin, and may affect lipid balance.

Chromium is available as an organic complex for enhanced absorption and bioavailability. The three most popular forms are high-chromium brewer's-type yeast, chromium picolinate, and chromium polynicotinate. Marketing claims to the contrary, all three forms are well utilized, and there is little evidence that one is better than the other.

Uses: Chromium works with insulin to control blood sugar levels and seems to be a valuable supplement for those with diabetes and hypoglycemia. It also

> *Indications:* Diabetes, cholesterol problems, weight loss, triglycerides (high), hypoglycemia.

seems to help in lowering elevated cholesterol levels.

There is also some interest in chromium supplementation for athletes, to enhance muscle formation and facilitate weight loss. Support for this use remains problematic, as some studies are positive and others are negative.

Dosage: Normal dosage is 200 micrograms daily. For those with problems managing glucose levels, and those with blood lipid problems, doses up to 400 micrograms daily may be appropriate. Higher levels are sometimes prescribed by health professionals, but caution should be observed at high doses, over 800 micrograms, even though some research has shown high levels to be beneficial and safe.

Products:

Solgar: Chromium Polynicotinate, 200 mcg, ChromeMate form of GTF chromium, 100 vegicaps.

CLA

See Conjugated Linoleic Acid.

CMO

See Cetyl Myristoleate.

Cobalamin

See Vitamin B$_{12}$.

Cod Liver Oil

Description: Cod liver oil is, as the name implies, derived from cod liver. It is rich in omega-3 oils, which is good. It is also rich in vitamin A and vitamin D, which can be good, up to a point.

Uses: Cod liver oil is an excellent source of vitamin A, vitamin D, and omega-3 oils (EPA and DHA). And it is now available in numerous, palatable variations—regular, emulsified, and flavored.

The problem is that some people might make the mistake of thinking cod liver oil is just another type of fish oil, and that it can be used the same way EPA-DHA fish oils are used. This can be a mistake.

One teaspoonful of cod liver oil supplies 4,600 IU of vitamin A (preformed vitamin A), and 460 IU of vitamin D. If you are already getting up to 4,000 or 5,000 IU of preformed vitamin A, or 400 IU of vitamin D in your daily multivitamin supplement, one teaspoonful of cod liver oil is the maximum amount that should be taken. More than that could result in too much A and D.

With omega-3 rich fish oil supplements, you can take as much as you want. While cod liver oil also contains omega-3 fatty acids, you are limited in how much cod liver oil you can use for that purpose.

Products:

Carlson: Cod Liver Oil Lemon Flavor, 2,250 IU vitamin A, 450 IU vitamin D, 480 mg EPA, 525 mg DHA per teaspoon, 8.9 oz liquid. Norwegian cod liver oil.
Sonne: Cod Liver Oil #5, 4,000 IU vitamin A, 400 IU vitamin D, 400 mg EPA, 400 mg DHA per 5 ml, 16 oz liquid.
Twinlab: Cod Liver Oil, 2,500 IU vitamin A, 164 IU vitamin D, 74 mg EPA, 77 mg DHA per 2 capsules, 250 capsules. Norwegian cod liver oil.

Coenzyme Q$_{10}$

See CoQ$_{10}$.

Coleus Forskohlii

Related Item: Forskolin.

Description: Coleus forskohlii (Makandi) is an herb native to India. It contains forskolin, a substance that exerts hypotensive and other cell-regulating actions through the activation of an enzyme called adenylate cyclase. This enzyme regulates the amount of cyclic AMP in cells, which, in turn, activates numerous other enzymes.

Uses: There has been a great deal of interest in this herb as a possible treatment for asthma, glaucoma, obesity, psoriasis, and various cardiovascular problems,

> *Indications:* Asthma, cardiovascular disease, glaucoma, psoriasis.

including hypertension, congestive heart failure, and cardiomyopathy.

Unfortunately, most of the research has been done with isolated forskolin, not coleus. In addition, some of the work involved topical application, injection, and inhalation, rather than oral administration.

There is good reason to think that oral administration of coleus preparations standardized to 18 percent forskolin will prove effective in many of these conditions.

Dosage: The usual dose of the standardized 18 percent coleus extract is 50 milligrams two or three times daily. Higher amounts are sometimes used.

Products:

America's Finest: Coleus Forskohlii, 100 mg coleus forskohlii extract (10%), providing 10 mg forskolin, 30 capsules.
Gaia Herbs: Coleus Forskohlii Liquid, 170 mg coleus forskohlii extract (2.5%), providing 4 mg forskolin, 2 oz.
Enzymatic Therapy: Coleus Forskohlii, 50 mg coleus forskohlii extract (18%), providing 9 mg forskolin, 60 capsules.

Colloidal Minerals

Description: Colloidal mineral supplements were dilute liquid suspensions of minerals derived from humic shale, inland sea beds, plants, or whatever other exotic source the marketing people could imagine. The minerals were supposed to be in colloidal suspension, but this was often not the case. It matters little, in fact. Despite claims shrouded in complex-sounding terminology and too-good-to-believe testimonials, the products were nothing more than very dilute suspensions or solutions of trace minerals. Very dilute is the key, for if all you have is a trace amount of any given mineral, it does not matter how well it may or may not be absorbed—you still have only a trace amount. Unfortunately, you also often had trace amounts of undesirable minerals as well, including aluminum, lead, and arsenic.

Use:s There is no valid use for this product.

Colostrum

Related Items: Lactoferrin, immunoglobulin.

Description: Colostrum is the liquid secreted by the mammary glands during the first day or two after giving birth. It is rich in immune factors, growth factors, proteins, and other nutrients designed to protect the newborn against infection and to stimulate growth.

Uses: Supplements contain bovine colostrum, which is derived from cows. Theoretically, these various immune-enhancing

> *Indications:* Immune system, diarrhea, weight loss.

and growth-stimulating factors might be effective in humans as well, but actual evidence for this remains scarce.

Products:

Jarrow: Colostrum Specific, 500 mg freeze-dried colostrum (491,000 cryptosporidium parvum binding Units), enteric coated, 60 capsules.
Symbiotics: New Life Colostrum, 120 capsules. Also available in powder form.

Conjugated Linoleic Acid

Description: Conjugated linoleic acid (CLA) refers to a group of fatty acids similar in structure to the essential fatty acid linoleic acid. They differ from linoleic acid in that each isomer contains a conjugated double bond (two double bonds separated by a single bond).

Uses: Based primarily upon animal studies and laboratory work, CLA is thought to be of value in preventing and treating

> *Indications:* Weight loss, cancer, cardiovascular disease, diabetes, athletic performance.

various types of cancer, cardiovascular disease, including elevated cholesterol and triglycerides, and Type 2 diabetes.

CLA seems to be uniquely beneficial in weight loss in that it seems to facilitate the redistribution of fat to lean body mass, or muscle.

People on low-fat diets may be inducing a subclinical deficiency of CLA, and supplementation may be appropriate.

Dosage: The typical dose is 1 to 2 grams daily; up to 6 grams daily have been used.

Products:

Twinlab: CLA Fuel, 1,000 mg, 1,000 mg CLA from pharmaceutical grade safflower oil, 120 softgels.
Jarrow: Tonalin® CLA, 750 mg, 750 mg CLA from 1,000 mg sunflower oil, 100 softgels.

Copper

Description: Copper is an essential trace mineral. It is involved in many key enzymatic reactions. Copper is required for the absorption and utilization of iron. It is needed for formation of collagen and elastin. It is a component of superoxide dismutase, an antioxidant enzyme.

Uses: Copper has antioxidant action in the body, and maintaining the proper balance of copper to other essential minerals is very important.

Indications: **Nutritional support, cardiovascular disease.**

There is no question that a deficiency of copper can contribute to cardiovascular disease. Deficiency may also result in impaired immune function and arthritic symptoms.

Supplementation with copper, however, should be limited to the correction or prevention of a deficiency. Use of higher doses of copper as a therapeutic agent in these conditions is not recommended, as high levels can be toxic.

Prolonged supplementation with high doses of zinc can cause a deficiency of copper.

Dosage: The usual dose of copper is 1 to 3 milligrams daily.

Copper is available in several forms in supplements. The one form that may be poorly absorbed is cupric oxide. Other forms, even inorganic forms such as copper sulfate, are better utilized. Chelated copper (glycinate) is also available, as is copper gluconate. These are excellent sources of copper.

However, in most instances, the 2 to 3 milligrams of copper that are necessary will be obtained from your balanced multivitamin supplement. Many reputable companies will add a small amount of copper to their higher-potency zinc-containing supplements. Check the label to see how much copper is present before you take additional copper.

Products:

Solgar: Chelated Copper, 2.5 mg copper as copper glycinate, 100 tablets.
Twinlab: Copper, 2 mg, copper as copper gluconate, 100 capsules.
Allergy Research: Copper Sebacate, 4 mg copper as copper sebacate, 75 capsules.

CoQ_{10}

Description: Coenzyme Q_{10} (CoQ_{10}) belongs to a group of compounds called ubiquinones. These are fat-soluble substances involved in electron transport and energy production in the cell's mitochondria.

Uses: There seems little doubt that CoQ_{10} is cardioprotective. It is useful in various types of cardiovascular disease, particularly congestive heart failure, angina, and hypertension. It has been shown to be beneficial in the treatment of periodontal disease.

> *Indications:* Cardiovascular disease, periodontal disease, angina, hypertension.

Certain drugs, such as HMG-CoA reductase inhibitors (Mevacor, Lipitor, and other "statin drugs"), used to lower cholesterol, also significantly lower the body's level of CoQ_{10}. Supplemental CoQ_{10} should be administered along with drugs of that type.

Other conditions that might benefit from CoQ_{10} supplementation are diabetes, cancer, and Alzheimer's disease. CoQ_{10} may also enhance athletic performance.

Dosage: The commonly used dosage now varies between 30 and 200 milligrams daily.

The product is available in a dry powder form (capsules and tablets), as well as oil-based softgels. Whereas CoQ_{10} is fat-soluble, the absorption of the oil-based softgel form is claimed to be significantly better than the dry form. On the other hand, if the dry form is taken with meals, the absorption will be facilitated as well. There are products that include a special black pepper extract (Bioperine) that seems to increase absorption of CoQ_{10} as well.

It should be pointed out, also, that it may take up to three weeks of supplementation to reach maximum blood levels of CoQ_{10}.

Products:

Country Life: Maxi Sorb CoQ$_{10}$, 30 mg, "Q-Gel" process, 90 softgels. Claims 4 times the absorption of powdered CoQ_{10} when taken on an empty stomach.

Jarrow: Q Sorb CoQ$_{10}$, 100 mg CoQ_{10}, 4 mg gamma-tocopherol, in "Q Sorb" delivery system, 60 softgels. Claims to raise plasma levels 28% more than dry CoQ_{10}.

Twinlab: Twinsorb CoQ$_{10}$, 50 mg, "Twinsorb" process, 60 softgels. Claims to be 9 times more absorbable than powdered CoQ_{10}.

Allergy Research: CoQ$_{10}$, with tocotrienols, 100 mg CoQ_{10} and 25 mg tocotrienols in rice bran oil, 60 softgels.

Carlson: CoQ$_{10}$, 50 mg, 60 softgels.

Doctor's Best: CoQ$_{10}$, 100 mg CoQ_{10} and 1.5 mg bioperine, which enhances the absorption of CoQ_{10}, 60 softgels.

Solgar: CoQ$_{10}$, 120 mg, vegetarian and kosher, dry-form CoQ_{10}, 60 vegicaps.

Jarrow: CoQ$_{10}$, 60 mg, dry-form CoQ_{10}, 60 capsules.

Twinlab: Mega CoQ$_{10}$, 30 mg, dry-form CoQ_{10}, 100 capsules.

Cordyceps

Description: Cordyceps (*Cordyceps sinensis*) is a type of mushroom that is highly prized in Chinese medicine. It was very rare in the past because it grows naturally on a particular species of caterpillar. But a method of cultivating it commercially, using a fermentation process, has allowed it to be mass produced.

Uses: In China, cordyceps is considered a longevity and vitality tonic. It is being used now to support respiratory system function and as a cancer treatment. It may also be of value in ameliorating the side effects of chemotherapy and radiation treatment.

Indications: Anti-aging, athletic performance, cancer, asthma, chronic fatigue syndrome, energy (low).

It is thought to have antioxidant activity, and may function as a detoxification agent, particularly through its support of kidney function.

Products:

Doctor's Best: Ultra Cordyceps Plus, 750 mg cordyceps, providing 8% (60 mg) cordycepic acid, 30 mg ginkgo ext, and 30 mg artichoke leaf ext (2–5% cynarin), 60 capsules.
Solaray: Cordyceps, 520 mg, 100 capsules.
Metabolic Response Modifiers: Cordyceps, 750 mg, 60 capsules.

Coriolus Versicolor Extract

Related Item: Trametes Versicolor.
Description: Coriolus versicolor extract is derived from a mushroom commonly known as the "turkey tail" in North America. It is also referred to as cloud fungus, and Trametes versicolor.

Uses: This product, also known as PSK, or crestin, is promoted in Japan as a treatment for cancer. It is claimed to have a nor-

> *Indications:* Cancer, immune system.

malizing effect on immune system function, and is thought to work synergistically with other immune-enhancing or cancer-fighting agents.

As is the case for many of the other mushroom extracts in this category, Coriolus versicolor is rich in beta-glucans.

PSK is a water-soluble extract of the mushroom, with beta-1, 4-glucan as the main component. Another extract, PSP, has been used as well, and it is referred to as coriolan.

Products:

Maitake Products: Turkey Tail, 500 mg fruit body powder, 300 mg (20:1), extract, ginger, maitake d-fraction, vitamin C, and bioperine per 4 capsules, 120 tablets.
JHS Natural Products: *Coriolus Versicolor* Extract, cell wall extract from 625 mg *Coriolus versicolor* fruit body, 150 vegicaps.

Cranberry

Description: Cranberry (*Vaccinium macrocarponum*) is a sturdy plant that grows wild in North America. It belongs to the same genus as blueberry and bilberry.

Uses: Cranberry has a long history of medicinal and food use by Native Americans. Its traditional use in treating urinary tract infections has now been substantiated by modern research. The explanation lies in its ability to prevent disease-causing bacteria from adhering to the walls of the urinary tract.

> *Indications:* Urinary tract infections, periodontal disease, kidney stones.

In addition, cranberry is very rich in flavonoid antioxidants, including proanthocyanidins and vitamin C. In fact, a recent study of the antioxidant properties of fruits revealed that cranberry had the highest level of activity.

The benefits of cranberry can be obtained from drinking cranberry juice, but unsweetened juice should be used, rather than the diluted, heavily sweetened products available in grocery stores. As an alternative, concentrated capsules are available.

Products:

Jarrow: Cran Clearance, 650 mg cranberry concentrate (10:1), 30 mg vitamin C, 100 capsules.
Solaray: Cran Actin, 400 mg "Cranactin Cranberry AF Extract," 120 capsules.

Creatine

Description: Creatine is a nitrogen-containing compound. In the body, it is formed in the liver and converted to phosphocreatine in muscle, where it serves as a source of high-energy fuel for muscle contraction.

Uses: Creatine supplementation seems to enhance short-term (anerobic) exercise performance. It has shown benefit in most, but not all, studies involving high in-

> *Indications:* Athletic performance, cardiovascular disease.

tensity, short duration physical activities. If creatine is the fuel used by muscle, supplemental creatine can be thought of as preventing the tank from hitting empty too quickly. This may allow athletes to train a little longer, for example, resulting in enhanced performance. It has also been shown to result in increased muscle mass. This may be due to enhanced training—that is, creatine allowing a weight lifter to work a little harder and longer, although some feel that this is more a result of hydration of muscle tissue, rather than actual generation of additional muscle. Perhaps there is some of both.

Creatine is available in supplements as creatine monohydrate powder.

Dosage: The usual dose is 20 grams a day for up to five days, followed by a maintenance dose of 2 to 5 grams daily. The initial, higher dose, is intended to "load" the muscle rapidly with maximum levels of creatine. Then, the lower dose maintains these levels. Some feel that taking creatine with a small amount of carbohydrate will enhance its uptake into muscle tissue.

Cautions: High doses should not be taken by those with compromised renal (kidney) function. Long-term effects of high doses of creatine have not been determined. The powder should be taken with ample amounts of water—six to eight glasses per day. Large amounts of caffeine may counter the beneficial effects of creatine.

Recent research has shown that creatine does not increase the risk of injury in athletes.

Products:

Jarrow: Creatine Powder, creatine monohydrate, 325 g.
Twinlab: Creatine Fuel Capsules, 4,200 mg creatine monohydrate in 6 capsules, 120 capsules.
NOW Foods: Creatine Crave Chewy Chocolate, 1,500 mg creatine monohydrate per chew, 60 chews.

Cryptoxanthin

See: Carotenoids.

Curcumin

Related Item: Turmeric.

Description: Curcumin is the principal medicinal component on the herb turmeric. Turmeric is a tropical plant native to south and southeast Asia. The curcuminoids in turmeric are deep yellow in color, and are what contribute to the yellow color of foods and spices such as mustard and curry.

Uses: Curcumin and turmeric extracts have powerful antioxidant and anti-inflammatory action. It is useful in treating arthritis, including rheumatoid

> *Indications:* Arthritis, cardiovascular disease, cancer, cataracts, digestive aid, immune system.

arthritis. It lowers cholesterol, prevents the oxidation of blood lipids, and inhibits platelet aggregation. Historically, it has been used for indigestion, and as a stimulant to bile production and liver function.

Considerable animal and laboratory research indicates that curcumin may have a significant anticancer activity and immune-stimulating capability.

Animal studies have even shown that curcumin may prevent the development of cataracts.

Dosage: Take 400 to 600 milligrams of curcumin three times daily, for maximum effect, with meals. Lower doses may be sufficient, and standardized turmeric extracts are often used, at two or three capsules daily, with meals.

Cautions: Curcumin may enhance the anticoagulant effect of anticoagulant medications.

Products:

Nature's Herb's: Curcumin Power, 300 mg curcumin (95% curcuminoids) and 145 mg turmeric root powder, 60 capsules.
Jarrow: Curcumin 95, 380 mg of an 18:1 concentrate of curcumin (95% curcuminoids), 60 capsules.

Cysteine

Related Items: NAC, N-acetyl-cysteine, glutathione.

Description: L-cysteine is a nonessential, sulfur-containing amino acid.

Uses: Cysteine is not considered "essential" because it can be made in the body from another amino acid, methionine.

Cysteine is an important constituent of connective tissue, hair, skin, and nails. It is an antioxidant, and a precursor to the formation of glutathione. It also seems to play a role in immune system function. As a supplement, cysteine has drawbacks. It readily absorbs moisture and oxidizes, and this leads to stability problems and a limited shelf life. Instead, a derivative of cysteine, N-acetyl cysteine (NAC), may be a better way to obtain supplemental cysteine. See N-acetyl cysteine for more information.

Products:

Solgar: Cysteine, 500 mg, vegetarian and kosher, 90 vegicaps.
Twinlab: Cysteine, 500 mg, 60 capsules.

Deglycyrrhizinated Licorice

Related Item: Licorice.

Description: Deglycyrrhizinated licorice (DGL) is an extract of licorice root from which one component, glycyrrhizinic acid, has been removed.

Uses: Licorice has many medicinal properties, and a long history of use in traditional Chinese medicine. It is an anti-inflammatory agent, antimicrobial, expec-

> *Indications:* Ulcer (peptic), GERD (gastroesophageal reflux disease), canker sores.

torant, and adrenal gland tonic. It has been shown to be effective in treating gastric and duodenal ulcers, and may even inhibit the growth of *Helicobacter pylori*.

Licorice, however, also has certain side effects that limit its usefulness. It can cause elevated blood pressure, water retention, and excess potassium loss in some people. The main component responsible for this is glycyrrhizinic acid. When this component is removed, you have deglycyrrhizinated licorice (DGL), which retains most of the benefits of licorice, without the side effects.

The primary use for DGL is to treat gastric and duodenal ulcers. It appears most effective as a chewable tablet. There is also some evidence that DGL protects the gastric lining from damage caused by aspirin and other NSAIDs (nonsteroidal anti-inflammatory drugs).

Dosage: Chew one wafer before each meal, and at bedtime.

Products:

Nature's Herbs: DGL Power, 760 mg DGL root, standardized to not more than 0.6% glycyrrhizinic acid, and 100 mg glycine, 40 wafers.

Enzymatic Therapy: DGL chewable, DGL root extract, 3:1, 760 mg DGL and 100 mg glycine per 2 tablets, 100 tablets. Sweetened with fructose.

Dehydroepiandrosterone

See DHEA.

Devil's Claw

Description: Devil's claw (*Harpagophytum procumbens*) is native to southern Africa. The fruit of the plant is covered with small claw-like barbs, leading to its unusual name. The secondary tubers are rich in iridoid glucosides (harpagoside, harpagide, and procumbide).

Uses: The German Com-
mission E has approved devil's
claw for loss of appetite, dyspepsia (or indigestion), and "degenerative disorders of the locomotor system."

Indications: Arthritis, indigestion, sports injuries, appetite (loss of).

Devil's claw seems to have anti-inflammatory action, and this may explain why it is a popular remedy for arthritis, tendinitis, low back pain, and similar problems.

Dosage: Follow the guidelines on the product label. For loss of appetite, use about one-third the dose indicated for joint inflammation.

Cautions: Devil's claw is helpful for indigestion, but since it might stimulate gastric acid secretion, it may not be appropriate for heartburn.

Products:

Nature's Herbs: Devil's Claw, 510 mg devil's claw secondary root, 100 capsules.
Nature's Answer: Devil's Claw, Devil's claw fluid extract (1:1), 2 oz liquid.

DGL

See Deglycyrrhizinated Licorice.

D-Glucarate

Description: D-glucarate is naturally found in some vegetables and fruits, including apples and cruciferous vegetables. It is available in supplement form as the calcium salt, that is, calcium D-glucarate.

Uses: D-glucarate is thought to have anticancer activity. The theory behind this is as follows. Many carcinogens are eliminated from the body when they are complexed, or chemically bound, to other substances. This is one of the liver's normal functions. This carcinogen, or toxin complex, can either be excreted or retained in the body if the complex is broken apart by certain enzymes. D-glucarate inactivates one of those enzymes, thus increasing the amount of toxin complex that is removed from the body. By enhancing the removal of potentially carcinogenic materials from the body, including estrogen, D-glucarate may help prevent cancer.

This has been shown to be the case in animal studies, and in the laboratory. When human studies

Indications: Cancer.

are forthcoming, we will have a better feel for its efficacy in this regard, as well as the appropriate dosage.

Dosage: The usual recommendation is 1,000 milligrams, twice a day, of calcium D-glucarate.

Products:

Tyler: Calcium D-Glucarate, 500 mg, 90 capsules.

DHA

Related Items: EPA (eicosapentaenoic acid), fish oil, omega-3 oils.

Description: DHA (docosahexaenoic acid) is an omega-3 fatty acid, present in relatively high levels in fish oil. It is abundant in the human brain, and seems to be essential to normal brain, visual, and nervous system development in the fetus. It is the predominant omega-3 fatty acid in breast milk.

A Comment from Dr. Abel

Cholesterol testing has given the term *fats* a bad name. There are actually two groups of fats: saturated and unsaturated. The saturated fats found in nature are derived from animals and have been called lard. The synthetic saturated fats called trans fats are from hydrogenated processed vegetable oils and contain no beneficial value. The unsaturated fats may be monounsaturated (one double bond) or polyunsaturated (containing more than one double bond) and are important structurally in our bodies. Polyunsaturated fatty acids with the important health benefits are defined as omega-3 and omega-6 fatty acids because of the location of the first double bond in the carbon chain. We can synthesize up to 16 carbons, but cannot make the jump to 18 carbons. We also have difficulty when supplied with the oils, nuts, or algae that contain the important 18 carbon fatty acids to build the longer-chain fatty acids, which are essential for brain and vision development. DHA is the end product of the omega-3 fatty acid line, and is present in every cell of our body; DHA also comprises at least 30 percent of our brain and our retina. Only the brains of humans and porpoises have an equal amount of omega-3 (DHA) and omega-6 fatty acids. The average American consumes at least six times as much omega-6 as omega-3. DHA is the best of the good fats. It is involved in heart function, the lining of blood vessels, skin, and even hair. Administration of DHA can reduce the likelihood of heart attacks, reduce blood pressure, reduce triglycerides, add to the production of "good" cholesterol, and improve inflammatory conditions such as rheumatoid arthritis. The brain and heart-healthy omega-3 fats are found primarily in algae, cold water fish, walnuts, and to a limited degree, grain. Fish oil, which is 80 percent EPA, a 20-carbon omega-3, leads to development of some inflammatory components, whereas the longer-chain (22-carbon) DHA produces noninflammatory products, which confer numerous health benefits. Furthermore, DHA is an important way to prevent and even combat depression and multiple sclerosis. DHA and arachidonic acid, when added to infant formulas during the first seventeen weeks of a baby's life, have been shown to result in better vision and increased IQ. This may decrease the incidence of learning disabilities as well. I have counseled many parents in terms of supplementing with DHA even in high school, and witnessed wonderful results. The essential fatty acids, or essential oils, need to be a part of everyone's diet.

Uses: DHA has been shown to lower elevated triglycerides. In this regard, its actions seems to be

| Indications: Triglycerides (high). |

equivalent to other omega-3 supplements, such as EPA and fish oil (containing both EPA and DHA). There is some concern, however, over its effect on LDL cholesterol, and while it may lower total triglycerides, it may not exert a beneficial effect on the ratio of desirable to undesirable cholesterol fractions. Administration of other LDL-lowering supplements, such as water-soluble fiber, niacin, garlic, and gum guggul, along with the fish oil may ameliorate this concern.

DHA is more uniquely indicated in other situations. It appears to be essential during pregnancy and nursing, and is now being added to infant formulas.

Research is ongoing to verify the role of DHA in treating several specific problems—attention deficit disorder, cystic fibrosis, dyslexia, Alzheimer's disease, Zellweger's syndrome, rheumatoid arthritis, depression, and autoimmune disorders such as lupus and psoriasis.

Many nutritionists believe that there is a relative deficiency of EPA and DHA in the general population owing to the increased intake of omega-6 oils (processed vegetable oils) and trans fatty acids. This can suppress the normal conversion of omega-3 oils to EPA and DHA. These conversions can be further impaired if there is a deficiency of certain nutrients, such as vitamins C, B_6, niacin, and zinc.

DHA can be obtained in supplement form derived from fish oil, or from phytoplankton (algae). It can also be formed in the body, with varying degrees of efficiency, from alpha-linolenic acid, which is converted first to EPA and then to DHA. Flaxseed oil is often recommended as a rich source of alpha-linolenic acid (ALA). Most fish oil supplements contain about 12 percent DHA.

Dosage: For elevated triglycerides, 1 to 2 grams daily.

Cautions: All omega-3 oils have some antithrombotic activity. This is generally advantageous. Those already taking anticoagulant medications (Coumadin), however, should exercise caution.

Products:

Solgar: DHA, 100 mg, Neuromins®, 100 mg DHA derived from 500 mg DHA-rich oil, 60 softgels.
Source Naturals: DHA, 200 mg, Neuromins®, 200 mg DHA derived from algal oil, 60 softgels.
Jarrow: MaxDHA, 500 mg sardine oil providing 250 mg DHA and 100 mg EPA, 180 softgels.
Carlson: Super-DHA, 1,000 mg fish body oil concentrate providing 500 mg DHA and 200 mg EPA, 60 softgels.

DHEA

Related Item: Androstenedione.

Description: Dehydroepiandrosterone (DHEA) is a hormone normally produced by the adrenal glands. It circulates throughout the bloodstream and is converted by the body into other steroid hormones, such as testosterone, androstenedione, and estrogen.

Uses: The use of DHEA as a dietary supplement remains controversial. It is a hormone, or hormone precursor, not a nutrient.

> *Indications:* Sexual performance, anti-aging, chronic fatigue syndrome.

Original claims by some that Mexican or wild yam was a dietary source of DHEA or DHEA precursors were false.

There is no question that DHEA is a key component in the body's complex regulatory mechanism. We know, for example, that levels of DHEA (or more correctly, DHEAS) are lower in individuals with chronic disease. And we know that levels of DHEA peak at age 25 and then steadily decline up to age 70. What we do not know for sure is whether or not it is beneficial to artificially boost levels of DHEA in an older person to what they were before. Nor do we know what the ramifications are of boosting levels over what they would normally be during the younger years. And we do not know what long-term effects might result from boosting DHEA levels through supplementation. In fact, there is quite a bit we do not know about the effects and possible side effects of DHEA supplementation. For this reason, many feel that supplementation with DHEA should be undertaken only under the direct supervision and monitoring of a physician.

In spite of this, the lure of DHEA's possible benefits has proven irresistible to many, including many researchers. Is DHEA really the miraculous anti-aging compound that some claim it is? It remains to be seen. Its effects differ, depending on gender and age. There is some evidence that DHEA supplementation may help those with depression, erectile dysfunction, fatigue, depressed immune system function, and certain symptoms associated with menopause. Other studies support the contention that DHEA supplementation results in increased lean body mass, improved mood, and an increased sense of well-being.

Dosage: The usual dosage is 25 to 50 milligrams daily for men, and perhaps less for women.

Cautions: Prudence dictates that DHEA supplementation is best undertaken only on the advice and guidance of a physician. Higher dosage levels should definitely not be used without medical supervision. The long-term effects of DHEA supplementation are unknown.

Those who are at risk for prostate, breast, uterine, or ovarian cancer should not take DHEA.

The most common adverse reactions seem to be androgenic effects, such as acne and increased facial hair.

Products:

Jarrow: DHEA, 50 mg, pharmaceutical grade, 90 capsules. NOTE: Products are available from various manufacturers in dosages of 5 mg, 10 mg, 15 mg, 25 mg, 25 mg TR, 25 mg sublingual, 50 mg, 50 mg TR.
Natrol: DHEA, 25 mg, 90 capsules.
Natrol: DHEA, 10 mg, 30 tablets.

Dibencozide

Related Items: Cobalamin, vitamin B_{12}, methylcobalamin.

Description: Dibencozide is a name for one of the two coenzyme forms of vitamin B_{12}, adenosylcobalamin (5-deoxyadenosylcobalamin). The other coenzyme form of vitamin B_{12} is methylcobalamin.

Uses: This particular form of B_{12} is sometimes marketed to body-builders and athletes, apparently as an energy aid and muscle-building agent. Unfortunately, the support for this is mostly anecdotal.

Dibencozide, or adenosylcobalamin, is a cofactor for the enzyme L-methylmalonyl coenzyme A mutase, while the other coenzyme form of B_{12}, methylcobalamin, is a cofactor for the enzyme methionine synthase.

If the only purpose of supplementing with this nutrient is muscle building and energy, perhaps there is some justification for using only the dibencozide form of vitamin B_{12}. Even though, again, the effectiveness of this is based primarily on theoretical and anecdotal evidence. But if the purpose is to obtain an effective, well-absorbed dose of vitamin B_{12}, we question the advisability of using only one of the two coenzyme forms. Instead, taking a high dose of cobalamin (or hydroxocobalamin) might be more beneficial.

Products:

Source Naturals: Dibencozide, 10,000 mcg, sublingual, 60 tablets. Dibencozide provides 6,800 mcg of vitamin B_{12}.
Country Life: Active B_{12} Dibencozide, 3,000 mcg with folic acid, 3,000 mcg vitamin B_{12} from dibencozide and 200 mcg folic acid, 60 lozenges.
Solgar: B_{12} Megasorb Nuggets, 5,000 mcg, 5,000 mcg cobalamin and 100 mcg dibencozide, 60 tablets.

Dimethylglycine

See DMG.

DLPA

See DL-Phenylalanine.

DL-Phenylalanine

Related Item: L-Phenylalanine.

Description: DL-phenylalanine, also referred to as DLPA, is a racemic mixture consisting of equal amounts of D-phenylalanine and L-phenylalanine. These are both amino acids, but only the L-form is used in protein synthesis.

Uses: DL-phenylalanine is thought to have analgesic and antidepressant activity. The antidepressant action is probably due to the presence of L-phenylalanine, while the analgesic activity results from the D-form.

> *Indications:* Pain, depression.

L-phenylalanine is a precursor to L-tyrosine, which in turn is a precursor to the neurotransmitters norepinephrine and dopamine. Increased levels of these neurotransmitter substances are thought to be associated with mood elevation and antidepressant effects.

D-phenylalanine may block pain by interfering with the degradation of natural enkephalins.

DLPA seems to be most useful as a long-term adjunct to the treatment of chronic pain.

Dosage: Typically, between 375 and 2,500 milligrams can be used, preferably under the supervision of a health professional. Take between meals.

Cautions: DL-phenylalanine is contraindicated in those with phenylketonuria, and those taking nonselective monoamine oxidase (MAO) inhibitors.

Products:

Solgar: DLPA, 500 mg, vegetarian and kosher, 100 vegicaps.
Country Life: DLPA, 1,000 mg, 1,000 mg DLPA and 10 mg vitamin B$_6$, 60 capsules.

DMG

Description: Dimethylglycine (DMG) is a nonprotein amino acid, found naturally in animal and plant tissue. Its proper chemical name is N,N-dimethylglycine, although in the past it has been known as pangamic acid, calcium pangamate, and vitamin B_{15}.

Uses: DMG was initially popular as a supplement because of claims that it enhanced cellular oxygenation, increased stamina, and boosted energy. Subsequent research has failed to support these claims. On the other hand, there is some preliminary evidence supporting DMG as an immune system enhancer. Of course, we have many other supplements that enhance the immune response, and their efficacy is well documented.

Cautions: DMG is not the same as TMG (betaine, or trimethylglycine), although DMG can be formed in the body from TMG.

Products:

Country Life: DMG, 125 mg, 90 tablets.
Da Vinci: Gluconic DMG, 125 mg, 90 tablets.

Docosahexaenoic Acid

See DHA.

Dolomite

Related Item: Calcium.

Description: Dolomite is a mineral containing calcium and magnesium carbonate, along with other naturally occurring trace and heavy metals. It is also known as magnesium limestone.

Uses: Dolomite was once popular as a nutritional supplement. However, it contains naturally high levels of lead, mercury, and other toxic minerals. With so many other calcium and magnesium supplements available, there is no reason to use dolomite.

EPA

See Fish Oil.

Echinacea

Description: Echinacea, also known as "purple coneflower," is one of the most popular herbs used as an immune system stimulant. Its use dates back to the American Indians. Three species are commonly used: *Echinacea purpurea, Echinacea angustifolia,* and *Echinacea pallida.*

Marketing claims to the contrary, there is no evidence that one species is more effective than another, and there is also no evidence that one part of the plant (roots, leaves) is more effective than another. There is also no evidence that wild echinacea is any better or worse than cultivated echinacea.

Uses: Echinacea has been shown to enhance immune system activity. It is thought that it exerts this effect primarily through stim-

> *Indications:* Cold and flu, immune system.

ulating the action of white blood cells, which attack and destroy invading organisms (phagocytosis).

When taken at the first signs of infection, echinacea will shorten the duration and severity of cold and flu symptoms.

Echinacea has also been used to treat wounds and other skin ailments.

Cautions: Some suggest that echinacea should not be used by those with autoimmune diseases, but there is some controversy as to whether or not this is a valid concern.

Products:

Nature's Herbs: Echinacea Power, 250 mg echinacea root extract (3.2–4.8% echinasides), 50 mg *echinacea angustifolia,* 50 mg *Echinacea purpurea,* and 680 mg Parthenium root per 2 capsules, 60 capsules.

Nature's Answer: Echinacea Liquid, 500 mg *echinacea angustifolia* root, 500 mg *Echinacea purpurea* whole plant in 28 drops, contains 20 mg of total phenols, 2 oz.

Solgar: Echinacea Vegicaps, 65 mg *Echinacea purpurea* root extract (4:1), 265 mg raw echinacea aerial powder, 135 IU vitamin A, vegetarian and kosher, 250 vegicaps.

Nature's Way: Echinaguard, 2 ml Echinaguard liquid, the expressed juice from the stem, leaf, and flower of *Echinacea purpurea* per 2.5, ml, 4 oz liquid.

Effervescent Vitamin C

Related Item: Buffered vitamin C.

Description: When a mixture of ascorbic acid, citric acid, and mineral bicarbonate is added to water, the citric and ascorbic acids react with the bicarbonate, releasing carbon dioxide, that is, it "fizzes." To some degree, the ascorbic acid will be converted to mineral ascorbates.

Uses: Some find this a more palatable alternative to tablets and capsules as a source of supplemental vitamin C. To the extent that the vitamin C is converted to mineral ascorbates, the acidic nature will be neutralized, creating a "buffered vitamin C."

Products:

Allergy Research: Buffered Vitamin C Powder, 900 mg vitamin C as calcium, magnesium, and potassium ascorbates per ½ teaspoon, 240 grams. This product contains vitamin C and mineral carbonates, which react when added to water. It is hypoallergenic and produces a moderate fizz. This same formulation is available in capsule form.

Alacer: Emergen-C, 1,000 mg vitamin C as mineral ascorbates and all the B vitamins, per packet, 36 packets. This product is a mixture of bicarbonates, vitamin C, and citric acid, resulting in a pronounced fizz. It comes in numerous flavors.

Elderberry

Description: Supplements of elderberry (*Sambucus nigra*) contain extracts of the flower or berry of the elder tree. Its medicinal use dates back to Rome and Greece. It is rich in flavonoids, including quercetin and rutin.

Uses: Elderberry extract has been used widely in Europe to treat colds and flu, especially when accompanied by fever and

> *Indications:* Cold and flu, immune system.

congestion. Studies in Israel support its supposed antiviral activity.

Products:

Nature's Way: Sambucol, 2 teaspoons contain 3.8 g elderberry extract, 4 oz liquid.

Nature's Way: Sambucol Lozenges, 130 mg elderberry dried extract and 100 mg vitamin C, 30 lozenges.

Emu Oil

Description: Emu oil is obtained from the fat of the emu, a bird native to Australia.

Uses: Enthusiastic claims were made that this oil would cure arthritis, heal wounds, relieve muscle pain, and eliminate wrinkles. It almost seemed too good to be true. Apparently, it was. There is no valid use for this product.

Ephedra

Description: Ephedra, or ma huang, is a plant found in desert regions throughout the world. It has been used as a medicinal herb for over 5,000 years, and is one of the stalwarts of traditional Chinese medicine. Its two most important medicinal constituents are the alkaloids ephedrine and pseudoephedrine.

Uses: There is no question that ephedra is a valuable, effective medicinal herb. Traditionally, it has been used for respiratory conditions (asthma, hay fever, cough-

> **Indications: Cold and flu, obesity, weight loss, allergies, sinusitis.**

ing, emphysema, congestion), colds, fevers, and other problems (nephritis, headache). During this long history of successful use, safety and toxicity have never been considered a problem.

Over the last few years, however, the safety of ephedra supplements has been one of the main concerns of various regulatory agencies. Some have demanded that the availability of ephedra-containing products be severely restricted.

Why would an herb with such a long history of safety and efficacy now be under regulatory attack?

The problem stems primarily from irresponsible marketing and use of two types of ephedra-containing products. One is the "recreational" ephedra product, which is designed for nonmedical purposes (creating a "high," euphoria and enhancing sexual pleasure). The other is the weight loss supplement, where ephedra or ephedra alkaloids are combined with caffeine to exert a powerful thermogenic effect.

When used responsibly, the benefits of ephedra far outweigh any concerns over safety. But when used improperly, the potential for problems is significant.

These problems are most likely of lesser concern when the whole herb is used, as it has been in traditional herbal medicine. The whole herb contains the two major alkaloids ephedrine and pseudoephedrine, along with numerous other compounds. When taken in this form, the alkaloids in the whole herb are absorbed more slowly and have a more prolonged effect than the isolated alkaloids.

Many of the products being promoted irresponsibly contain added ephedra alkaloids. When products are spiked with extra alkaloids and with other central nervous system stimulants such as caffeine or caffeine-rich herbs (guarana, kola nut), they exert amphetamine-like action and are more like drugs than herbs.

The major component of ephedra is ephedrine. Ephedrine is categorized as a "sympathomimetic," a substance that stimulates the sympathetic nervous system. If you think back to your early lessons in biology, you might remember the "fight or flight" syndrome. This is a way of describing what happens when you stimulate the sympathetic nervous system, releasing adrenalin from the adrenal gland. Body functions that might hinder your ability to fight or flee are depressed. This would include reducing stomach and gastrointestinal motility, constricting the urinary sphincter, dilating the pupil of the eye, and constricting systemic blood vessels. At the same time, other functions would be stimulated, such as heart rate and contraction strength, coronary blood vessel dilation, and bronchiole dilation.

Well, this is all very nice, but what does it have to do with ephedra? If you have hay fever, and nasal congestion, the sympathomimetic action of ephedra (constricting the tissue in the nose) is something you benefit from. If you have asthma, or emphysema, the bronchiole-dilating actions of ephedra is something you benefit from. But if you have high blood pressure, constriction of peripheral blood vessels may make it worse. If you have benign prostatic hyperplasia, the last thing you want is to take something that might further constrict the urinary sphincter. Thus, the concern with side effects.

The more pronounced the activity of any herb (or drug), the more potential for side effects. The likelihood that whole-herb ephedra, or ma huang, will cause these problems is slight, but when additional ephedra is added to the product, the likelihood increases.

Responsible manufacturers should indicate on the label whether or not additional ephedra has been added, and the product should indicate the level of ephedra alkaloids. Currently, standardized ephedra products are available, usually at a level of 6 to 8 percent ephedra alkaloids, and such products are preferred to those with no quantitative information.

There are two primary uses for ephedra supplements that merit consideration. As a treatment for respiratory problems, nasal congestion, sinusitis, and perhaps mild asthma, we see no problem with using reasonable amounts of standardized ephedra supplements. There is little question that a combination of ephedra and caffeine can facilitate weight loss. It seems to exert a pronounced thermogenic action, and, to some degree, an appetite suppressant effect. But this combination more closely resembles a drug than an herb, and should be used only if necessary, preferably under the guidance of a health professional. It should not be considered a "miracle" pill, replacing the need for exercise, behavior modification, and dietary changes.

Dosage: Ephedra is available in capsule and tablet form, standardized and unstandardized, as well as extracts and tinctures. A prudent dose should not exceed the equivalent of 12 to 25 milligrams total alkaloids (as ephedrine), two or three times a day. It is also available as a tea.

Note: An herb identified as "Mormon tea" (*Ephedra nevadensis*) is available, but it contains little or no ephedrine. Also, ephedra root does not contain ephedrine. It actually may contain components that counter the action of ephedrine.

Cautions: Responsible manufacturers should include warnings similar to this on the product label:

> Ephedra should not be taken by patients with heart disease, high blood pressure, thyroid disease, diabetes, or difficulty in urination due to enlargement of the prostate. It should not be taken by patients taking antihypertensive and antidepressant medications. Discontinue use if you experience rapid heartbeat, dizziness, severe headache, shortness of breath, or similar problems.

On the other hand, responsible consumers should not take products that claim to produce euphoric sexual enlightenment or melt away 10 pounds a day while you sleep off a Häagen-Dazs-induced soporific coma.

Products:

Nature's Answer: Ma Huang Twig Extract, 100 mg ma huang twig extract, providing 8% (8 mg) ephedrine alkaloids, vegetarian and kosher, 100 vegicaps.

Nature's Answer: Ma Huang Liquid, 1,000 mg ma huang twig extract, providing 2 mg ephedrine alkaloids per 28 drops, 1 oz.
Solaray: Ephedra Capsules, 375 mg ephedra aerial parts, providing 3.75–7.5 mg ephedrine alkaloids, 100 capsules.

Essiac Tea

Description: Essiac is an herbal mixture developed by a nurse, Rene Caisse, containing burdock root, sheep sorrel, slippery elm, and Turkey rhubarb.

Uses: This product, and the variations thereof, are claimed to be "cures" for cancer. While convincing evidence of its "curative" properties remains lacking, there is an impressive array of anecdotal reports of improvement when used by cancer patients.

It is difficult to separate fact from fiction when it comes to competing marketing claims by various companies marketing their versions of the "original" formula. Most likely, such differences are of minimal relevance. The basic formula is agreed upon, and more important, as is the case for all supplements, is the integrity, quality, and reproducibility of the product.

While essiac may not be a "miracle cure" for cancer, as many have claimed, it certainly seems to have some value to those with cancer. It may help—that is, reduce pain, cause some degree of tumor regression, promote an increased sense of well-being, and so on—and seems to cause no harm. There is little reason not to include essiac as part of a comprehensive supplement regimen for the patient with cancer.

Products:

Flora: Flor Essence Dry, "improved" formula, adds watercress, kelp, blessed thistle, and red clover to original formula, 2.2 oz powder. Needs to be brewed into a tea.
Flora: Flor Essence Liquid, "improved" formula, adds watercress, kelp, blessed thistle, and red clover to original formula, 17 oz liquid. Ready to use.
Essiac Int: Essiac Herbal Remedy, "original" Rene Caisse formula made by Resperin Corp. Burdock root, sheep sorrel, slippery elm, and Indian rhubarb root, 1.5 oz powder. Needs to be brewed into a tea.

Ester-C

Related Item: Vitamin C.
Description: Ester-C refers to a mineral ascorbate and vitamin C

metabolite complex. The mineral ascorbate is typically a calcium salt of ascorbic acid (calcium ascorbate), and the predominant metabolite seems to be threonic acid, or calcium L-threonate.

Uses: Ester-C is a patented ascorbate-metabolite complex, and it is claimed to enhance the delivery of vitamin C into the cells of the body. The product is buffered and well tolerated.

The claims of superior utilization are supported primarily by animal and test-tube studies, however.

For those who feel they do not tolerate vitamin C products well, or for those to whom optimal absorption is important, an ester-C supplement may be the appropriate choice.

Products:

Natrol: Ester C 1,000 with Bioflavonoids, 1,000 mg vitamin C as calcium ascorbate, 200 mg lemon bioflavonoids, 180 tablets.
Natrol: Ester C 500 with Bioflavonoids, 500 mg vitamin C as calcium ascorbate, 200 mg citrus bioflavonoids, 240 capsules.
Allergy Research: Ester C Magnesium, 500 mg vitamin C as magnesium ascorbate, 100 capsules.
Twinlab: Ester-C, 1,000 with citrus bioflavonoid complex, 1,000 mg of vitamin C as calcium ascorbate, 200 mg citrus bioflavonoid complex, 100 tablets.

Evening Primrose Oil

Related Items: Borage oil, black currant seed oil.

Description: Evening primrose oil is derived from the seed of the evening primrose plant, *Oenthera biennis*, which is native to North America. It contains gamma-linolenic acid (GLA), the precursor to the inflammation-suppressing series 1 prostaglandins.

Uses: Evening primrose oil was the first commercially available source of a GLA-rich oil. Therefore, most of the initial research on the therapeutic value of GLA supplementation was done

Indications: Arthritis (rheumatoid), diabetes, skin disorders, eczema, fibrocystic breast disease, premenstrual syndrome.

with evening primrose oil. Later, more potent sources of GLA were brought to market (borage oil, black currant oil), but many nutritionists still recommend evening primrose oil.

GLA (gamma-linolenic acid) is an omega-6 oil. Not all omega-6 oils are bad. The predominant omega-6 oils in the diet—linoleic, linolenic, and arachidonic—can be both detrimental and beneficial. Linoleic acid is essential to life. In the body, these oils are converted into powerful, hormone-like substances called prostaglandins. The omega-6 oils can form two types. One type, the 2 series, is usually detrimental, causing inflammation. The other type, the 1 series, is beneficial, reducing inflammation. The GLA type of omega-6 oil leads to the beneficial, series 1 type of prostaglandin. The beneficial actions of series 1 prostaglandins are similar to those of the series 3 prostaglandins derived from omega-3 oils, ALA (flaxseed oil) and EPA (fish oil). Thus, GLA, from borage, black currant, and evening primrose oil, provides much the same benefit as the omega-3 oils from fish and flaxseed.

Dosage: The dose can vary widely, with the equivalent of 270 to 540 milligrams of GLA being a common range.

Products:

Nutricia: Efamol Evening Primrose Oil, 1,000 mg, 120 mg gamma-linolenic acid (12%), 700 mg linoleic acid per capsule, 60 softgels.
Health from the Sun: EPO Liquid Gold, 200 mg gamma-linolenic acid per dose, 4 oz liquid.
Jarrow: Primrose 1300, 117 mg gamma-linolenic acid per capsule, 60 softgels.

Fenugreek

Description: Fenugreek (*Trigonella foenum-graecum*) is an annual herb native to the Mediterranean, the Ukraine, China, and India. The part used therapeutically is the ripe, dried seed, which contains high amounts of mucilaginous fiber, proteins rich in lysine and tryptophan, and various other compounds.

Uses: Traditionally, fenugreek was used to treat anorexia, dyspepsia, gastritis, and convalescence. The German Commission E has approved it for loss of appetite. But the current interest in fenugreek is based on studies that have shown it can regulate blood sugar and lower cholesterol and triglycerides. It may be an ideal dietary supplement for diabetics, preventing elevated blood lipids and atherosclerosis, while helping to normalize blood glucose levels.

> *Indications:* Diabetes, cholesterol problems, appetite (loss of).

Dosage: For diabetes and cholesterol control, between 5 to 30 grams with each meal can be used. The typical dosage indicated for capsules is two to three capsules with each meal. In tincture form, 3 or 4 millileters can be taken two or three times a day.

Products:

Fenugreek Nature's Herbs: Fenugreek, 620 mg, 100 capsules.
Fenugreek Nature's Answer: Fenugreek Seed, 2,000 mg fenugreek seed fluid extract per 2 ml, 2 oz liquid.

Feverfew

Description: Feverfew *(Tanacetum parthenium)* can be found throughout North America and Europe. The leaves are used medicinally.

Uses: Feverfew is best known as a treatment for migraine headaches. Its ability to reduce the frequency, severity, and duration of

> *Indications:* Migraine headaches.

migraine attacks has been confirmed by several published scientific studies. Feverfew also has general anti-inflammatory and antiplatelet aggregation activity. It is rich in substances known as sesquiterpene lactones, with parthenolide being the most common.

Products:

Solaray: MigraGard, 350 mg feverfew, std to 0.7% (2.45 mg) parthenolide, 60 capsules.
Nature's Answer: Feverfew Leaf Alcohol Free, 2,000 mg feverfew leaf fluid extract per 2 ml, 1 oz liquid.

Fiber

Related Items: Pectin, psyllium.

Description: Fiber, or dietary fiber, can be defined in different ways. One definition for dietary fiber is undigestible plant compounds. Another is undigestible carbohydrate.

There are two main types of fiber—insoluble fiber and soluble fiber. The best-known example of insoluble fiber is wheat bran. There are a number of types of soluble fiber—hemicelluloses, mucilages, gums, and pectins. Some well-known examples are oat bran, guar gum, and psyllium.

Uses: Certain types of fiber are thought to be more beneficial for certain conditions than other types. Soluble fiber, for example, is thought to be more effective in lowering cholesterol and modu-

> *Indications:* Cholesterol problems, constipation, diarrhea, irritable bowel syndrome, weight loss, cardiovascular disease, cancer (colon), diabetes.

lating blood sugar levels. Insoluble fiber is thought to be more effective as a stool softener, laxative, and anti–colon cancer agent. Ongoing research, however, is leading to a blurring of these distinctions in many cases. For this reason, we are more inclined to recommend blends of various types of dietary fiber, rather than individual types.

Dietary fiber decreases intestinal transit time, reducing the amount of time toxins remain in contact with the intestinal wall. Dietary fiber slows gastric emptying time, moderating blood glucose levels. Dietary fiber, especially the soluble types, lowers serum cholesterol and triglyceride levels. The fermentation of dietary fiber by intestinal microorganisms produces short-chain fatty acids, such as butyric acid, which is a source of energy for the cells lining the colon, and may contribute to fiber's anticancer action. Dietary fiber fills the stomach, contributing a feeling of satiety that may aid in weight loss. Dietary fiber can alleviate constipation and diarrhea and may be helpful in conditions such as irritable bowel syndrome. Dietary fiber increases stool weight, stool softness, and eases elimination, which may reduce diverticular disease and hemorrhoids.

Dosage: Typical dosage is from 5 to 15 grams daily, before meals or at bedtime.

Cautions: If you are not accustomed to supplementing with dietary fiber, be sure to start out with small doses and gradually increase the amount. Always drink ample quantities of water when taking fiber supplements.

Products:

Solgar: Apple Pectin Powder, 8 oz.
Yerba Prima: Psyllium Whole Husks, 4.5 g fiber per tablespoon, 12 oz powder.
Yerba Prima: Psyllium Husk Vegicaps, 625 mg psyllium per capsule, 2.2 grams fiber per 4 vegicaps, 180 vegicaps.

Fish Oil

Related Items: EPA (eicosapentaenoic acid), omega-3 oils, DHA (docosahexaenoic acid).

Description: Fish oil supplements are derived from cold water fish, rich in omega-3 oils containing EPA and DHA.

Uses: EPA is a fatty acid used by the body to produce certain types of prostaglandins that have beneficial actions, such as reducing inflammation, reducing the stickiness of platelets, preventing

> *Indications:* Triglycerides (high), cardiovascular disease, hypertension, arthritis (rheumatoid), Crohn's disease, ulcerative colitis, depression, psoriasis.

clot formation, and dilating blood vessels. Prostaglandins are powerful, short-lived hormone-like substances produced in the body from various fatty acids. DHA is an important component of cell membranes, particularly in the brain, nervous system, and retina.

A COMMENT FROM DR. ABEL

Get those dry eyes working again. Remember the combination of blink, drink, and essential fatty acids. This can be cod liver oil, fish oil, or better yet, DHA (docosahexanoic acid). Also remember to keep a humidifier in your bedroom, especially during the winter. Lastly, cleaning out the ductwork in your house every four or five years will provide a measurable relief for both your eyes and your respiratory system.

Fish oil supplements contain both EPA and DHA, typically in the ratio of 1.5:1 (i.e., 180 milligrams of EPA and 120 milligrams of DHA). Other variations are available, however (see below).

Supplements of EPA and DHA are usually used to treat elevated triglyceride levels and other cardiovascular system problems, including high blood pressure, atherosclerosis, arrhythmias, and Raynaud's disease. The anti-inflammatory action is used to alleviate the discomfort of conditions such as rheumatoid arthritis, asthma, ulcerative colitis, and Crohn's disease. The EPA and DHA in fish oil seem to exert an immune system–modulating action as well and are recommended by some for a wide variety of problems, including eczema, psoriasis, lupus, depression, bipolar disorder, and schizophrenia. While fish oil supplements certainly may be helpful to some degree in these and similar conditions, more research is needed to verify this.

Fish oil supplements are available in several forms. The natural form usually provides 30 percent EPA and DHA. A softgel capsule containing 1,000 milligrams of fish oil would provide 300 milligrams of EPA and DHA. A 1,200-miligram softgel would contain 360 milligram of EPA and DHA. It is important when reading the label of fish oil supplements to look at the actual EPA and DHA content, rather than the total amount of oil in the capsule. This is the only way to properly compare one product to another, and is the basis on which you should determine the required dosage. If you have been told to take 2 grams of EPA/DHA per day, for example, that would mean you need about seven 1-gram capsules if the capsule was 30 percent EPA/DHA. In other words, each capsule may contain 1 gram of fish oil, but the fish oil only contains 30 percent EPA/DHA, or 300 milligrams.

The total number of capsules, therefore, can easily build up to an unwieldy level. Thus, the lure of more concentrated versions of EPA/DHA has led to the development of some natural oils that reach 50 percent EPA/DHA potency, as well as semisynthetic ethyl ester derivatives that provide as much as 85 percent EPA/DHA.

In deciding which type of product might be appropriate for you, the therapeutic value and convenience of a high-dose EPA/DHA supplement has to be weighed against the lower cost of less-concentrated products.

A product with a higher ratio of EPA might be appropriate when the intended use involves treating cardiovascular problems or inflammatory disorders such as rheumatoid arthritis. A product higher in DHA would not be appropriate under those conditions. A higher DHA-containing product would be preferable if treating problems relating to the central nervous system, attention deficit disorder, retinal problems, or cognitive impairment.

Enteric-coated fish oil supplements are available, and are especially useful when treating ulcerative colitis or Crohn's disease. They are also less likely to result in a fishy aftertaste.

Small amounts of vitamin E are usually added to fish oil supplements to act as an antioxidant, preventing the fish oil from deteriorating during storage.

Cautions: All omega-3 oils have some antithrombotic activity. This is generally advantageous. Those already taking anticoagulant medications (Coumadin), however, should exercise caution.

Cod liver oil is a fish oil that contains some EPA and DHA. However, cod liver oil also contains substantial amounts of vitamin A and vitamin D. It is inappropriate to use cod liver oil as a source of EPA/DHA because of the danger of overdosing on vitamin A and vitamin D.

Products:

Solgar: MaxEPA, 600 mg omega-3 polyunsaturates, 360 mg EPA, 240 mg DHA per 2 capsules, 120 softgels.

Solgar: Omega-3 700, 700 mg omega-3 polyunsaturates, 360 mg EPA, 240 mg DHA, 100 mg other fatty acids per capsule, 60 softgels. Note: This is twice the potency of regular MaxEPA.

Twinlab: Super MaxEPA Capsules, 750 mg omega-3 polyunsaturates, 450 mg EPA, 300 mg DHA per 2 capsules, 100 softgels.

Twinlab: Emulsified Super MaxEPA Liquid, 1,000 mg EPA, 670 mg DHA per tablespoon (15 ml), 12 oz liquid.

Tyler: Eskimo-3 Liquid, 1,500 mg omega-3 fatty acids, 720 mg EPA, 480 mg DHA per teaspoon, 105 ml liquid. No fishy taste. Free of heavy metals and PCBs and other contaminants.

Tyler Eskimo-3 Capsules, 500 mg omega-3 fatty acids, 240 mg EPA, 160 mg DHA per 3 capsules, 105 softgels.

Carlson: Salmon Oil, 750 mg omega-3 fatty acids, 360 mg EPA, 250 mg DHA per 2 capsules, 120 softgels.

Nature's Way: Fisol Enteric Coated, 500 mg omega-3 fatty acids, 150 mg EPA, 100 mg DHA per capsule, enteric coated, 90 softgels.

Twinlab: TwinEPA, 600 mg EPA, 240 mg DHA per capsule, 60 softgels.

European Reference Lab: Coromega, 650 mg omega-3 fatty acids, 350 mg EPA, 230 mg DHA per orange-flavored packet, 28 packets.

Flavonoids

Related Items: Quercetin, proanthocyanidins, rutin, hesperidin, bioflavonoids.

Description: In the broad sense, *flavonoids* is a term that covers a broad group of plant pigments. Chemically, there are several subgroups, but all have a 2-phenylchromane skeleton. There are, in fact, over 3,000 known flavonoids, and they include flavonols (quercetin), flavan-3-ols (catechin), chalcones, anthocyanidins, isoflavones (genistein), polyphenols (green tea), citrus bioflavonoids (rutin, hesperidin), and more.

The nomenclature can be confusing, because different authors group them differently.

Uses: The powerful antioxidant action of flavonoids protect the cell membranes of both the red blood cells and the cells lining the capillary walls. This prevents those cells, the endothelial cells, from become brittle and damaged. This condition, sometimes called capillary fragility, can lead to poor circulation, easy bruising, varicose veins, spider veins, and hemorrhoids. When fluid leaks from fragile capillaries, you have swelling and inflammation.

Similarly, when the cell membranes of red blood cells remain strong and elastic, they can more readily squeeze through the elastic capillary bed, carrying oxygen to the various tissues of the body.

The anthocyanoside flavonoids in plants such as bilberry, for example, probably exert their beneficial effect on the retina of the eye by this very mechanism.

Historically, flavonoids are associated with "vitamin P" activity. This was a term originally applied by Albert Szent-Gyorgyi, who discovered vitamin C, because of his observation that this group of compounds reduced capillary permeability.

We now feel that the most important biochemical, or therapeutic, action of the flavonoids as a group is their powerful antioxidant activity. Some have referred to them as "biological response modifiers," owing to their anti-inflammatory, antiviral, anticarcinogenic, and anti-allergy properties.

Products: The products listed here are the citrus bioflavonoids. Other flavonoid supplements are listed under their respective headings.

Solgar: Citrus Bioflavonoids, 1,000 mg, 1,000 mg citrus bioflavonoid complex, 100 tablets.
Twinlab: Citrus Bioflavonoid Capsules, 1,400 mg citrus bioflavonoid complex and 100 mg rutin per 2 capsules, 100 capsules.
Nature's Answer: Citrus Bioflavonoid Liquid with Rose Hips, 5,000 mg citrus bioflavonoids per teaspoon, 8 oz.

Flaxseed Oil

Related Item: Linseed oil.
Description: Flaxseed oil *(Linium usitatissimum)* differs from most

other vegetable oils in that it contains very high levels of alpha linolenic acid (ALA), an omega-3 fatty acid. Flaxseed and flaxseed oil also contain lignans. Another name for flaxseed oil is linseed oil.

Uses: The average American diet is too rich in omega-6 fatty acids, and lacking in omega-3 fatty acids. Flaxseed oil is a rich source of omega-3 oils in general,

> *Indications:* Cholesterol problems, triglycerides (high), arthritis.

and ALA specifically. ALA is unique in that it can be metabolized directly to eicosapentaenoic acid (EPA).

Supplementation with flaxseed oil is certainly going to alter the ratio of omega-3 to omega-6 oils, but it may not be as effective as EPA or fish oils as a therapeutic agent. EPA serves as a precursor in the body to beneficial prostaglandins, the powerful hormone-like agents that reduce inflammation and protect against heart disease. Not all of the ALA in flaxseed oil is converted into EPA, however. In fact, 1 gram of EPA would require about 15 to 20 grams of ALA to achieve the same effect. Converting this to actual supplement quantities, if flaxseed oil contains about 50 percent ALA and fish oil contains 18 percent EPA, that would mean one needs about four times as much flaxseed oil as fish oil to achieve the equivalent EPA-like activity. Other estimates indicate an even higher ratio. Add to this the question of whether or not the conversion from ALA to EPA becomes less efficient with age, and the value of flaxseed oil as an alternative to fish oil or EPA/DHA is less convincing.

As a general dietary source of omega-3 oils, flaxseed oil is sufficient. For those who prefer to avoid the taste of fish oil, flaxseed oil is an appropriate substitute. But for those with cardiovascular problems or arthritis, who need to achieve maximum therapeutic benefit, fish oil or similar omega-3 supplements should be used.

On the other hand, flaxseed oil may have a benefit that fish oil does not. In its natural state, flaxseed oil contains lignans. Lignans are valuable in their own right, exerting antioxidant, phytoestrogen, and antithrombotic activity. There is some evidence that the lignans in flaxseed may have anticancer activity, blocking the effects of endogenous estrogen much the same way as does soy.

Flaxseed oil is available in two forms. The clear, golden yellow oil has had the lignans and other fiber components removed, while the "high-lignan" version has a darker, muddy appearance. The former has been filtered, and the latter is the unfiltered type.

To achieve maximum therapeutic value, we suggest the high lignan, or unfiltered type of flaxseed oil whenever possible.

Cautions: All omega-3 oils have some antithrombotic activity. This is generally advantageous. Those already taking anticoagulant medications (Coumadin), however, should exercise caution.

High-lignan flaxseed oil should be avoided during pregnancy or any other time when the use of phytoestrogens is contraindicated.

Flaxseed oil is easily oxidized. It must be kept under refrigeration and used in a relatively short time. The addition of antioxidants, such as vitamin E, is recommended. If the oil develops a bitter flavor, it should be discarded. Shake well before each use.

Products:

Barlean: Hi Lignan Flaxseed Oil Liquid, 6,200 mg ALA, 2,660 mg flax particulates, plus omega-6 and omega-9 fatty acids, 16 oz.
Solgar: Flaxseed Oil, 1,250 mg, 1,250 mg organic flaxseed oil, 100 softgels.

Flower Pollen

Related Item: Bee pollen.

Description: Flower pollen is an extract of pollen collected directly from plants, rather than from bees. Pollen is the male germ seed of plants. The commercial product is then processed to enhance absorption.

Uses: Studies have shown that flower pollen is effective in treating benign prostatic hyperplasia and prostatitis. There are also reports that flower pollen has liver protective activity, and that it may be of some value in preventing cancer, cardiovascular disease, and rheumatoid arthritis.

Indications: Benign prostatic hypertrophy, prostatitis.

Products:

Graminex: Cernilton, 250 mg pollen extract from rye *(Secale cereale),* std. 20:1, 200 tablets.

Folic Acid

Description: Folic acid is an essential B vitamin. It is involved in a number of key biological processes, including the synthesis of DNA,

RNA and proteins. It is needed for proper blood cell function and nervous cell development.

Uses: A marginal deficiency of folic acid can lead to increased risk of cardiovascular disease, certain types of cancer, Alzheimer's disease, depression, and

> *Indications:* Pregnancy, cardiovascular disease, Alzheimer's disease, depression, cancer.

in pregnant women, can result in increased risk of birth defects (neural tube defects).

Folic acid is actually one of those vitamins that is absorbed better from supplements than in its natural food state.

An elevated homocysteine level is now thought to be associated with increased risk of cardiovascular disease. Folic acid is involved in controlling homocysteine levels by facilitating the conversion of homocysteine to methionine. The enzyme that metabolizes this conversion, methionine synthase, uses folic acid and vitamin B_{12} as cofactors.

When folic acid is used in response to elevated homocysteine levels, it is best combined with vitamin B_{12} and vitamin B_6. Some also recommend added trimethylglycine (TMG).

A folic acid mouth rinse is thought to be of help in treating gingivitis.

Dosage: The usual dose is 400 micrograms per day, with those at risk of the indicated conditions often taking up to 800 micrograms daily.

Cautions: Vitamin B_{12} should be included with folic acid supplementation because folic acid can mask an underlying vitamin B_{12} deficiency.

Products:

Twinlab: Folic Acid, 800 mcg, 200 capsules.
Solgar: Folic Acid, 400 mcg, vegetarian and kosher, 250 tablets.
Scientific Botanicals: Folirinse, 5 mg folic acid, USP per drop, 1 oz liquid. As a mouthwash/rinse, dilute 5 drops in a quarter cup warm water.

Forskolin

Related Item: Coleus forskohlii (Makandi).

Description: Coleus forskohlii is an herb native to India. It contains a substance, forskolin, that exerts hypotensive and other cell-regulating actions through the activation of an enzyme called adenylate cyclase.

This enzyme regulates the amount of cyclic AMP in cells, which, in turn, activates numerous other enzymes.

Uses: There has been a great deal of interest in forskolin as a possible treatment for asthma, glaucoma, obesity, psoriasis, and various cardiovascular problems, including hypertension, congestive heart failure, and cardiomyopathy. Most of the research has been done with isolated forskolin, not the herb coleus. In addition, some of the work involved topical application, injection, and inhalation rather than oral administration. There is good reason to think that oral administration of coleus preparations standardized to 18 percent forskolin will prove effective in many of these conditions.

Dosage: The usual dose of the standardized 18 percent coleus extract is 50 milligrams, two or three times daily. A dose of 100 milligrams of a 10 percent extract would be approximately the same. Higher amounts are sometimes used.

Products:

America's Finest: Coleus Forskohlii, 100 mg coleus forskohlii extract (10%), providing 10 mg forskolin, 30 capsules.
Gaia Herbs: Coleus Forskohlii Liquid, 170 mg coleus forskohlii extract (2.5%), providing 4 mg forskolin, 2 ounces.
Enzymatic Therapy: Coleus Forskohlii, 50 mg coleus forskohlii extract (18%), providing 9 mg forskolin, 60 capsules.

FOS

Related Item: Inulin.

Description: Fructo-oligosaccharides (FOS) is a particular type of carbohydrate, composed of 3 to 5 monosaccharide units, that is resistant to human digestive enzymes. In this respect, it can be considered a type of fiber, that is, a nondigestible carbohydrate. But it can be digested, or fermented, by certain bacteria.

Uses: FOS is said to be a prebiotic, a material that may promote the growth of beneficial bacteria. In providing "food" for beneficial bacteria, FOS is thought to improve colon function and boost

> *Indications:* Immune system, cancer (colon), irritable bowel syndrome, gastrointestinal disorders, diarrhea, constipation.

gastrointestinal immunity, helping perhaps to even protect against colon cancer.

When FOS is broken down by friendly bacteria, it forms short chain fatty acids, such as butyrate, which are thought to have anti-cancer activity.

In facilitating the growth of beneficial bacteria, FOS suppresses the growth of detrimental, or pathogenic bacteria. FOS also shares many of the advantages of dietary fiber in general.

Some have suggested that FOS can be helpful in lowering elevated cholesterol and triglyceride levels, but the quantities needed are as high, if not higher, than other forms of water-soluble fiber. So it would seem to make no sense to use FOS for this purpose when other forms of fiber (psyllium, oat bran, guar gum, etc.) are available.

Products:

Twinlab: Nutraflora FOS Powder, 4 oz.

Fructo-Oligosaccharides

See FOS.

Garcinia Cambogia

Related Item: Hydroxycitric acid (HCA).

Description: Garcinia cambogia is a fruit native to southeast Asia, also called Brindle berry or Malabar tamarind. It is rich in a substance called hydroxycitric acid.

Use: Extracts of garcinia cambogia have been promoted as an aid to weight loss. In animal stud-

| Indications: Obesity, weight loss. |

ies it has been shown to suppress appetite and enhance weight loss when used in conjunction with a calorie-restricted diet. It may exert this action by blocking an enzyme (ATP citrate lyase) involved with the conversion of carbohydrates to fat.

Unfortunately, clinical studies on humans have yielded mixed results. For those who are overweight, the use of garcinia cambogia in conjunction with other measures, certainly merits consideration. On the other hand, an expectation that this supplement alone is going to make fat disappear, with no additional effort on your part, is unrealistic. However, the same can be said for all weight loss supplements.

Products:

Natrol: Citrimax Capsules, 250 mg hydroxycitric acid from the rind of garcinia cambogia fruit, 90 capsules.

Twinlab: Mega Citrimax, 750 mg garcinia cambogia rind extract, 100 mcg chromium picolinate, 100 capsules.

Garlic

Description: Garlic (*Allium sativum*) is an herb that has been used as a medicinal agent and food seasoning for many centuries. In fact, its medicinal use may predate its food use. Almost all commercially available garlic is cultivated, not wild.

Uses: Describing the medicinal uses of garlic is easy. It has been shown to exert vasodilation and diuretic properties, making it useful to those with high blood pressure and congestive heart failure.

> *Indications:* Cancer, cardiovascular disease, cholesterol problems, hypertension, immune system, parasites, stroke, triglycerides (high).

It has been shown to contain components that reduce blood clotting, making it useful to those with thrombotic types of heart disease. It has been shown to lower cholesterol levels. And it has demonstrated varying degrees of germicidal activity, antioxidant action, and immune system stimulation.

Describing the best form of supplemental garlic, on the other hand, is not so easy. There are over 1,900 scientific studies published on the activities of garlic, and these studies have utilized all the various forms—fresh, powdered, oil, aged, etc. In most cases, all forms seem to work well. But fueled by the various marketing arms of the companies selling garlic supplements, controversy of which type of supplements is best rages on.

The difference between the forms is related primarily to the presence, or absence, of one component in fresh garlic—allicin. Garlic contains about 1 percent alliin. When alliin is activated, in the presence of the enzyme alliinase, it converts to allicin. Allicin, a thiosulfinate, is thought to be responsible for most of the beneficial actions of garlic. Unfortunately, the allicin content is what gives garlic its characteristic odor.

Aged, or deodorized garlic, may not provide as much allicin (or allicin potential) as other forms of garlic, but it may be more socially acceptable. The best-known brand of aged garlic is Kyolic. Other methods of avoiding the odor involve enteric coating the product, which will prevent the release of allicin in the upper part of the digestive tract. This is the principle utilized by Kwai. Other companies focus on allicin content, or allicin-potential, and produce supplements with as high a level of allicin as possible.

Which is best? An easy answer would be to say they are all good, and the best one for you is the one you tolerate best. This would actually not be a bad answer, for as stated above, there is research supporting the efficacy of all forms of garlic supplements. If there is any difference, it might be that the aged form (Kyolic) seems to be better documented for its anticancer action, while higher allicin-containing products may be preferable for those with cardiovascular, immune, and microbial problems.

It is our recommendation, then, that in general, a standardized garlic preparation is preferable to a nonstandardized, with a reasonably high alliin content. Alliin itself will not cause odor, but on enzymatic hydrolysis, will release allicin. But personal tolerances have to be taken into account, and in the case of garlic supplements, some degree of experimentation may be necessary.

While allicin content, or potential, is an easy marker to be used in standardization, it should be pointed out again that allicin may not be the only active ingredient in garlic. Both aged and cooked garlic, as well as distilled garlic oil, have low allicin content but show clinical activity.

Dosage: Ten milligrams of alliin is equivalent, potentially, to 4,000 micrograms of allicin. This is said to be equivalent to one clove (4 grams) of fresh garlic, and is the recommended dose unless advised otherwise.

Products:

Kwai: Kwai Garlic, "Unique Coating," 4 tablets provide 600 mg concentrated garlic powder, 120 tablets.
Kyolic: Kyolic Reserve, 600 mg aged garlic extract, 120 capsules.
Enzymatic Therapy: Garlinase, 4,000, enteric-coated, 320 mg, yielding 5,000 mcg allicin, 30 tablets.
Nature's Way: Garlicin, enteric-coated, 350 mg, releasing 3,200 mg allicin, 90 tablets.
Natrol: Garlipure, Once Daily Potency, enteric-coated, 600 mg, yielding 6,000 mcg allicin, 30 tablets.
Solgar: MaxGar Garlic, 280 mg, garlic oil macerate (2.4:1 concentrate), odor controlled, 180 softgels.

Genistein

Related Item: Soy isoflavones.

Description: Genistein is the isoflavone-type of flavonoid found in soybeans. It is categorized as a phytoestrogen, a plant-derived non-steroidal compound that exhibits estrogen-like biological activity. Genistein occurs naturally in soy as genistin, a glycoside.

Uses: Genistein can be thought of as having both weak estrogenic and weak anti-estrogenic action. It is an antioxidant, and may have anticarcinogenic, anti-osteoporotic, and anti-atherogenic activity.

> *Indications:* Benign prostatic hypertrophy, cancer (breast), cancer (prostate), cholesterol problems, menopause.

Dosage: Owing to the wide variety of products, generalization is difficult. Read the product label. For example, 125 milligrams of soy isoflavone concentrate may contain about 50 milligrams of soy isoflavones, and 25 milligrams of that might be genistin.

Products:

Twinlab: Mega Soy, 200 mg soy bean extract (40% isoflavones, 80 mg), providing 40 mg genistin, 31 mg diadzin, and 8 mg glycetin, 60 capsules.

Jarrow: Isoflavone 50, 50 mg isoflavonoid complex providing 25 mg genistin, 18 mg diadzein, and 7 mg glycetein, 60 capsules.

Solgar: Super Concentrated Isoflavones, 38 mg total isoflavones from soy isoflavone extract, 120 tablets.

Germanium

Description: Germanium is a mineral found in the earth's crust. It is present in grains, vegetables, and seeds. It is not considered an essential nutrient for humans.

Uses: Germanium has been claimed to exert anticancer and antioxidant activity. It can be highly toxic, under certain circumstances, and is not recommended for general supplement use. The form used in supplements is known as Ge-132, germanium-132, germanium sesquioxide, or bis-carboxyethyl germanium sesquioxide.

Cautions: We recommend avoiding germanium supplementation unless done under the guidance or direction of a qualified health professional. The Ge-132 form is thought to be relatively nontoxic.

Products:

Allergy Research: Germanium, 150 mg, bis-carboxyethyl germanium sesquioxide, 150 mg, 36 capsules.
Jarrow: Germanium, 150 mg, Ge-132, 150 mg, 30 capsules.

Ginger

Description: Ginger *(Zingiber officinale)* is a large root (rhizome, actually) native to southern Asia, but now cultivated in almost all tropical areas. It has been used as a medicine since ancient times.

Uses: Ginger has been used for thousands of years to treat stomach, diarrhea, nausea, and other gastrointestinal disorders. Considerable attention in recent years

Indications: Gastrointestinal disorders, motion sickness, nausea, arthritis.

has focused on its effectiveness in treating morning sickness, motion sickness, and other types of nausea.

Ginger may also be of some value to those with cardiovascular and inflammatory problems. As is the case with many herbs (ginkgo, feverfew, garlic, turmeric), ginger inhibits PAF (platelet-activating factor), which is involved in blood clotting and inflammation.

Ginger is considered a gastrointestinal tonic, protecting the stomach lining from damage.

Most recently, Ginger's powerful antioxidant and anti-inflammatory action has been linked to its ability to inhibit COX-2, just as NSAIDs do, without their serious side effects.

Cautions: The Commission E contraindicates ginger usage for morning sickness during pregnancy. According to most other experts, however, there is no basis for this. Also, ginger has been widely used for morning sickness in other cultures (Chinese medicine) for quite some time.

Products:

Nature's Answer: Ginger Root Fluid Extract, 1,000 mg of ginger root per 28 drops, 2 fl oz.
Enzymatic Therapy: Gingerall, ginger 100 mg, 20% pungent compounds, as 6-gingerol and 6-shogaol, 90 softgels.
New Chapter: Gingerforce, 150 mg, ginger, super critical extract, 30% pungent compounds, 8% zingiberene, 60 capsules.
Nature's Herbs: Ginger Root, ginger from India, 100 capsules.

Ginkgo Biloba

Description: Ginkgo is the world's most ancient tree. The dry extract from the ginkgo leaf is a 50:1 extract, with 22 to 27 percent flavonone glycosides (quercetin, kaempferol), 5 to 7 percent terpene lactones (ginkgolides A, B, and C, bilobalide), and less than 5 parts per milligram ginkgolic acid.

Uses: There have been over 400 scientific studies on standardized ginkgo extract over the past thirty years. Ginkgo biloba has been shown to enhance cerebral and peripheral circulation. It has been used to prevent or treat

> *Indications:* Alzheimer's disease, age-related cognitive decline, intermittent claudication, depression, macular degeneration, erectile dysfunction, vertigo, tinnitus, asthma, retinopathy.

Alzheimer's disease and other types of age-related cognitive decline, memory problems, intermittent claudication, vertigo, tinnitus, erectile dysfunction, peripheral arterial occlusive disease, and altitude sickness.

The impressive body of research supporting these uses of ginkgo is not limited to foreign medical journals. A placebo-controlled, double-blind, randomized, multicenter trial on ginkgo's effect on Alzheimer's disease was published in the *Journal of the American Medical Association* in 1997. The ginkgo group showed either improvement or a delay in the progression of the disease.

Clearly, ginkgo biloba is an herb that should be part of the supplement program for anyone with impaired cerebral or peripheral circulatory function.

Dosage: The usual dose is 120 to 240 milligrams of standardized extract per day, in divided doses.

Cautions: This item has a slight "thinning" effect on the blood. This, generally, is a good thing. But if you are taking blood-thinning medications, check with your doctor.

Products:

Nature's Way: Ginkgold, 60 mg, 60 mg ginkgo leaf std. (24% ginkgo flavone glycosides and 6% terpene lactones) extract, providing 20 active and co-active compounds, 100 tablets.
Natrol: Ginkgo Biloba Extract, 60 mg std. ginkgo leaf extract per dropper, 2 oz liquid.
Solgar: Super Ginkgo, 60 mg ginkgo biloba leaf extract (50:1), std to 24% (14 mg ginkgoflavoglycosides), and 375 mg ginkgo leaf powder, 100 vegicaps.

Ginseng

Related Items: Siberian ginseng, American ginseng.

Description: Ginseng is a slow-growing perennial herb native to northeastern China, Korea, and part of Russia. The main active ingredient is ginsenosides.

There are several types of ginseng. Asian, or Korean, ginseng *(Panax ginseng)* is available in a red (steamed and cured) form as well as the regular white (unprocessed) form. The red form is considered more stimulating. And American ginseng *(Panax quinquefolus)* is considered less stimulating, or "yang," than Asian ginseng.

Uses: A summary of the numerous studies on ginseng is far beyond the scope of this book. An explanation of the various nuances of using one type of ginseng over another and its role in traditional Chinese medicinal philosophy is also inappropriate.

> *Indications:* Immune system, athletic performance, energy (low), antiaging, cold and flu, erectile dysfunction, fertility (male), chronic fatigue syndrome, cancer, diabetes.

Instead, suffice it to say that ginseng has retained a reputation as one of the premier general tonic herbs for over 5,000 years. In Asian medicine, it is used as a tonic to revitalize and replenish vital energy. This does not mean you should expect the type of energy jolt you get from a dose of caffeine. The effect is more subtle. It is a tonic that revitalizes the function of the organism as a whole, building resistance, reducing susceptibility to illness, and promoting health and longevity.

Commission E approves ginseng as a tonic for invigoration and fortification in times of fatigue and debility or declining capacity for work and concentration.

Dosage: Standardized extracts: 200 to 500 milligrams per day. The dose for nonstandardized concentrates is higher. For liquid tinctures, follow the directions on the label, or use 2 to 3 milliliters three times a day.

Cautions: Asian and American ginseng may be contraindicated in those with hypertension.

Products:

Nature's Way: Korean Ginseng Root, 510 mg Panax ginseng (2% ginsenosides) per capsule, 100 capsules.
Solgar: Korean Ginseng Root Extract, 250 mg Panax ginseng

root extract (8% ginsenosides, 20 mg), 200 mg panax ginseng powder, 60 vegicaps.
Nature's Way: Korean Ginseng Extract, 535 mg Panax ginseng root extract (7% ginsenosides), 50 mg Panax ginseng root powder, 60 capsules.
Root to Health: American ginseng, 500 mg Panax quinquefolius per capsule, 100 capsules.
Solgar: American Ginseng Extract, 100 mg Panax quinquefolius root extract (10% ginsenosides), 200 mg Panax quinquefolius powder (5% ginsenosides), 15 mg ginsenosides total, 60 vegicaps.
Nature's Answer: Ginseng, American, Root, 2,000 mg American ginseng root fluid extract per 2 ml (75 mg total ginsenosides), 1 oz liquid.
Nature's Answer: Ginseng, Chinese White, Root Alcohol Free, 1,000 mg White Chinese ginseng root (75 mg total ginsenosides) per ml, 1 oz. liquid.
Prince of Peace: Panax Ginseng Extractum, 2,000 mg Red Panax ginseng root extract (3:1) per vial, 30 10-ml vials. Ready-to-drink single-dose vials.

Glucosamine

Related Items: Cartilage, chondroitin.

Description: Glucosamine is the building block from which the body makes cartilage, collagen, and all the other components of connective tissue. Specifically, it is an amino sugar, and is involved in the synthesis of proteoglycans such as chondroitin.

Usage: Glucosamine is used to repair damaged joints, reduce inflammation, enhance wound healing, induce the regeneration of

> *Indications:* **Arthritis, sports injuries.**

connective tissue, and maintain the proper viscosity of synovial fluid, to cushion the joint area.

Glucosamine is available in several forms—glucosamine sulfate, glucosamine hydrochloride, and N-acetyl-glucosamine.

The glucosamine sulfate form is the one most widely studied, and may be the preferred form. One problem is that it needs to be stabilized by the inclusion of sodium chloride or potassium chloride. The sodium chloride form is the type most often used in the research studies, but because some people are concerned about their total daily intake of salt, the potassium chloride form is available as well.

The glucosamine hydrochloride form does not need to be stabilized, and can provide more actual glucosamine per unit dose. Most of the research, however, has been done on the sulfate form of glucosamine.

Some claim that another reason the sulfate form of glucosamine may be preferred is that the sulfate itself is used as part of the tissue-regenerating process. But when absorbed, the sulfate is split from the glucosamine molecule, and there is no evidence that the sulfur necessary for its subsequent action cannot be obtained from existing cellular stores.

The fact that the sulfate form was the form most often used in the published research does not necessarily mean that that form is the best. It does mean, however, that the sulfate form is known to work.

Likewise, the fact that a researcher reported positive results when using a combination of glucosamine and chondroitin does not mean that glucosamine alone, or chondroitin alone, would not work even better. The book popularizing the use of the combination did not do a comparison between the combination and the individual components.

Combination products sometimes seem to work better, but this may be because the total amount of chondroitin and glucosamine in those combinations is greater than the amount usually taken individually.

Products:

Enzymatic Therapy: GS-500, 150 mg of sodium in three capsules, 120 capsules.
Jarrow: Glucosamine Sulfate, 1,000, Sodium-free. Stabilized with potassium chloride.
Twinlab: Glucosamine Sulfate, 750 mg, 100 tablets. 90 capsules sodium-free. Stabilized with potassium chloride.

Glutamine

Description: L-glutamine is an amino acid. It is not categorized as "essential" because it can be made in the body in sufficient amounts under normal health conditions. When the body is under stress (trauma, cancer, infections, burns, healing), the value of L-glutamine increases, and the quantity needed may increase as well.

Uses: L-glutamine serves many roles in the body. It helps regulate the acid-base equilibrium of the body. It provides nitrogen to various tissues of the body, and is involved in protein synthesis and

Indications: Nutritional support, healing, immune system, gastrointestinal disorders, athletic performance.

carbohydrate metabolism. L-glutamine is involved in energy production, and supports immune system function. It can serve as a source of glucose when necessary, and is involved in the synthesis of glutathione, one of the body's most important antioxidants. L-glutamine is thought to be helpful in treating various infections and disorders of the gastrointestinal tract, perhaps owing to its seeming ability to decrease intestinal permeability and mucosal atrophy in the small intestine.

For these reasons, L-glutamine is considered an important dietary supplement when the body has been exposed to various types of trauma and stress.

Products:

Solgar: Glutamine, 500 mg vegetarian and kosher, 250 vegicaps.
Jarrow: Glutamine Powder, 8 oz.
Twinlab: Glutamine, 1,000 mg, 50 tablets.

Glutathione

Related Items: GSH, cysteine, NAC (N-acetyl cysteine).

Description: Glutathione is a tripeptide, a small protein composed of the amino acids cysteine, glutamic acid, and glycine. It can occur in two forms, a monomer (commonly referred to as reduced glutathione or GSH) and a dimer (commonly referred to as oxidized glutathione, or glutathione disulfide). The reduced form, or GSH, is the type that is used in nutritional supplements.

Uses: Glutathione is a powerful antioxidant. It exerts this antioxidant function is several ways, as a cofactor in various enzyme systems and helping maintain and regenerate other antioxidant nu-

Indications: Cancer, cataracts, detoxification, diabetes, lung (pulmonary) disease, HIV, Parkinson's disease, infertility (men).

trients. It appears to play an important role in the body as a detoxifier and immune system modulator.

One problem with glutathione as a supplement is that it may not be absorbed well when taken orally. This casts some doubt on the advisability of taking glutathione in supplement form. Instead, taking supplements of glutathione precursors such as N-acetyl-cysteine, cysteine, and methionine may be a more efficient way of increasing glutathione levels in the body. Studies have shown that other nutrients, such as vitamin C, alpha-lipoic acid, SAMe, and whey protein result in increased glutathione levels. Selenium, vitamin B_6, and riboflavin are involved in optimal glutathione function as well.

A Comment from Dr. Abel

NASA knows all about glutathione boosters. For more than thirty years, astronauts have been taking 3,000 mg of N-acetyl-cysteine (NAC) daily. The reason is that cysteine is one of the three amino acids in the tripeptide glutathione (cysteine, glutamine, and glycine). Glutathione is a very powerful antioxidant with multiple beneficial effects throughout your body.

The astronauts were taking the cysteine as a glutathione booster as the best prevention for radiation toxicity in space. Considering that the ozone layer is thinning, we are all being subjected to more UV light. Our skin, our eyes, and perhaps even our internal organs need the added protection. Therefore, supplementing with glutathione boosters, such as cysteine, N-acetyl-cysteine, alpha-lipoic acid, MSM, or SAMe, and perhaps melatonin (but I don't recommend taking a hormone) would be important.

Products:

Twinlab: Mega Glutathione, 250 mg, reduced glutathione, 60 capsules.
Jarrow: Reduced Glutathione 500, Pharmaceutical grade, 60 capsules.
Solgar: L-Glutathione, 250 mg, vetetarian and kosher, 60 vegicaps.
Tyler: Recancostat 100, 200 mg L-glutathione, reduced, 100 mg, "AnthoRedoxin Blend," 40 mg L-cysteine, 90 capsules.
"AnthoRedoxin Blend" has been shown to recycle glutathione from the oxidized to the reduced form.
Jarrow: ThioNac, 500 mg NAC, 100 mg lipoic acid, 60 tablets. *Glutathione precursors.*
Allergy Research: Thiodox, 250 mg NAC, 150 mg lipoic acid, 200 mg glutathione, plus selenium, riboflavin, vitamin C, and thiamine, 60 tablets. *Glutathione and precursors.*

Goldenseal

Related Item: Berberine.
Description: Goldenseal *(Hydrastis canadensis)* is a plant that is na-

tive to eastern North America. It contains small amounts of the alkaloids berberine and hydrastine.

Uses: Goldenseal has a reputation as a powerful antibiotic, a treatment for the common cold, and an ability to mask the presence of illicit drugs in the urine. Unfortunately, this reputation remains, even though evidence supporting it is lacking.

> *Indications:* Canker sores, gastrointestinal disorders, parasites.

There is little to be gained in using a combination of echinacea and goldenseal, for example, rather than echinacea alone for treating a cold.

Goldenseal seems to exert its anti-infective and healing action best when used topically, for example, as a mouthwash (for canker sores), a gargle (for sore throat), or an eyewash (for conjunctivitis or blepharitis). It also appears to work when taken internally for gastrointestinal problems, including bacterial parasites. In situations where there is either increased mucous production, or not enough, goldenseal is thought to exert a corrective or "alterative" action.

Products:

Nature's Way: Goldenseal Root, 570 mg goldenseal root providing 5% total alkaloids, 100 capsules.

Nature's Answer: Goldenseal Root Drops, 500 mg goldenseal in 28 drops, 1 oz liquid.

Grape Seed Extract

Related Items: PCO, OPC, Pycnogenol.

Description: Grape seed extract is a rich source of a certain type of plant flavonoids, the proanthocyanidins.

Proanthocyanidin is a term used to define a certain group of flavonoid composed mostly of catechin and epicatechin. When catechin, epicatechin, and in the case of grape seed, gallic acid esters form complexes, or oligomers, you have proanthocyanidins, or procyanidins. These procyanidin polymers are also known as OPCs, which stands for oligomeric procyanidins or PCOs, which stands for procyanidolic oligomers. While it is not necessary for you to understand the chemistry behind this nomenclature, it is important because products are labeled in terms of their PCO or OPC content.

Uses: The type of flavonoids present in grape seed extract are thought to function as powerful antioxidants, protecting tissues, glands, and organs throughout the body from the deleterious effects of free radical damage. In addition, these flavonoids have an ability to strengthen collagen. This explains its value in enhancing the integrity of skin, blood vessels, and

> *Indications:* Vision problems, anti-aging, arthritis, cancer, allergies, cardiovascular disease, cataracts, macular degeneration, night blindness, retinopathy, sports injuries, vision problems, hemorrhoids, varicose veins, chronic venous insufficiency.

connective tissue. It exerts an anti-inflammatory action, perhaps by inhibiting the release of pro-inflammatory prostaglandins. There is also compelling evidence that the proanthocyanidins in grape seed have anticarcinogenic activity.

Products containing PCO or OPC flavonoids are considered by many to be some of the most valuable and inclusive antioxidants available, and should be part of any comprehensive supplement programs.

Note: There are two types of supplements available that are rich in OPCs. One is grape seed extract, and the other is a trademarked product called Pycnogenol, which is derived from pine bark. There have been claims and counterclaims as to which is better. Much of this was a result of the initial multilevel marketing involvement with Pycnogenol. Marketing hyperbole to the contrary, they are similar in composition and function. Grape seed extract contains between 92 and 95 percent PCO while the Pycnogenol products contain only 80 to 85 percent PCO. Considerable research has been performed on the grape seed extract, and in Europe, it is the more popular of the two supplements. Finally, the grape seed extract is often less expensive.

Products:

Seagate Gold: Grape Seed Extract, 250 mg, 150 mg red grape seed extract, 100 mg red grape skin extract, 90 capsules. Note that this product contains not only an extract of the grape seed, but also an extract of grape skin. (See "Resveratrol.")
Jarrow: OPCs+95, 100 mg grape seed extract (100:1), 95% polyphenols, 100 capsules.

THE PHARMACIST SAYS

And as Larry Siegel, the chief pharmacist at Willner Chemists, likes to point out, "Grapes are a normal part of human nutrition, while pine bark is a normal part of termite nutrition!"

Grapefruit Seed Extract

Description: Grapefruit seed extract is a natural antiseptic.

Uses: This material is caustic and potentially irritating to the skin and mucous membranes. Although when properly diluted, it has been recommended as an antifungal or antibacterial for sinus, vaginal, and topical infections, the desirability of such applications is questionable. There is some speculation that its antimicrobial activity is due more to the inclusion of certain other nonnatural preservatives than the GSE itself.

The only justifiable internal use, when properly diluted, is as a treatment for certain chronic intestinal infections. The liquid has been used as a fruit and vegetable wash.

Do not confuse grapefruit seed extract with grape seed extract.

Cautions: This product should be used only under the guidance of a health professional. Be sure to wash your hands after use, and avoid getting it near your eyes.

Products:

Allergy Research: Paramicrocidin, 250 mg, citrus seed extract, 250 capsules.
Nutribiotic: Grapefruit Seed Concentrate.

Green Foods

Related Items: Spirulina, chlorella, wheat grass, barley grass, chlorophyll, blue green algae

Description: All green-food supplements are relatively rich in protein, chlorophyll, and carotenoids. Marketing claims to the contrary, there is little documented therapeutic difference among them.

Uses: Green-food concentrates of this type are claimed to have anticancer activity, modulate immune system function, lower cho-

> *Indications:* Nutritional support, detoxification, immune system, cancer.

lesterol, treat gastrointestinal problems, and function, generally, as detoxification agents.

While convincing proof of all these actions may be lacking, there is certainly no reason not to include one of the green-food concentrates in a comprehensive supplement program. They are all rich in phytonutrients, antioxidants, and varying amounts of trace nutrients. The problem with these supplements is that exaggerated marketing claims often accompany the products, and consumers may overestimate their value. As a general rule, they should be considered adjuncts to other supplements, not replacements or alternatives to them.

Cautions: Green-food supplements may be rich in vitamin K, so caution should be exercised if you are taking anticoagulant medication.

Products:

Green Foods: Veggie Magma, mixture of 13 dried juices including barley, carrot, alfalfa, tomato, kale, broccoli, and 7 others. 9 oz powder.

Gary Null: Green Stuff Powder, "Green Mix" containing 8 juices including kamut, barley green, wheat grass, and alfalfa, 200 g.

Green Tea Extract

Related Item: Theanine.

Description: Green tea *(Camellia sinensis)* and black tea are derived from the same plant, but green tea is less extensively processed. To prepare black tea, the leaves are allowed to oxidize. During this "aging" process, some of the beneficial components, such as the polyphenols, are enzymatically converted to ingredients with less therapeutic value. Green tea is especially high in the particular type of polyphenol flavonoids known as catechins. (See the discussion of grape seed extract for more information.) Unique to green tea is the high level of one catechin in particular, EGCG, or epigallocatechin gallate.

The predominant amino acid found in green tea is L-theanine. *See* Theanine for more information.

Use: Green tea has powerful antioxidant and anticancer properties. High consumption of green tea in Japan is thought to be one of the main reasons for their low cancer rate. The EGCG in green tea appears to be the component responsible for its anticancer activity. It seems to exert this anticarcinogenic action through a variety of different mechanisms, and it is still a matter of intense, ongoing research.

Indications: Cancer, prostate cancer, arthritis, cardiovascular disease, obesity, weight loss.

The antioxidant properties of green tea catechins may explain its anti-inflammatory and anti-atherosclerosis action. There is also some evidence that green tea extract is an effective thermogenic agent, and may therefore be helpful in weight loss.

For those concerned about reducing their risk of cancers of almost any type, taking green tea extract and drinking green tea seems prudent and reasonable.

Dosage: The amount of polyphenols, or EGCG, necessary for therapeutic benefit is thought to range from 250 to 750 milligrams per day.

Note: While green tea may theoretically be richer in certain of the components thought to be cancer-protective, research has shown that black tea is not without benefit in this regard as well.

Cautions: Green tea contains less caffeine than black tea, and most research now indicates that small amounts of caffeine are benign. But decaffeinated products are available for those who wish to avoid even small amounts of caffeine.

Products:

Nature's Herbs: Green Tea Power, Caffeine Free, 383 mg green tea extract (20% polyphenols, 75 mg), 75 mg grapeskin extract (18% polyphenols), 60 capsules.
Solgar: Green Tea Leal Extract, 400 mg green tea extract (50% polyphenols, 200 mg), 100 mg green tea leaf powder, 60 vegicaps.
Jarrow: Green Tea 5:1 Powder, 50% polyphenols, 33% catechins, 16.5% EGCG, 100 g.

Green-Lipped Mussel Extract

Related Items: Cartilage, shark cartilage, bovine cartilage.

Description: Cartilage is the gristle or connective tissue attached to the ends of bones. It is a component of joints, and helps cushion and support the bones. In general terms, cartilage is composed of collagen and proteoglycans, which in turn contain glycosaminoglcans (GAGs) or mucopolysaccharides, which in turn contain chondroitin sulfate, which in turn contains glucosamine. There is considerable argument and debate in the nutritional-supplement industry over which of the forms of cartilage—shark cartilage, bovine cartilage, glocosamine sulfate, chondroitin sulfate, or another mucopolysaccharide-rich substance such as green-lipped mussel extract or sea cucumber—is most effective. There is no clear answer, as there is some degree of support for each argument, and there is clinical evidence supporting the efficacy of each supplement.

Uses: A source of muco-polysaccharides, from the New

Indications: Arthritis.

Zealand green-lipped mussel, which has been shown in at least one study to help reduce the inflammation and joint damage in arthritis.
Products:

Da Vinci: Perna, 1,000 mg *Perna canaliculus* (green-lipped mussel), 200 mg alfalfa leaf, 2 mg cinnamon oil, 180 capsules.

GSH

See Glutathione.

Guarana

Description: Guarana is a plant indigenous to the Amazon basin. It contains caffeine and related alkaloids.

Uses: Guarana is used as a source of caffeine, as a stimulant, or in combination with ephedra as a thermogenic agent.

Cautions: Guarana has been a major ingredient in many weight loss products over the years. Many of the people taking these products were not aware that the primary use of guarana in these products is as a source of caffeine.

Products:

Natrol: Guarana Capsules, 200 mg guarana seed extract (4:1), 90 capsules.

Guggul

Description: Guggul *(Commiphora mukul)* is the gum resin of the Indian myrrh tree. The resin contains guggulsterones, which are thought to be responsible for its hypolipidemic effects, that is, they lower blood lipids.

Uses: Gum guggul has long been used in Ayurvedic (Indian) medicine for its usefulness in treating obesity and inflamma-

Indications: Cholesterol problems.

tion. Current interest in gum guggul, however, is related to its ability to lower cholesterol, triglycerides, and LDL cholesterol, while raising HDL cholesterol.

Crude powdered guggul contains between 0.5 and 1 percent gug-

gulsterones. A purified powder contains between 2 and 5 percent guggulsterones, but an extract of gum guggul, called gugulipid, contains 5 percent guggulsterones and is the form most often used in research.
Products:

Doctor's Best: Ultra Guggulow, 1,000 mg gum guggul ext (resin), providing 2.5% (25 mg) guggulsterones, and 5 mg black pepper ext, 90 tablets.
Nature's Herbs: Gugulmax, 50 tablets.

Gymnema Sylvestre

Description: Gymnema is a plant that is native to the tropical forest of central and southern India.

Uses: Gymnema has been shown to improve blood sugar control in diabetes. It seems to work in both Type I and Type II diabetes, apparently by enhancing the production of endogenous insulin.

> *Indications:* Diabetes.

Several studies have shown that Type II diabetics are able to reduce or discontinue their oral hypoglycemic medications, and Type I diabetics on insulin therapy can reduce their insulin requirements.

Dosage: The usual dose is 400 milligrams daily.

Products:

Nature's Herbs: Gymnesyl Ayurvedic, 250 mg gymnema leaf ext (75% gymnemic acid) and 280 mg gymnema leaf, 50 capsules.
Natrol: Gymnema Sylvestre with Pullulan, 300 mg gymnema leaf ext (5:1, 25% gymnemic acid) and 150 mg pullulan, 90 capsules.

Hawthorn

Description: Hawthorn *(Crataegus oxyacantha)* is a spiny shrub that is native to Europe. The leaves, berries, and flowers are very rich in flavonoids, including the proanthocyanidins, quercetin, catechin, and epicatechin.

Uses: Hawthorn has long been used as a heart tonic. Specifically, it is thought to be valuable in treating congestive heart failure,

> *Indications:* Cardiovascular disease, hypertension, cholesterol problems.

angina, and high blood pressure. Hawthorn strengthens heart muscle (an inotropic agent), dilates the coronary vessels, and seems to prevent cholesterol from forming deposits in the arterial walls. It is thought that the proanthocyanidins in Hawthorn actually have an ACE-inhibiting action.

Dosage: 100 to 300 milligrams of standardized extract, three times a day.

Products:

Nature's Way: Heart Care, 80 mg hawthorn leaf and flower extract (18.75% oligomeric procyanidins), 120 tablets.

Nature's Answer: Hawthorn Berries, 2,000 mg hawthorn berry, leaf and flower fluid extract per 2 ml, 2 oz liquid.

Solgar: Hawthorn Berry Extract, 150 mg hawthorn leaf and flower extract (1.8%, 3 mg vitexin), 250 mg hawthorn berry powder, 60 vegicaps.

HCA

See Garcinia Cambogia.

Hemp Oil

Related Item: Flaxseed Oil.

Description: Hemp seed oil is derived from the seed of *Cannabis sativa.* It is rich in ALA (alpha-linolenic acid) and also contains small amounts of GLA (gamma-linolenic acid).

Uses: Hemp seed oil, because it is rich in ALA and GLA fatty acids, may serve as an alternative to flaxseed oil. *(See* Flaxseed Oil for more information.) These two types of fatty acids serve as precursors to prostaglandins with beneficial actions such as reduction of inflammation, inhibition of platelet aggregation, vasodilation, etc.

Hemp seed oil may eventually be shown to exert the same benefits as flaxseed oil and other omega-3 rich oils, but the research has not yet been published. There is also the concern that small amounts of tetrahydrocannabinol and similar psychoactive substances may be present. For the moment, there seems little reason to use hemp seed oil rather than other omega-3-containing oils such as flaxseed, fish oil, black currant oil, etc.

Products: The availability of hemp oil products is currently restricted due to an ongoing debate with the FDA as to their legal status.

Hesperidin

Related Items: Flavonoids, citrus bioflavonoids.

Description: Hesperidin is a flavonoid, often a component of the "citrus bioflavonoid" type of supplement. On hydrolysis, hesperidin yields hesperetin (methyl eriodictyol), rhamnose, and glucose.

Uses: Hesperidin is an antioxidant, as are most flavonoids. It exerts anti-inflammatory, anti-allergic, vasoprotective and lipid-lowering action. There is also

> *Indications:* Cardiovascular disease, varicose veins, hemorrhoids, cholesterol problems, allergies.

interest in hesperidin as an anticancer agent, based on numerous animal and laboratory studies. Of the various flavonoids, hesperidin and catechin *(see* OPCs) seemed to be the most powerful.

Hesperidin's antioxidant and vasoprotective actions are well recognized. Less well appreciated, however, is the fact that hesperidin seems to be effective in raising HDL cholesterol, while lowering total cholesterol and triglyceride levels.

Products:

Thorne Research: HMC Hesperidin, 250 mg hesperidin methyl chalcone, 60 capsules.

HMB

Description: (beta-hydroxy beta-methylbutyrate) (HMB) is a metabolite of the amino acid leucine.

Uses Leucine is an essential amino acid. Amino acids function as the building blocks of protein.

> *Indications:* Athletic performance.

HMB is claimed to enhance the synthesis of muscle protein and to inhibit the breakdown of muscle tissue that occurs during and immediately after weight training. Human research in support of this is inconclusive. Some studies do suggest greater muscle gain when supplementing with HMB, while others do not.

Dosage: The usual dose seems to be 3 grams daily, in conjunction with weight training.

Products:

EAS Labs: HMB, 250 mg HMB per capsule, 120 capsules.
Twinlab: Mega HMB Fuel, 750 mg, 750 mg HMB per capsule, 60

capsules. Note that the Twinlab product has a much higher HMB content.

Horse Chestnut

Description: Horse chestnut *(Aesculus hippocastanum)* seed extract is derived from a deciduous tree native to the central Balkan peninsula. The seed contains 3 to 6 percent of a mixture of triterpene saponins referred to as escin. The dry extract, used in supplements, should contain 16 to 20 percent escin (aescin).

Uses: In Germany, the consensus among physicians is that horse chestnut is an effective treatment for varicose veins, chronic venous insufficiency, and related vascular disorders.

> *Indications:* Chronic venous insufficiency, varicose veins, hemorrhoids, leg cramps.

A survey of 800 German physicians concluded that horse chestnut seed extract improved or resolved symptoms (pain, tiredness, tension and swelling in the legs, itching, edema, etc) of chronic venous insufficiency.

Chronic venus insufficiency is the term used to describe what happens when veins become chronically swollen and inflamed. It results in an aching, tired feeling in the legs. There may be pain, itching, leg ulcers, and changes in skin pigmentation. It is commonly associated with varicose veins. The standard treatment for CVI (chronic venous insufficiency) is compression using bandages or support stockings, drugs, or surgery. Compliance is typically poor. Compliance when using herbal therapies such as horse chestnut and butcher's broom is significantly improved.

Dosage: The usual dose is around 300 milligrams (corresponding to about 50 milligrams escin, or aescin), taken twice a day.

Products:

Pharmaton: Venastat Sustained Release, 300 mg sustained release horse chestnut seed extract (HCE50), as triterpene glycosides calculated as escin (16%), 60 capsules.
Nature's Herbs: Veno Care, 257 mg horse chestnut seed extract (18.22% triterpene glycosides) with ginger, rutin, and butcher's broom, 60 capsules.
Nature's Answer: Horse Chestnut Seed Extract, 250 mg horse chestnut seed extract (20% B-aescin), 90 vegicaps.

Horsetail

Related Item: Silicon.

Description: Horsetail *(Equisetum arvense)* is a plant found throughout the northern temperate regions of Asia, Europe, and North America. It is also known as bottlebrush and shave grass.

Uses: Horsetail is rich in silicon and flavonoids. It is used traditionally as a treatment for various genitourinary tract problems—infections and inflammations. It has mild diuretic properties. More recently, horsetail is of interest because of its purported value in strengthening hair and nails, and perhaps bone.

Indications: Urinary tract infections, hair, skin, and nails.

Products:

Nature's Herbs: Silica Power, 300 mg horsetail (aerial part) extract, standardized to 10% silicic acid, eqivalent to 7.7% silica, 150 mg horsetail (aerial part) powder, 60 capsules.
Alta Health: Alta Silica, 500 mg horsetail herb extract, Pure ortho form of soluble/colloidal silica, 120 tablets.

Huperzine A

Description: Huperzine A is a plant alkaloid derived from a type of moss that grows in China called huperzia.

Use: Huperzine A seems to be as effective in treating Alzheimer's disease and age-related cognitive decline and memory loss as certain prescription medications. It functions as an inhibitor of the enzyme acetylcholinesterase. Acetylcholine is the primary neurotransmitter in the brain. Acetylcholinesterase is the enzyme that breaks down this neurotransmitter. When huperzine A, or drugs such as Donepezil or Tacrine, inhibit this enzyme, the net result is higher levels of acetylcholine, and enhanced brain function.

Indications: Alzheimer's disease, anti-aging, mental function.

There seems to be little question that huperzine A works. In fact, it works so well that it has to be used with caution. (See below.)

Dosage: 50 to 200 micrograms, two or three times a day.

Cautions: If you are taking medication, huperzine A should be used only with your doctor's approval. If used with other acetylcholinesterase inhibitors, the effect could be additive. The same could prove true if used with cholinergic drugs, or choline-boosting nutritional supplements (i.e., phosphatidylcholine, CDP choline).

Persons with seizure disorders, asthma, and cardiac arrhythmias should avoid using huperzine A without a doctor's approval.

Huperzine A, on the other hand, has been widely used for centuries in China for the treatment of fevers, inflammation and irregular menstruation, without reports of serious side effects.

Products:

Solaray: Hup A, 50 mcg huperzine A from Chinese moss, 285 mg gotu kola, 100 mg lecithin, 60 capsules.

Hydroxycitric Acid

See Garcinia Cambogia.

Indole-3-Carbinol

Related Item: Broccoli.

Description: Indole-3-carbinol is a substance found in cruciferous vegetables, such as cabbage and broccoli. It is actually released from the plant when it is crushed or cooked.

Uses: Indole-3-carbinol may have anticancer activity, especially relative to breast and cervical cancer. This may be due to its

Indications: Cancer (cervical), cancer (breast).

effect on estrogen metabolism. It also affects several other enzymes, some of which are directly involved in detoxification functions.

While the majority of studies support its value as a promising anticancer agent, some have pointed out that not all studies have been positive, and in some instances, it may have promoted cancer rather than suppressed it. This may be an aberration, and of little concern when using it to treat cancer. But some suggest that taking an extract, or concentrate, of cruciferous vegetables, may be a preferable approach at this time when used as a preventative agent.

Dosage: The amount being used ranges from 200 to 800 milligrams daily.

Products:

Solaray: Indole-3-Carbinol, 100 mg I-3-C, plus 50 mg each of cabbage, Brussels sprouts, kale, broccoli, and cauliflower powders, 100 capsules.
America's Finest: Indole-3-Carbinol, 100 mg, 60 capsules.

Inosine

Description: Inosine is substance (a purine ribonucleoside) widely found in all living matter. It is involved in purine synthesis, and is a precursor to adenosine, which is involved in energy production.

Uses: Inosine has been marketed as an ergogenic aid—a substance that will improve endurance and enhance athletic performance. This was based on some anecdotal reports from Russian and Eastern European athletes. Studies have shown, however, that inosine is not effective for this purpose.

On the other hand, inosine is used in certain pharmaceutical preparations in Europe, and may have some effect in cardiovascular disease, inflammatory conditions, and immune system disorders. It will be interesting to see if any of these uses show any validity.

At this time, there is no reason to supplement with inosine.

Cautions: Those with gout should avoid this supplement.

Inositol

Related Items: IP_6 (Inositol hexaphosphate).

Description: Inositol is a vitamin-like substance that is not considered "essential" for humans. No inositol deficiency condition has been found, probably because it is so readily available in various foods. It is a primary component of cell membranes, functioning similar to choline.

Uses: While deficiencies of inositol are not a problem, some doctors have used high doses to treat certain types of depression and anxiety.

> **Indications: Anxiety, depression, obsessive-compulsive disorder, diabetes, liver disorders.**

Inositol may be of benefit to diabetics in treating neuropathy. Inositol is also a common component of "lipotropic formulas," to treat liver disorders and enhance the metabolism of fat in the liver.

Inositol, when obtained from the diet, is in the form of inositol hexaphosphate (phytate, or IP_6) in plants and myo-inositol in animal products. Bacteria normally present in the intestine release the inositol from inositol hexaphosphate.

Dosage: For general liver-supporting, lipotropic activity, 100 to 500 milligrams daily are a common dose. For diabetics, amounts ranging from 1,000 to 2,000 milligrams can be used. For depression and anxiety, amounts in the 12-gram to 15-gram-per-day range are used, but this should be done under the supervision of a health professional.

Products:

Jarrow: Inositol Powder, 600 mg inositol per quarter-teaspoon, 8 oz (227 gm).
Solgar: Inositol, 650 mg, vegetarian and kosher, 100 tablets.

Inositol Hexanicotinate

See Niacin, No-Flush.

Inositol Hexaphosphate

See IP_6.

Inulin

Related Item: FOS.

Description: Inulins are a group of oligosaccharides, found naturally in several vegetables and fruits, including Jerusalem artichoke. Like fiber, inulins are poorly digested in the human digestive system, but are fermented by beneficial bacteria in the colon. Thus, inulin functions as a prebiotic.

Uses: Inulin, like FOS, is said to be a prebiotic, a material that may promote the growth of beneficial bacteria. In providing "food" for beneficial bacteria, inulin is thought to improve colon function and boost gastrointestinal immunity, perhaps even helping to protect against colon cancer.

In facilitating the growth of beneficial bacteria, inulin suppresses the growth of detrimental, or pathogenic, bacteria. Inulin also shares many of the advantages of dietary fiber in general. Some have suggested that inulin may be helpful in lowering elevated cholesterol and triglyceride levels, but the quantities needed are as high, if not higher, than other forms of water-soluble fiber. So it would seem to make no sense to use inulin for this purpose when other forms of fiber (for example, psyllium, oat bran, or guar gum) are available.

Products:

NOW Foods: Inulin Powder, derived from chicory root, 8 oz powder.
Naturally Vitamins: Inuflora, 1,000 mg, derived from Jerusalem artichoke root, 120 tablets.

THE PHARMACIST SAYS

The term *probiotic* refers to friendly, or beneficial, bacteria. The best known example is *Lactobacillus acidophilus.* Probiotic bacteria favorably influence the intestinal-microflora balance, inhibiting the growth of harmful bacteria, promoting good digestion, and boosting immune function. A *prebiotic,* on the other hand, refers to a substance that enhances or supports the growth of probiotic bacteria. An example of a popular probiotic substance is FOS, or fructo-oligosaccharides.

Iodine

Description: Iodine is a trace element. In the thyroid gland, iodine is combined with the amino acid tyrosine to form the thyroid hormones.

Uses: A deficiency of iodine can lead to hypothyroidism and goiter. Overt iodine deficiency is now very rare in developed countries, however. For those with hy-

> *Indications:* **Goiter, hypothyroidism, fibrocystic breast disease.**

pothyroidism, supplementing with iodine will be of benefit only if the condition is caused by or related to a deficiency in dietary iodine. Lacking such a deficiency, supplemental iodine is of dubious value.

Those who are strict vegetarians, however, may be at risk for iodine deficiency. Exclusion of fish, seaweed (sea vegetables), and iodized salt will result in a diet very low in iodine. Supplementation may be appropriate under these circumstances.

Some research indicates that iodine can be helpful to those suffering from fibrocystic breast disease.

Dosage: The usual dose is 150 micrograms of potassium iodide. In nutritional supplements, the source of iodine is usually a kelp concentrate.

Products:

Thorne: Iodine 225, 225 mcg iodine from potassium iodide, 60 capsules.

IP$_6$

Related Items: Inositol, phytic acid.

Description: Inositol hexaphosphate (IP$_6$) is a substance composed of inositol and phosphate. It is also known as phytic acid.

Uses: Inositol hexaphosphate is the form of inositol found in cereal grains and seeds. It is high in

> *Indications:* Cancer (colon).

phosphate, and is a strong chelating agent, readily binding divalent metals such as calcium, magnesium, and zinc.

There is interest in IP$_6$ as a possible treatment for some cancers, especially colon cancer, and perhaps breast cancer. Most of this is based on laboratory and animal studies, however. It remains to be seen if it exhibits the same anticancer activity in humans.

Because of its potential interference with the availability of essential minerals, including iron, it should not be taken with meals or supplements, and should not be used as a general immune system modulator.

Products:

Jarrow: IP$_6$, 500 mg, 500 mg IP$_6$ from 615 mg calcium magnesium inositol hexaphosphate, 120 capsules.
Enzymatic Therapy: Cell Forte with IP$_6$, 400 mg inositol hexaphosphate and 110 mg inositol, 120 capsules.

Ipriflavone

Description: Ipriflavone is a semisynthetic derivative of plant isoflavones. It is similar in action to the isoflavones genistein and daidzein from soy, but without the phytoestrogen activity.

Uses: Ipriflavone has been shown in numerous studies to be helpful in preventing osteoporosis and bone loss. Ipriflavone is actually approved as a drug for preventing

> **Indications:** Osteoporosis.

osteoporosis in several European countries and Japan.

It does not have weak estrogenic activity, and may therefore be more suitable in certain instances than other isoflavones for men, as well as for women who are concerned about taking natural isoflavones with weak estrogenic properties.

Ipriflavone works best when used along with adequate calcium supplementation.

Dosage: The usual dose is 600 micrograms daily, in divided doses.

Cautions: Numerous studies have shown ipriflavone to be effective and free of side effects. One study, however, much to everyone's surprise, yielded contradictory results, (*JAMA* March 2001). In addition, this study found that women taking the ipriflavone had lower levels of lymphocytes than the placebo group. While this study has been criticized, and is only one negative study among a large number of positive studies, we feel obligated to report it.

Products:

Enzymatic Therapy: Ostivone, 200 mg ipriflavone, 60 capsules.
Solgar: Ipriflavone, 200 mg, 60 vegicaps.

Iron

Description: Iron is an essential element. It is a key component of hemoglobin, the oxygen-carrying component of red blood cells.

Uses: Too little iron is bad, as is too much. Too little iron leads to anemia, a life-threatening disorder. Iron deficiency is the most

> **Indications:** Anemia (iron deficiency).

common nutritional disorder in the world. Too much iron on the other hand, can lead to serious problems as well.

Some nutritionists, concerned about the problems caused by too much iron, have become alarmists. Some consumers have become so frightened, they avoid multivitamin supplements that contain iron.

This may be a serious mistake. Iron is essential, and iron deficiency is a very common problem, and a serious one.

Once the body gets iron, it holds on to it very efficiently. This is by design. The biggest source of iron excretion is in menstrual blood loss. For this reason, men and postmenopausal women are less likely to become iron-deficient than are premenopausal women.

Does this mean that men and postmenopausal women do not require a regular source of dietary iron? Not at all. They just require less.

The Reference Daily Intake (RDI) for iron is 18 milligrams. The Dietary Reference Intake for iron is also18 milligrams. The Upper Limit (UL), the upper level of intake considered to be safe for use by adults, is 45 milligrams.

Teenagers and premenopausal women should take supplements that contain as least the recommended daily level of 18 milligrams. Men and postmenopausal women can take a smaller amount if they prefer, perhaps in the 9- to 10-milligram range. Those who are concerned about iron should have their physician include the appropriate blood tests when they have their next scheduled exam. Those with elevated serum ferritin levels should be cautious in the use of iron-containing supplements.

There are a number of conditions beside overt iron-deficiency anemia that may benefit from iron supplementation: fatigue, depression, athletic performance, cold sores, immune system function, celiac disease, and restless leg syndrome. In each of these conditions, however, iron supplementation may help only if the condition is influenced by an iron deficiency. Excess iron intake over the amount needed to correct the deficiency is not recommended, unless under the guidance of a health professional.

There are a number of forms of iron used in supplements. One form, reduced iron, is commonly used in food fortification, but it is poorly absorbed and should be avoided. The other forms used in supplements—ferrous gluconate, ferrous fumarate—are well absorbed. Ferrous sulfate is often recommended by physicians, but may be the most irritating and constipating form or iron. Carbonyl iron is well absorbed but only when sufficient stomach acid is present. Vitamin C enhances the absorption of iron.

Dosage: For general supplementation, a daily dose of between 9 and 18 milligrams is recommended. Greater amounts may be necessary during pregnancy, and for premenopausal women in general.

Note: For more information on the necessity for iron supplementation, refer to www.bestsupplementsforyourhealth.com.

Cautions: Those with a rare inherited condition called hemochromatosis must avoid iron supplements. Iron supplements should not be

used for treatment of any type of anemia other than iron deficiency anemia; treatment of all anemia conditions should be under a physician's supervision.
Products:

Twinlab: Iron, 18 mg, 18 mg iron from ferrous fumarate, 100 capsules.
Solgar: Gentle Iron, 25 mg, 25 mg iron as "non constipating" iron bis glycinate, 180 vegicaps.
Natrol: Iron Liquid, 14.5 mg iron from iron bis glycinate, plus 100 mg vitamin C, B complex, and herbs, 8 oz liquid.

Kava Kava

Description: Kava *(Piper methysticum)* is a member of the pepper family. It is a popular drink in the Pacific Islands, used in ceremonies and celebrations, because of its calming and relaxing action. The main active constituent is kavalactones.

Uses: Kava is used as a treatment for anxiety, nervousness, and stress. Studies have shown kava to be as effective as certain antianxiety drugs, without the serious side effects.

> *Indications:* Anxiety, stress, insomnia, muscle spasm, nervousness, pain.

While not as well documented, there is some evidence that kava also has muscle-relaxing and analgesic action. Kava is also under investigation for its possible anticonvulsant activity.

Kava seems to exert its relaxing, anti-anxiety action without as much sedating activity as some drugs. It has less effect on mental alertness and function. Caution should still be exercised, however, when driving.

Cautions: At the time this was written, kava products were being withdrawn from the market in certain European countries, owing to reports of liver toxicity. Based on the widespread and longtime use of this product, with little indication of safety problems, it would seem to be an overreaction, but an investigation is ongoing.

Products:

Natrol: Kavatrol, 400 mg kava kava ext (30% kavalactones), 400 mg blend of passion flower, chamomile, hops, schizandra, per 2 capsules, 60 capsules.

Enzymatic Therapy: Kava-55, 150 mg kava kava ext, 55% kavalactones (82.5 mg), 60 softgels.

Kombucha

Description: Kombucha is a tea prepared from a mixture of bacteria and yeasts.

Uses: Kombucha will cure just about any disease known to man. Or at least that is what many people were ready and willing to believe. We hear frequently from people who are afraid to use a supplement because the inner seal on the bottle may not be completely attached. Others will worry themselves to the brink of mental paralysis because they are not sure if "take with meals" means before the meal, after the meal, or with dessert. And yet these same people were willing to accept a "starter culture" of mysterious fungal gloop, grow it in the remote dank recess of their basement, and then drink the stuff. All because someone said it cures everything from AIDS to baldness. Amazing, isn't it?

Cautions: Avoid this product. First, most people thought kombucha was a mushroom, but it is not. Second, none of the claims were substantiated. And third, the material was easily contaminated with pathogenic bacteria, fungi, and possibly lead contamination from the ceramic containers it was often brewed in. Bottles of the product have a tendency to explode on store shelves.

If we are being overly subtle in our evaluation of this product, forgive us.

Kudzu

Description: Kudzu *(Pueraria lobata)* is a vine that is found throughout China and the Southeastern United States. The root has long been used in traditional Chinese medicine. The root contains high levels of isoflavones.

Uses: Interest in kudzu was stimulated by one study that suggested it may have some value as a treatment for alcoholism. Unfortunately, subsequent research has so far failed to support this function.

Products:

Nature's Herbs: Kudzu Power, 1 mg kudzu root extract (1% diadzin), 100 mg, kudzu root 450 mg, 60 capsules.

Nature's Way: Kudzu, 610 mg kudzu root and kudzu root extract (1 mg diadzin), 50 capsules.

Lactoferrin

Related Item: Colostrum.

Description: Lactoferrin is an iron-binding protein, normally found thoroughout the body. It is found in high concentrations in colostrum and breast milk.

Uses: Lactoferrin's use as a supplement is based upon its ability to support immune system function. There are many explanations as to how it exerts this function, but the main action seems to be related to its ability to bind excess iron in the body. This deprives disease-causing microbes of iron, which is necessary for their growth and replication.

It seems to also have a beneficial effect on intestinal health, inflammatory conditions, and may prove to have anticancer activity as well.

Lactoferrin is present in colostrum, but high-potency lactoferrin supplements are usually derived from whey protein.

Products:

Allergy Research: Laktoferrin, 350 mg lactoferrin (95% purity), derived from the milk of free-range cattle, 100 capsules.
Jarrow: Lactoferrin, 250 mg, 250 mg low-iron lactoferrin from whey, 60 capsules.
Jarrow's Lactoferrin contains 250 mg of purified, low-iron lactoferrin, a glycoprotein from whey protein. One of the biological activities of lactoferrin comes from its powerful ability to bind iron (300 times that of serum transferrin). Low-temperature processing ensures this potency. Digestion of lactoferrin liberates the immune-supporting peptide lactoferricin B. Lactoferrin benefits intestinal health by promoting the growth of lactobacilli and bifidobacteria.

Larch, Western

Description: The western larch *(Larix occidentalis)* is used as a source of arabinogalactan (Larch arabinogalactan), which is a water-soluble polysaccharide composed of D-galactose and L-arabinose units.

Uses: Larch arabinogalactan is a type of dietary fiber, and may enhance the growth of friendly

Indications: Immune system.

bacteria in the intestinal tract. If this is correct, Larch arabinogalactan functions as a prebiotic, and this may explain its apparent immune-enhancing action.

Arabinogalactan is also present in echinacea and certain species of mushroom. Some speculate that this may contribute to their immune activity as well.

Although there is considerable interest in this products' immune-enhancing activity, published studies at this time are limited to animal and test-tube research. The final determination as to how this supplement compares to other more well-established products remains to be demonstrated.

Products:

Eclectic Institute: Larix Powder, 3 oz.
Jarrow: Larix 1000, 60 tablets.

L-Carnitine

See Carnitine.

Lecithin

Related Items: Choline, phosphatidylcholine, CDP-choline.

Description: Lecithin is a phospholipid—a mixture of fatty acids, glycerol, phosphoric acid, and choline. It is the choline content or, more specifically, the phosphatidyl choline content of lecithin that makes it so valuable as a nutritional supplement.

Uses: In the food industry, lecithin is used as an emulsifying agent. It is this emulsification action that led early health food advocates to think it might dissolve

> *Indications:* Cholesterol problems, Alzheimer's disease, liver disorders.

cholesterol deposits in the blood. While some studies indicate it helps those with elevated cholesterol levels, this action remains somewhat speculative.

More important is the fact that lecithin is a natural source of phosphatidylcholine.

Lecithin is available in several different forms. In the liquid form, as liquid lecithin, it contains about 38 percent oil and 62 percent phosphatides, of which only one-third is phosphatidylcholine. Liquid lecithin, then, provides only approximately 20 percent phosphatidylcholine at best. Liquid lecithin is available as an oil, or in softgel capsules.

Dry or granular lecithin has had the oil removed, and thus contains about 95 percent phosphatides. This would result in a phosphatidylcholine content close to 30 percent.

If higher levels of choline are necessary, there are other types of supplements available, including phosphatidylcholine, CDP-choline, and choline. Please refer to those listings for more information.

Even though lecithin is not the most concentrated source of supplemental choline, it still has value. It is perhaps the best tolerated form, least likely to result in a fishy body odor, gastrointestinal upset, or other side effects sometimes associated with choline. For those with elevated cholesterol, other more powerful supplements may be available and better documented. But lecithin can be a useful component of a comprehensive cholesterol-lowering regimen.

Dosage: The dose can vary widely.

Products:

Solgar: Lecithin "95" Granules, 260 mg choline per tablespoon, 16 oz granules.
Solgar: Lecithin, 1,200 mg, 33 mg choline per capsule, 100 softgels.

Linseed Oil

See Flaxseed Oil.

Lipoic Acid

Related Items: Alpha-lipoic acid, thioctic acid.

Description: Lipoic acid is a fat-soluble, vitamin-like substance that works along with certain B vitamins in the metabolism of carbohydrates and other nutrients to produce energy.

Uses: Lipoic acid helps in the metabolism of carbohydrates, and can be of benefit to those with diabetes. It is especially valuable in the treatment of diabetic neuropathy.

> *Indications:* Diabetes, diabetic neuropathy, glaucoma, anti-aging.

Lipoic acid is also a powerful antioxidant. Lipoic acid functions to protect and regenerate both water-soluble and fat-soluble antioxidants (glutathione, vitamin C, vitamin E, and CoQ_{10}).

Preliminary work suggests it might be of benefit to those with glaucoma.

Cautions: Lipoic acid may cause diabetics to require a reduction of their dosage of insulin or other antidiabetic drugs.

Products:

Medical Research Institute: Glucotize, 300 mg time-release lipoic acid per tablet, 60 tablets.
Solgar Lipoic Acid, 120 mg, 60 vegicaps.
Jarrow: Lipoic Acid, 100 mg, pharmaceutical grade, 180 tablets.

L-Phenylalanine

Related Item: DL-phenylalanine.

Description: L-phenylalanine is an essential amino acid.

Uses: L-phenylalanine is thought to have antidepressant activity.

| *Indications:* Depression. |

L-phenylalanine is a precursor to L-tyrosine, which in turn is a precursor to the neurotransmitters norepinephrine and dopamine. Increased levels of these neurotransmitter substances are thought to be associated with mood elevation and antidepressant effects.

Dosage: Typically, between 375 and 2,500 milligrams can be used, preferably under the supervision of a health professional. Take between meals.

Cautions: L-phenylalanine is contraindicated in those with phenylketonuria, and those taking nonselective monoamine oxidase (MAO) inhibitors.

Products:

Solgar: L-Phenylalanine, 500 mg, 500 mg free-form L-phenylalanine, vegetarian and kosher, 100 vegicaps.

Lutein

Related Items: Carotenoids, zeaxanthin.

Description: Lutein, a carotenoid, is a fat-soluble, yellowish pigment found in plants, algae, and photosynthetic bacteria. Lutein and a related carotenoid compound, zeaxanthin, are found in the macula of the human retina and the lens of the eye.

Uses: It is thought that lutein and zeaxanthin function to protect the retina of the eye from age-related macular degeneration and cataract formation.

> **Indications:** Cataracts, macular degeneration.

Dosage: Optimal dosage is yet to be determined, but between 6 and 20 milligrams per day are commonly used. Look for products containing flora glo lutein.

Cautions: Lutein and zeaxanthin should not be used for vitamin A deficiency as they are not converted to vitamin A.

Products:

Twinlab: Lutein, 20 mg, dry, water dispersed, from marigolds, 60 capsules.
Jarrow: Lutein, 20 mg, 20 mg lutein and 1 mg zeaxanthin, 60 softgels.

Lycopene

Related Items: Carotenoids, beta-carotene, lutein.

Description: Lycopene is one of the carotenoids, a fat-soluble, red-colored pigment found in certain plants and microorganisms. The best-known source of lycopene is tomatoes and processed tomato products.

Uses: Lycopene seems to be es-pecially useful in relation to prostate cancer and lung cancer. Lycopene seems to be the most powerful antioxidant of all the carotenoids, but it is not clear if this totally explains its action against these cancers, or its antiatherogenic activity.

> **Indications:** Cancer, cardiovascular disease, cholesterol problems, prostate cancer.

Dosage: The optimal dose is not known, but between 5 and 15 milligrams daily are often used. In a clinical trial of men with prostate cancer, two 15-milligram capsules daily was the dose utilized.

Lycopene is oil soluble, and its absorption might be enhanced when given in a preparation that is oil based, or with emulsifiers.

Products:

Jarrow: Lyco-Sorb, 10 mg lycopene, 4 mg gamma-tocopherol in a phospholipid delivery system, 60 softgels.

Nature's Answer: Lycopene Alcohol Free, 28 drops contain 1,000 mg tomato extract providing 5 mg lycopene, 1 oz liquid.
Natrol: Lycopene, 15 mg, 15 mg "LycoMato" lycopene, and 535 mg tomato powder, 30 tablets.

Lysine

Description: L-Lysine is an essential amino acid.

Uses: Herpes simplex virus proteins are rich in L-arginine. It is thought that altering the ratio of lysine to arginine may inhibit

> *Indications:* Herpes simplex virus, shingles, cold sores.

the replication of the herpes simplex virus. Lysine supplementation may therefore reduce the frequency and severity of cold sore, genital herpes, and shingles outbreaks. There is some preliminary evidence that lysine may enhance the absorption of calcium.

Cautions: There may be some connection between high levels of lysine and elevated cholesterol.

Products:

Solgar: Lysine, 500 mg, vegetarian and kosher, 100 vegicaps.
Solgar: Lysine, 1,000 mg, vegetarian and kosher, 100 tablets.
Twinlab: Lysine, 500 mg, 100 capsules.

Ma Huang

See Ephedra.

Magnesium

Related Items: Magnesium oxide, magnesium citrate, magnesium glycinate (chelated).

Description: Magnesium is an important essential mineral, involved in almost every aspect of the body's function. Magnesium deficiency is very common in America, partly due to our increasingly high intake of refined foods. The problem is especially serious in the elderly.

> *Indications:* Cardiovascular disease, osteoporosis, asthma, migraine headaches, hypertension, diabetes, chronic fatigue syndrome.

Uses: Magnesium deficiency is associated with ischemic heart disease, congestive heart failure, cardiac arrhythmias, diabetes mellitus, and hypertension. Magnesium supplementation is important in preventing and treating osteoporosis, and may be effective to some degree in asthma, migraine headaches, kidney stones, and strokes.

Calcium and magnesium are different from most other essential vitamins and minerals. In what way? The required amounts of most vitamins are in the milligram range, usually from 2 to 20 milligrams daily. The same can be said for the trace minerals, like zinc and copper. Others, like selenium, chromium, and biotin, are required in microgram quantities. It's easy to get these vitamins and trace minerals in one or two multivitamin capsules a day. But not calcium and magnesium. For most of us, we are looking at a requirement of 1,200 milligrams calcium and 400 to 600 milligrams of magnesium. You cannot squeeze that into a one-a-day multivitamin!

Many doctors do their patients a disservice by telling them to "take a calcium supplement" or "take Tums." What happens is that now the patient may go out, and in addition to taking a daily multivitamin, she takes a calcium supplement as well. . . . and grumbles about having to "take so many pills!" What about magnesium? It's not in the daily multivitamin, and it's not in the calcium supplement. You're not even getting the minimal government recommended daily quantity.

Calcium gets the headlines, but magnesium deficiency is more likely a bigger problem. And magnesium is extremely important to good health.

THE PHARMACIST SAYS

Larry Siegel, chief pharmacist at Willner Chemists, points out that magnesium is very important for heart function, specifically for heart muscle relaxation (after contraction). Vasospastic heart attacks, where the coronary arteries have little plaque buildup, have been linked to a magnesium deficiency.

The conventional guideline is that you should take half as much magnesium as calcium. So if you take 1,000 milligrams of calcium, you should try to take at least 500 milligrams of magnesium. The current "Daily Value" is 400 milligrams.

For convenience, we usually recommend a supplement that contains a combination of calcium and magnesium, in a 2 to 1 ratio, although magnesium supplements are available as well. Many nutritionists recommend a higher ratio of magnesium to calcium. Those who have the health problems indicated here, for example, may want to add additional magnesium to their calcium/magnesium blend.

When increasing the amount of magnesium, be aware that high levels of magnesium may exert a mild laxative action for some people. Taking magnesium supplements with food, and in divided doses, will lessen that problem.

The most common form of magnesium in supplements is magnesium oxide. This is an inorganic form, and may not be absorbed as well as other forms, such as magnesium citrate, magnesium gluconate, and magnesium aspartate.

Dosage: At least 320 to 420 milligrams per day.

Products:

Ecological Formulas: Magnesium Taurate, 125 mg magnesium as magnesium taurate (this product especially useful for those with heart problems), 60 capsules.
Thorne: Magnesium Aspartate, 90 mg magnesium as magnesium aspartate (well absorbed, but low in potency), 90 capsules.

Magnesium Citrate

Related Item: Magnesium.

Description: Magnesium citrate is used as a source of magnesium in nutritional supplements.

Uses: Magnesium citrate is an "organic" magnesium compound thought to have improved absorption and tolerance over magnesium oxide.

Indications: Cardiovascular disease, osteoporosis, asthma, migraine headaches, hypertension, diabetes, chronic fatigue syndrome.

For general supplementation, magnesium oxide is adequate. For therapeutic purposes, when optimal absorption and tolerance are required, magnesium citrate, glycinate, or aspartate might be preferred.

Magnesium citrate is the supplement of choice in certain specific conditions. One example is kidney stones. The most common type of kidney stone is the calcium oxalate type. Magnesium and citrate together function to reduce the incidence of this type of kidney stone. Consult with your doctor to be sure you do not have a different form before using magnesium citrate, however.

Products:

Solgar: Magnesium Citrate, 200 mg magnesium from magnesium citrate, 120 tablets.
Allergy Research: Magnesium Citrate, 170 mg magnesium from magnesium citrate, 90 capsules.

Magnesium Glycinate

Description: Magnesium glycinate (chelated magnesium) is an organic amino chelate of magnesium used as a source of magnesium in nutritional supplements.

Uses: Magnesium glycinate is a form of magnesium better absorbed, and perhaps better tolerated, than magnesium oxide. For general supplementation, the oxide form is adequate. For thera-

> *Indications:* Cardiovascular disease, osteoporosis, asthma, migraine headaches, hypertension, diabetes, chronic fatigue syndrome.

peutic purposes, however, magnesium glycinate, magnesium citrate, or magnesium aspartate may be preferred.

The glycinate or chelated form is very effective, but it has a lower level of magnesium, so a higher number of tablets may be required.

Products:

Solgar: Chelated Magnesium, 100 mg magnesium from magnesium glycinate per tablet, 250 tablets.

Magnesium Oxide

Related Item: Magnesium.

Description: Magnesium oxide is an inorganic form of magnesium used as a source of magnesium in nutritional supplements.

Uses: Magnesium oxide contains 60 percent of "elemental" magnesium. It is inexpensive and commonly used as a source of magnesium. Even though it is inorganic, it is relatively well absorbed.

> *Indications:* Cardiovascular disease, osteoporosis, asthma, migraine headaches, hypertension, diabetes, chronic fatigue syndrome.

For general supplementation, magnesium oxide is adequate. For

therapeutic purposes, when optimal absorption and tolerance is re-quired, magnesium citrate, glycinate or aspartate, might be preferred.
Products:

Twinlab: Magnesium Capsules, 400 mg, 400 mg magnesium from oxide, 200 capsules.

Maitake Mushroom

Related Item: Medicinal mushroom.

Description: Maitake is a large mushroom found in the mountains of Japan, North America, and Europe. It is also called the "dancing mushroom."

Uses: Certain mushrooms, such as maitake, have been shown to have immunomodulatory activity, as well as possible anti-

> *Indications:* **Immune system, cancer, HIV.**

tumor, antimicrobial, lipid-lowering, and glucose-regulating actions. The components thought to be responsible for this are polysaccharide complexes found in the cell walls of the organism. The active consi-tituent is beta-D-glucan, or beta-glucans.

Maitake is rich in a certain type of beta-glucan, and has been shown to have a general immune system stimulatory action. It is used as a tonic and adaptogen. The regular maitake concentrate is also thought to be helpful in controlling cholesterol and lipid levels, as well as general immune problems.

The "D-fraction," a special beta-glucan-enriched maitake product, is a more potent immune-stimulating product, and is being investi-gated as an anticancer agent.

Dosage: Follow instructions on the bottle.

Products:

Nature's Answer: Maitake Bio Beta Glucan, 1 ml contains 14 mg of beta 1,6 glucan with beta 1,3 branches, 2 oz liquid.
Maitake Products: Maitake D Fraction, 20 drops contain 5.5 mg beta glucan, 4 oz liquid.
Maitake Products: Grifron Pro Maitake D Fraction, 6 drops con-tain 6.6 mg beta glucan, 1 oz liquid.
Maitake Products: Maitake Mushroom Grifron, whole maitake mushroom, a general immune tonic, 180 caplets.

Makandi

See Coleus Forskohlii.

Malic Acid

Description: Malic acid is an organic acid normally found in apples and other fruits. Malic acid is an intermediate in the energy-producing pathway in the cells (the Krebs Cycle).

Uses: There is some evidence that malic acid, in combination with magnesium, may be helpful to those suffering from fibromyalgia. This has not been verified by scientific study.

Products:

Source Naturals: Magnesium Malate, 1,000 mg, supplies 152 mg magnesium and 825 mg malic acid, 180 tablets.
Nature's Life: Magnesium Malate, 1,300 mg, supplies 200 mg magnesium and 1,100 mg malic acid, 100 tablets.
Nature's Life: Malic Acid, 800 mg, 100 capsules.

Manganese

Description: Manganese is an essential trace element. The recommended daily intake level for manganese is between 2 and 5 milligrams, and 10 milligrams are considered "safe," although levels in the 5- to 20-milligram range have been commonly used in nutritional supplements for some time now.

Uses: Manganese may be valuable as a dietary supplement owing to its role as an antioxidant (it is a component of the

> **Indications: Arthritis (osteo), osteoporosis.**

enzyme superoxide dismutase), and its anti-osteoporosis and anti-arthritic properties.

Supplemental manganese is available in several different forms—manganese glycinate (chelate), manganese gluconate, manganese sulfate, and manganese ascorbate. There is little reason to choose one over the other.

Do not confuse manganese with magnesium.

Dosage: Levels of 10 to 20 milligrams daily are common, but this is higher than the current government recommendations of 2 to 5 milligrams.

Products:

Solgar: Chelated Manganese Tablets, 50 mg manganese as manganese glycinate per 3 tablets, 250 tablets.
Twinlab: Manganese Caps, 10 mg manganese from manganese gluconate, 100 capsules.

MCHC

Related Item: Calcium.
Description: Microcrystalline hydroxyapatite (MCHC) is a type of purified bone meal.

Uses: Microcrystalline hydroxyapatite is used in supplements as a source of calcium.

Indications: Osteoporosis, cancer (colon), hypertension.

Theoretically, as is the case for bone meal, it might seem to be an ideal supplement, but clinical evidence is inconclusive. It is claimed that MCHC is less likely to have undesirable contaminants, such as lead. It obviously is not suitable for vegetarians.

It is inorganic, and the calcium is in the form of a phosphate.
Products:

Solaray: Calcium Hydroxyapatite, 4 capsules supply 1,000 mg calcium from 4,000 mg of calcium hydroxyapatite, 120 capsules.
Progessive Labs: MCHC Capsules, 250 mg, 4 capsules supply 1,000 mg calcium from calcium hydroxyapatite and calcium citrate, 120 capsules.
Ethical Nutrients: Bone Builder, 6 tablets supply 1,200 mg calcium from 3,000 mg calcium hydroxyapatite and 2,100 mg of dicalcium phosphate, 120 tablets.

MCT

See Medium-Chain Triglycerides.

Medicinal Mushroom

See Mushroom, Medicinal.

Medium-Chain Triglycerides

Description: Medium-chain triglycerides (MCTs) are more easy metabolized than the longer-chain fatty acids (oleic acid, linoleic acid). They contain between 6 and 12 carbon atoms. They do not require the digestive actions of pancreatic enzymes or bile salts. Nor is carnitine necessary for their transport into the mitochondria for energy production. MCTs yield slightly fewer calories than regular oils.

Uses: The most valid use of MCTs is as nutritional support for those with compromised digestive function.

> *Indications:* Nutritional support.

This could be due to serious illness, gastrointestinal disorders, carnitine deficiency, pancreatic disorders, liver disease, or problems with the lymphatic system.

Some have promoted this supplement as a weight loss aid or a means of enhancing athletic performance. These uses do not seem to be effective.

There is also some interest in the use of MCTs by those with epilepsy. This is based on the fact that MCTs are ketogenic. Ketogenic diets may reduce the frequency and severity of siezures.

Products:

Douglas Labs: MCT Oil, 8.4 g caprylic acid, 3.6 g capric acid per tablespoon, 8 oz liquid.

Melatonin

Description: Melatonin is a main hormone produced by the human pineal gland. It is involved in regulating the circadian rhythm (biological clock).

Uses: There have been a wide variety of claims made for melatonin supplements. Only one

> *Indications:* Insomnia, jet lag.

seems to have valid, practical application, and that is its use in treating sleeping problems and ameliorating the symptoms of jet lag. The human pineal gland normally secretes melatonin during periods of darkness. It is a signal to the body that it is time to sleep. Thus, taking supplemental melatonin sends a message to the body that it is time to sleep. Drowsiness should occur about thirty minutes after taking a melatonin supplement, and should last for at least one hour.

Melatonin also functions as an antioxidant, and has other possible roles as well. Claims have been made that it can be helpful in a great number of diverse conditions (cancers, headaches, depression, schizophrenia, tinnitus, aging, epilepsy, glaucoma, fibromyalgia, among others), but convincing proof of its value in these instances is lacking.

Dosage: A dose of between 1 to 3 milligrams seems to be sufficient. Those first starting out with melatonin should buy a 1-milligram strength, and then experiment with the dosage using from one to three capsules. Sustained-release products may be better for those who wake up after only an hour or two of sleep.

Cautions: The same commonsense cautions that apply to all medications and supplements that may cause drowsiness should apply as well to melatonin. Do not drive race cars, jet fighters, or heavy construction machinery after taking a melatonin supplement. Do not give melatonin to children. Do not take melatonin if you suffer from depression. Do not take melatonin if you are using alcohol or other sleep-inducing medications. Do not use melatonin if trying to become pregnant, if you are pregnant, or if you are nursing.

Products:

Source Naturals: Melatonin Liquid, orange flavor, 1 ml contains 1 mg melatonin, 2 oz liquid.
Allergy Research: S. Gard, 20 mg, highest-potency melatonin, 30 capsules.
Nature's Way: Melatonin, 500 mcg sublingual, low-dose melatonin, 100 tablets.
Twinlab: Melatonin, 1 mg, 100 capsules.
Source Naturals: Melatonin Sublingual, 5 mg, orange flavor, contains 5 mg melatonin, 100 sublingual tablets.
Natrol: Melatonin, 3 mg T.R., 60 timed-release tablets.

Methylcobalamin

Related Items: Vitamin B_{12}, cobalamin, dibencozide.

Description: Methylcobalamin is an active, or coenzyme, form of vitamin B_{12}, (cobalamin).

Uses: There are two coenzyme forms of vitamin B_{12}. Methylcobalamin is one, and adenosylcobalamin is the other. Adenosylcobalamin (dibencozide) is a cofactor for the enzyme L-methylmalonyl coenzyme A mutase, while methylcobalamin is a cofactor for the enzyme methionine synthase. Some claim that supplementation with methylcobalamin is preferable to supplementation with cobalamin, or vitamin B_{12}, presumably because it might be more readily absorbed. What about the other vitamin B_{12} coenzyme? We are not completely convinced that supplementing with either of the coenzyme forms of B_{12} alone is as effective as supplementing with cobalamin (or hydroxocobalamin) in high doses.

Products:

Jarrow: Methyl B_{12}, 1,000 mcg, 100 lozenges.
Jarrow: Methyl B_{12}, 5,000 mcg, 60 lozenges.

Methylsulfonylmethane

See MSM.

MGN_3

Related Items: Beta-glucan, medicinal mushroom.

Description: A combination of modified rice bran extract and shiitake mushroom. Chemically, an arabinoxylane, similar to beta-glucan. Thought to be a stimulator of NK cell activity, enhancing immune system function, with specific antiviral, anticancer and anti-HIV activity.

Uses: Anticancer; antiviral.

Products:

Lane Labs: MGN-3 Vegicaps, 2 capsules contain 500 mg of an Arabinoxylan Proprietary Complex, 50 capsules. Take 2 hours before or after other supplements.

Microcrystalline Hydroxyapatite

See MCHC.

Milk Thistle

Description: Milk thistle (*Silybum marianum*) grows wild, and is found throughout the world. The extract from the dried fruit (seeds) is used in preparing supplements.

Uses: Milk thistle has been shown to exert a protective effect on the liver, and is used as a treatment for hepatitis, liver cirrhosis, and alcohol-induced liver disease.

Indications: Hepatitis, cirrhosis (liver).

This well-studied herb should be used whenever exposure to liver toxins is anticipated. For example, we would recommend that anyone who works in a dry-cleaning business, photographic darkroom, or chemistry laboratory take milk thistle extract as part of their daily supplement regimen.

The main active ingredient in milk thistle is thought to be the flavonoid complex silymarin. Standardized milk thistle supplements are available, standardized to 80 percent silymarin.

The official European (Commission E) list of approved uses for the standardized extract includes toxic liver damage, and supportive treatment in chronic inflammatory liver disease and hepatic cirrhosis.

Dosage: For chronic liver disease, milk thistle may have to be considered long-term therapy. For other conditions, 420 milligrams of silymarin, from standardized milk thistle, should be taken daily, in divided doses. It should be taken for at least 6 to 8 weeks.

Products:

Solgar: Milk Thistle Herb Extract, 175 mg milk thistle extract (aerial, seed) standardized to 80% silymarin, 140 mg, plus 300 mg milk thistle powder (aerial), 60 vegicaps.
Nature's Answer: Milk Thistle Seed, 2,000 mg milk thistle seed fluid extract per 2 ml (56 drops), 1 oz liquid.
Nature's Way: Thisilyn, 175 mg "thisilyn" milk thistle seed extract standardized to 80% silymarin, 100 capsules.

Mixed Tocopherols

Related Item: Vitamin E.

Description: Mixed tocopherols consist of a mixture of all four tocopherols (alpha, beta, gamma, and delta). It can also contain the four tocotrienols. Each of the eight isomers has activity, and some have different actions.

Uses: Vitamin E is an important antioxidant. Because it is fat-soluble, it exerts its protective effect very efficiently at the cell-membrane (which contains a high proportion of fat) level. Vitamin E is now recognized, even by mainstream medicine, as protective against cardiovascular disease and some forms of cancer. It may also be of benefit to those with rheumatoid arthritis, asthma, neurological diseases, cataracts, diabetes, and premenstrual syndrome. It can protect against environmental toxins and enhances immune system function.

For maximum potency and the broadest spectrum of activity, we recommend using mixed tocopherols, with tocotrienols, as the supplement of choice for vitamin E.

Cautions: Those taking blood-thinning medication should be aware that vitamin E may also exert some blood-thinning action. Their prothrombin times should be monitored, and the amount of medication (Coumadin) should be adjusted accordingly.

Products:

Yasoo Health: Vitamin E Factor 400/400, 400 IU vitamin E as d-alpha tocopherol, 400 mg beta, gamma, and delta tocopherols, 31 mg gamma tocotrienol, 5 mg alpha, beta, and delta tocotrienols, 60 softgels.
Solgar: E 400 Mixed Tocopherols, 400 IU vitamin E as d-alpha tocopherol, plus beta, gamma, and delta tocopherols, 250 softgels.

Modified Citrus Pectin

Related Item: Pectin.
Description: Modified citrus pectin is citrus pectin that has been chemically hydrolyzed, that is, broken down to smaller molecular weight fragments. This may make it more absorbable.

Uses: Modified citrus pectin is thought to possibly have anti-cancer activity, particularly for

Indications: Cancer (prostate).

prostate cancer. This is based primarily on test-tube and animal studies. Just how applicable this is to humans remains to be demonstrated.
Products:

Allergy Research: Modified Citrus Pectin, 1 teaspoon contains 5 g of modified citrus pectin, 16 oz powder.
Allergy Research: Modified Citrus Pectin, each capsule contains 500 mg of modified citrus pectin, 120 capsules.

Molybdenum

Description: Molybdenum is an essential trace mineral. It plays a role in certain enzyme systems, including the enzyme sulfite oxidase, which is necessary to detoxify sulfites.

Uses: A deficiency of molybdenum can have life-threatening consequences. Fortunately, overt deficiency is rare. It is most often

> *Indications:* Asthma (sulfite sensitivity), cancer

seem when patients are placed on total parenteral nutrition (TPN), or when they live in areas where the soil is low in molybdenum. In one such instance, in northern China, it was determined that low soil molybdenum levels was responsible for the unusually high incidence of esophageal cancer.

Molybdenum is antagonistic to copper, and there is some interest in the use of high doses of molybdenum to suppress copper, and thus suppress tumor growth.

Another possible effect of molybdenum supplementation is to prevent sulfite sensitivity. Sulfites, as preservatives, are no longer used as commonly as in the past, but those with sulfite sensitivity remain susceptible to allergic reactions. Molybdenum deficiency can enhance this problem.

Dosage: The recommended daily intake of molybdenum is 75 micrograms. In supplements, the amount used can vary from 50 to 250 micrograms.

Molybdenum is easily absorbed, and the form used does not seem to be overly important. In fact, molybdenum seems to be more efficiently absorbed from supplements than from food.

Products:

Solgar: Chelated Molybdenum, 150 mcg molybdenum as molybdenum amino acid chelate, 100 tablets.
Allergy Research: Liquid Molybdenum, 25 mcg molybdenum as ammonium molybdate, 1 oz liquid.

MSM

Description: Methylsulfonylmethane (MSM) is an organic sulfur-containing mineral supplement found naturally in a wide variety of foods. It is a metabolite of DMSO (dimethyl sulfoxide).

Uses: MSM is recommended as a treament for disorders such as osteoarthritis. Sulfur is a component of the amino acids methionine and cysteine, and may be involved in maintaining the integrity of joints and connective tissue. Many report that it reduces the pain and discomfort associated with various types of musculoskeletal problems.

MSM is widely used, and anecdotal reports of benefit abound. But scientific support is lacking.

Products:

Doctor's Best: Best MSM, 1,000 mg, 180 capsules.
Jarrow: MSM Powder, 200 g.
Twinlab: MSM, 1,000 mg, 120 tablets.
Natrol: MSM, 500 mg, 200 capsules.

Mushroom, Medicinal

Related Items: Maitake, reishi, shiitake

Description: A mushroom is a type of fungus. Some mushrooms are edible and some are poisonous. Others have been used for centuries as medicinal agents.

Uses: Certain mushrooms have been shown to have immunomodulatory activity, as well as possible antitumor, antimicrobial, lipid-lowering, and glucose-regulating actions. The components thought to be responsible for this are polysaccharide complexes found in the cell walls of the organism. The active consitituent is beta-D-glucan, or beta-glucans.

There are a number of mushrooms currently being used medicinally. In addition to maitake, reishi, and shiitake, there is cordyceps, coriolus, and others.

Products:

Maitake Products: Super Tremella, 700 mg tremella fruit body, 300 mg tremella 8:1 extract, plus maitake D-fraction, vitamin C, and bioperine. (Tremella fuciformis), 120 tablets.
Maitake Products: Super Royal Agaricus, 500 mg agaricus fruit body, 400 mg agaricus 12:1 extract, plus maitake D-fraction, vitamin C, and bioperine (Agaricus blazei), 120 tablets.
Maitake Products: Super Shiitake, 700 mg shiitake fruit body, 300 mg shiitake 12:1 extract, plus maitake D-fraction, vitamin C, and bioperine (Shiitake edodes), 120 tablets.
New Chapter: Reishi 5, combination of reishi, shiitake, maitake, cordyceps, and coriolus mushroom extracts, 60 vegicaps.

NAC

See N-Acetyl-Cysteine.

N-Acetyl-Cysteine

Related Items: Cysteine, glutathione.

Description: N-acetyl-cysteine (NAC) is a derivative of the non-essential, sulfur-containing amino acid cysteine. It is more stable than cysteine, and may be better absorbed.

Uses: N-acetyl-cysteine is an antioxidant. As a source of cysteine, it is a precursor to glutathione, a powerful antioxidant.

NAC is known to function as a mucolytic, liquifying overly viscous mucus.

Indications: Liver disorders, hepatitis, lung disease, detoxification, cardiovascular disease, bronchitis, immune system.

It exerts a strong protective action on the liver, owing most likely to its antioxidant and glutathione regeneration activities.

NAC is used, in high doses, to counteract acetaminophen poisoning.

Products:

Jarrow: NAC, 600 mg, Sustain, sustained release formula, 100 tablets.
Solgar: NAC, 600 mg vegicaps, vegetarian and kosher, 120 vegicaps.
Source Naturals: NAC, 1,000 mg, 120 tablets.

NADH

Description: Nicotinamide adenine dinucleotide (NAD) is a natural substance found throughout the body and involved in energy production. It is the active, coenzyme form of niacin (vitamin B$_3$). NADH is the reduced form of NAD. Some products contain NAD and some contain NADH. Because the two substances are converted from each other as part of normal redox reactions (oxidation-reduction) related to metabolic energy production, many people think that they are effective. But it seems that NADH, in an enteric-coated form, is the more active of the two—especially in supplement form.

Uses: Supplemental NADH is being used as a treatment for Parkinson's disease, chronic fatigue syndrome, and Alzheimer's disease. Early indications are that it may be effective, but scientific evidence of its efficacy in this form is lacking.

Enteric-coated or otherwise modified forms are claimed to provide better stability.

Products:

Menuco: Enadalert, 10 mg, sublingual, 8 tablets. For jet lag, take 1 hour before traveling between time zones.
Menuco: Enada, 5 mg, patented enteric-coated formula, 30 tablets.

Niacin

Related Items: Niacinamide, no-flush niacin.

Description: Niacin is one of the B vitamins. It is also called nicotinic acid and vitamin B_3. *Niacin* is sometimes used as a general term to include niacinamide. Both niacin and niacinamide have similar vitamin activity, but they differ in certain other respects. (Niacinamide is discussed below.) A deficiency of niacin causes the disease pellagra. Medical students remember the signs of pellagra as the four D's, i.e., dermatitis, diarrhea, dementia, and death.

Uses: Beyond its role in preventing deficiency symptoms, niacin currently receives most attention as a result of its role in lowering serum cholesterol, LDL

Indications: Cholesterol problems, Raynaud's phenomenon, intermittent claudication.

cholesterol, VLDL cholesterol, and triglycerides, while increasing serum levels of HDL cholesterol. Many studies have shown niacin to be as good as, or better than, many of the commonly used prescription drugs used for lowering elevated cholesterol.

The only drawback to the use of niacin for this purpose is that at high doses, it causes a skin flush reaction over the face, neck, and chest. By starting with a lower dose, and gradually increasing the dose over a period of weeks, this problem can be alleviated. Also, taking the niacin with meals will reduce the problem.

In an attempt to avoid the skin flush problem, some turned to a time-release or delayed form of niacin. This did indeed reduce the skin flush problem. There was some initial concern that this form might have been more likely to cause liver problems, but this is no longer an issue. If anything, it might be a little more likely to cause gastric discomfort.

Another solution is "no-flush" niacin, or inositol hexanicotinate. This form of niacin has been used for many years in Europe, seems to have the desired effect on cholesterol, does not cause liver problems, and does not cause a flush. (*See* Niacin, No-Flush, for additional information.)

Dosage: For general nutritional supplementation, niacin or niacinamide is usually included in multivitamin supplements at levels of 50 to 200 milligrams. The recommended daily intake level is 20 milligrams.

For lowering cholesterol, the daily dose can vary between 1,500 and 3,000 milligrams. Regardless of the form of niacin used, when taking this high an amount, it should be done under the supervision of a health professional.

Cautions: High doses of niacin, over 1.5 grams daily, may impair glucose tolerance, both in diabetics and nondiabetics.

Products:

Carlson: Niacin Time, 500 mg, 100 tablets. Gradual release over 5 to 7 hours.
Solgar: Niacin, 500 mg, vegetarian and kosher, 250 vegicaps.

Niacin, No-Flush

Related Item: Niacin.

Description: Niacin is one of the B vitamins. It is also called nicotinic acid and vitamin B_3. *Niacin* is sometimes used as a general term to include niacinamide. Both niacin and niacinamide have similar vitamin activity, but niacinamide does not have the same cholesterol-lowering action. To lower cholesterol, niacin, or the form of niacin known as inositol hexanicotinate, must be used.

Uses: Niacin has been shown to be an effective agent in lowering serum cholesterol, LDL cholesterol, and triglycerides. Niacin, when used at the high dose re-

Indications: Cholesterol problems, Raynaud's phenomenon, intermittent claudication.

quired to achieve this effect, can cause an uncomfortable skin flush reaction on the face, neck, and chest.

Inositol hexanicotinate, or no-flush niacin, exerts the same cholesterol-lowering effect, without the annoying skin flush reaction.

Dosage: The recommended dosage can range from 500 to 4,000 milligrams daily, with meals.

Cautions: Even though there are no reports of liver toxicity with this product, caution is recommended. Some are concerned that, theoretically, since it behaves similarly to time-release niacin, liver function should be carefully monitored. It should be used at these dosages only under the supervision of a health professional.

Products:

Twinlab: No Flush Niacin, 800 mg, 640 mg of niacin per capsule, 100 capsules.
Solgar: No Flush Niacin, 500 mg, 450 mg of niacin per capsule, 100 vegicaps.

Niacinamide

Related Item: Niacin.

Description: Niacinamide is one form of vitamin B$_3$ (niacin). Both forms have the same vitamin activity, but they differ in their nonvitamin actions.

Uses: While niacin is a powerful cholesterol-lowering agent, niacinamide does not have this activity. Nor does niacinamide

Indications: Diabetes, arthritis (osteo).

cause a skin flush. For this reason, niacinamide is the preferred form of vitamin B$_3$ for use in multivitamin formulas.

Niacinamide is the precursor to NAD/NADH and is involved in the production of energy and the synthesis of fatty acids, cholesterol, and steroids.

There is considerable interest in niacinamide as a possible agent useful in preventing or delaying the onset of Type 1 diabetes mellitus (insulin-dependent diabetes mellitus, or IDDM).

Dosage: For general vitamin supplementation, the dosage range is 20 to 100 milligrams daily. For therapeutic purposes, i.e., diabetes, osteoporosis, higher dosages are used, but this should be done under the supervision of a health professional.

Products:

Twinlab: Niacinamide, 100 mg, 100 mg niacin from niacinamide, 100 capsules.
Solgar: Niacinamide 550, 550 mg niacin from niacinamide, 100 vegicaps.

Nicotinamide Adenine Dinucleotide

See NADH.

Nicotinic Acid

See Niacin.

No-Flush Niacin

See Niacin, No-Flush.

Octacosanol

Related Item: Policosanol.
Description: Octacosanol is a waxy substance found in various vegetable or plant waxes, including wheat, sugar cane, yams and wheat germ.
Uses: Octacosanol is the main long-chain alcohol found in policosanol.
This would lead to speculation that it might have some cholesterol-lowering activity, but this has not been confirmed.
The main interest in octacosanol supplements is the claim that it can boost energy, athletic performance, and male sexual performance. This is an outgrowth of work done back in the early 1970s by Cureton, using an extract of wheat germ oil. Unfortunately, in over thirty years, no research has been produced to substantiate these early claims.
Claims that it may be of some benefit in Parkinson's disease are preliminary, and yet to be confirmed.
Products:

Solgar: Octacosanol 2000, 2,000 mcg of octacosanol from wheat germ oil, 90 vegicaps.

Twinlab: Octcosanol 8000, 8,000 mcg of octacosanol from spinach, 60 capsules.

OKG

See Ornithine Alpha-Ketoglutarate.

Olive Leaf Extract

Description: The olive tree is a small evergreen native to the Mediterranean region. Olive oil, of course, is well known and highly respected. But olive leaf has unique medicinal value. The leaf contains oleuropein and various flavonoids.

Uses: Olive leaf has been used for various cardiovascular problems, especially high blood pressure. It is popular in Europe as a treatment for mild to moderate hypertension. There is also speculation that the oleuropein in olive leaf may inhibit the oxidation of LDL cholesterol.

Indications: Hypertension, immune system.

Historically, olive leaf has been used as a treatment of wounds and infection. Currently, this use has gained a good deal of support as a result of a number of studies supporting the antimicrobial activity of various components of olive leaf. Under certain conditions, the oleuropein in olive leaf is converted to elenolic acid, which has antiviral activity.

While there has been considerable interest in the use of olive leaf extract as a treatment for various viral, fungal, and bacterial infections, most of the research in support of this is based on test-tube and animal studies. A study on the antiviral activity of calcium elenolate on parainfluenza infection in hamsters, for example, does not necessarily mean that olive tree extract will have antiviral activity in humans.

Dosage: Most commonly, 250 to 500 milligrams of standardized extract, three times a day.

Products:

Solaray: One Daily Olive Leaf, 1,000 mg of olive leaf extract (17% oleuropein), providing 170 mg of oleuropein, 30 capsules.
Allergy Research: Prolive, 500 mg of olive leaf extract (10% oleuropein), providing 50 mg of oleuropein, 60 tablets.
Nature's Answer: Oleopein Vegicaps, 400 mg of olive leaf extract

and 20 mg of olive leaf powder providing 30 mg of oleuropein, 60 vegicaps.

Seagate: Olive Leaf Extract Vegicaps, olive leaf extract prepared by a water extraction process; oleuropein content not provided, 90 vegicaps.

Omega-3 Oils

See Fish Oil.

OPC

Related Items: Grape seed extract, Pycnogenol.

Description: OPC (oligomeric proanthosyanidin) is a type of flavonoid found in grape seed extract and maritime pine extract (Pycnogenol). OPCs are also found in cocoa (and chocolate), bilberry, grape skin, green tea, black tea, black currant, cranberry, apples, peanuts, and almonds.

Use: OPCs, also called PCOs, represent a type of flavonoids thought to function as a powerful antioxidant, protecting tissues, glands, and organs throughout the body from the deleterious effects of free-radical damage. In addition, they have an ability to strengthen collagen. This explains their value in enhancing the integrity of skin, blood vessels, and connective tissue. They exert an anti-inflammatory action, perhaps by inhibiting the release of pro-inflammatory prostaglandins. There is also compelling evidence that the proanthocyanidins have anticarcinogenic activity.

Products containing OPC flavonoids are considered by many to be the most valuable and inclusive antioxidants available and should be part of any comprehensive supplement program.

Note: There are two types of supplements available that are rich in OPCs. One is grape seed extract and the other is a trademarked product called Pycnogenol, which is derived from pine bark. There have been claims and counterclaims as to which is better. Much of this is a result of an initial multilevel program involving Pycnogenol. Marketing hyperbole to the contrary, they are similar in composition and function. Grape seed extract contains between 92 and 95 percent OPCs, while Pycnogenol products contain only 80 to 85 percent OPCs. Considerable research has been performed on grape seed extract, and in Europe, it is the more popular of the two supplements. Finally, grape seed extract is often less expensive.

Products:

Seagate Gold: Grape Seed Extract, 250 mg, 150 mg red grape seed extract, 100 mg red grape skin extract, 90 capsules.
Jarrow: OPCs+95, 100 mg grape seed extract (100:1), 95% polyphenols, 100 capsules.

Oregano Oil

Description: Oregano (Origanum vulgare) has a long history as a food spice and medicinal herb.

Uses: Oregano is an aromatic herb, containing volatile oils. Volatile oils are known to possess antimicrobial properties, and

> *Indications:* Fungal infections (topical).

their antifungal and antibacterial action is easily demonstrated in the test tube. There is little question but that this action can be utilized to advantage in topical products, for the treatment of fungal infections and similar problems.

The claims being made that oral oregano supplements can cure almost any disease known—or soon to be discovered—by man is not justified. In most cases, the basis for such claims are test-tube experiments that may or may not reflect similar action when oregano is taken orally by humans.

Alcohol is a powerful antimicrobial agent in a test tube. But that does not mean that two shots of vodka three times a day will cure systemic candidiasis.

In small doses, oral ingestion of oregano oil seems harmless, and the same can be said for larger doses of dried oregano herb. Perhaps its value as a systemic antibacterial, antifungal and antiparasitic agent will be demonstrated eventually, but at this time we are more comfortable with its use as a topical treatment.

Products:

NAH: Oregamax Capsules, 100% wild oregano, 2 caps contain 1,100 mg of a proprietary blend of oregano, Rhus coriaria, garlic, and onion, dry powder, 90 capsules.
NAH: Super Oregano Oil, 2 drops contain 60 mg of a proprietary blend, 1 oz liquid.

Nature's Answer: Oregano Oil Alcohol Free, 4 drops supply 13 mg oil of oregano leal extract containing 7 mg of carvacrol, 1 oz liquid.

Nature's Herbs: Oregano Power, oregano leaf oil, 20 mg, and rosemary leaf extract, 20 mg, 60 softgels.

NOW Foods: Oregano Oil, 0.2 ml oil of oregano containing 55% carvacrol, 90 softgels.

Oregon Grape

Description: Oregon grape (*Berberis aquifolium*) root contains berberine alkaloids, similar to goldenseal and barberry. It is an evergreen shrub, native to northwest North America.

Uses: Oregon grape is used for many of the same conditions as is goldenseal. In addition, it has been shown to be of some value in treating chronic skin conditions (acne, psoriasis, and eczema).

Indications: Immune system, skin disorders, psoriasis, canker sores, gastrointestinal disorders, parasites.

Products:

Nature's Answer: Oregon Grape Drops, 1,000 mg of Oregon grape root in 28 drops, 1 oz liquid. Do not use for longer than 4 weeks.

Solaray: Oregon Grape Root, 400 mg, 100 capsules.

Ornithine

See Ornithine Alpha-ketoglutarate.

Ornithine Alpha-Ketoglutarate

Description: L-ornithine is a nonessential, nonprotein amino acid. Ornithine can serve as a precursor to L-arginine, L-glutamine, and proline.

Uses: Ornithine, especially in combination with arginine, is thought to promote increased levels of growth hormone and in-

Indications: Wound healing, athletic performance.

sulin, and promote muscle growth. Just how valid this claim might be is somewhat questionable, especially at reasonable dosage levels.

A form of ornithine, ornithine alpha-ketoglutarate (OKG) is used medically to support burn and trauma patients, the chronically malnourished, and postsurgical elderly. It seems to enhance wound healing and may have some immunomodulating action.

Dosage: The use of either ornithine or ornithine alpha-ketoglutarate for medical conditions should be done under medical supervision. Athletes typically use 2 or 3 grams several times a day, although there is little evidence that this is beneficial.

Products:

Twinlab: Ornithine, 500 mg, as L-Ornithine HCl, 100 capsules.

Orthosilicic Acid

Related Item: Silicon.

Description: Orthosilicic acid is a soluble form of silicon. Other forms of silicon, from horsetail or silicon dioxide, have to be converted to orthosilicic acid before being absorbed.

Uses: Silicon is an essential mineral thought to be required for the strength and elasticity of bones, joints, connective tissue, hair, skin, nails, mucous membranes, and arteries.

> *Indications:* Hair, skin, and nails, osteoporosis.

A 2 percent stabilized solution of orthosilicic acid may be the best utilized form of silicon.

Dosage: The liquid form contains about 1 milligram silicon, as orthosilicic acid, per drop. The recommended dosage is 6 to 20 drops daily, mixed with juice or water.

Products:

Jarrow: Biosil Liquid, 6 drops contain 6 mg silicon from orthosilicic acid, 1 oz liquid.

Oyster Shell Calcium

See Calcium Carbonate.

Pantethine

Related Item: Pantothenic acid.

Description: Pantethine is an active metabolite of pantothenic acid (vitamin B_5), the precursor to coenzyme A.

Uses: Pantethine seems to have a lipid-lowering action not shown by pantothenic acid. It may be useful in lowering total cholesterol, LDL cholesterol, and triglyceride levels while increasing HDL cholesterol.

> *Indications:* Cholesterol problems, cataracts, cardiovascular disease, detoxification.

Dosage: The typical dose for treating elevated cholesterol seems to be 300 milligrams, three times a day.

Cautions: Exceptionally safe and nontoxic.

Products:

Atkins: Mega Pantethine, 450 mg, 30 softgels.
Jarrow: Pantethine, 300 mg, 60 softgels.

Pantothenic Acid

Related Item: Pantethine.

Description: Pantothenic acid (vitamin B_5) is one of the water-soluble, B-complex vitamins. It is essential for the metabolism of fatty acids, amino acids, and carbohydrates. A clinical deficiency is rare but usually involves the skin, liver, adrenals, and nervous system.

Uses: Pantothenic acid works together with the other B vitamins for proper energy production and lipid synthesis. It is thought to be useful in treating stress, owing to

> *Indications:* Arthritis (rheumatoid), stress, skin disorders.

its support of adrenal hormone production, and to be helpful in rheumatoid arthritis, acne, and lupus.

The usual form of pantothenic acid used in nutritional supplements is D-calcium pantothenate. The corresponding free alcohol form, dexpanthenol, is also available, but is typically used in topical products.

There is another form of pantothenic acid, pantethine. Pantethine is a metabolite of pantothenic acid, which differs in one very significant way—pantethine has a marked lipid-modulating action, while pantothenic acid does not. *See* Pantethine for more information.

Dosage: The recommended daily value is 10 milligrams, but the amounts found in supplements typically run between 25 and 50 milligrams, or more.

Products:

Solgar: Pantothenic Acid, 550 mg, 550 mg calcium pantothenate providing 500 mg pantothenic acid, 100 vegicaps.
Twinlab: Pantothenic Acid, 500 mg, 550 mg calcium pantothenate providing 500 mg pantothenic acid, 100 capsules.

PCO

See OPC.

Pectin

Related Items: Fiber, modified citrus pectin.

Description: Pectin is a soluble fiber. It is found commonly in citrus fruits and apples. When obtained from citrus peel, it is referred to as citrus pectin.

Uses: Pectin is used in foods as a gelling or thickening agent. It is used in combination with kaolin, a clay, for the management of diarrhea.

> *Indications:* Cholesterol problems, constipation, diarrhea, weight loss.

As a nutritional supplement, it may be helpful in lowering elevated cholesterol.

Dosage: Typical doses range from 5 to 15 grams daily, before meals or at bedtime.

Cautions: If you are not accustomed to fiber supplementation, start out with small doses and gradually increase the amount.

Products:

Solgar: Apple Pectin Powder, 8 oz.
Twinlab: Apple Pectin USP Capsules, 500 mg apple pectin, USP, 10 mg vitamin C, 100 capsules.

Peppermint Oil

Description: Peppermint (*Mentha piperita*) is a perennial aromatic herb. It is a natural hybrid of water mint and spearmint. The main volatile oil in peppermint is menthol.

Uses: Peppermint oil is used internally as a antispasmodic, carminative, and cholagogue. An interesting external use involves application of peppermint oil to the temples as a treatment for headaches.

Indications: Irritable bowel syndrome, gastrointestinal disorders, digestive aid.

The use of enteric-coated peppermint oil capsules, either alone or mixed with caraway oil, seems to be an effective treatment for irritable bowel syndrome and other gastrointestinal problems.

Dosage: For irritable bowel and similar problems, take one or two enteric-coated capsules, two or three times daily. For digestive disorders, use peppermint tea as needed, or take one or two regular capsules, two or three times daily.

Cautions: Use caution when giving peppermint to small children, especially as a tea. Also, use caution when obstruction of the bile ducts, gallbladder inflammation, or liver damage is a possibility.

Products:

Enzymatic Therapy: Peppermint Plus, 0.4 ml peppermint oil, plus thyme and rosemary oils in 2 capsules, 60 softgels.
Nature's Way: Pepogest, 0.2 ml peppermint oil per capsule, 60 softgels.

Phosphatidylcholine

Related Items: Choline, lecithin, CDP-choline.

Description: Phosphatidylcholine is a form of choline used in dietary supplements.

Uses: Choline is important for the formation and maintenance of normal cellular membranes, brain function, cardiovascular function, and liver function.

Indications: Alzheimer's disease, cholesterol problems, liver disorders, hepatitis, manic depression, mental function, Parkinson's disease, tardive dyskinesia.

Choline is available alone, as choline bitartrate, choline citrate, or choline chloride. While these forms provide the highest level of choline per dose, they are not as well tolerated as phosphatidylcholine, which is obtained from lecithin. High doses of phosphatidylcholine, for example, will not cause the fishy odor that results from high doses of choline.

Dosage: The amount taken as a supplement can vary over a wide range. The new "dietary reference intake" is 550 milligrams daily and the suggested "upper limit" is 3,500 milligrams daily. The usual dose of phosphatidylcholine is 500 to 1,000 milligrams daily.

It is important to note that the amount of actual "choline" varies with the source. Phosphatidylcholine contains about 13 to15 percent choline. A 500-milligram phosphatidylcholine capsule, therefore, provides only about 70 milligrams of actual choline. The potency of phosphatidylcholine supplements (not lecithin supplements) can vary, however, from 55 to 90 percent phosphatidylcholine, so it is necessary to read the label carefully. Liquid concentrates are available as well.

Cautions: At levels of over 3 grams per day, some people experience gastrointestinal discomfort.

Products:

Solgar: Phosphatidylcholine, 1,200 mg, 400 mg phosphatidyl choline from 1,200 mg phosphatidylcholine complex, 100 softgels.
American Lecithin: Phos Chol 900, contains 900 mg pure phosphatidylcholine, 100 softgels.
American Lecithin: Phos Chol Concentrate, 1 tablespoon contains 9 G pure phosphatidylcholine, 8 oz liquid.

Phosphatidylserine

Description: Phosphatidylserine is a phospholipid that is an integral component of the cell membrane in all life forms. It is found in high concentrations in brain tissue. Other phospholipids are phosphatidylcholine and phosphatidylethanolamine.

Uses: Phosphatidylserine has been shown to be useful in treating conditions such as Alzheimer's disease, age-associated memory impairment, and other types of dementia.

Indications: Age-related cognitive decline, Alzheimer's disease, depression, Parkinson's disease.

Most of the research on phosphatidylserine has been done with material derived from bovine brain tissue. The material available in the United States for use in supplements is derived from soy lecithin. It is not exactly the same as the material in animal brain tissue, but seems to have the same effect.

Dosage: The usual dose is about 300 milligrams daily.

Products:

Progessive Labs: Phosphatidylserine Licaps (Liquid Vegetable Capsules), 100 mg phosphatidylserine, 50 mg phosphatidylcholine, 60 softgels.

Jarrow: PS-100, 100 mg phosphatidylserine, 45 mg phosphatidyl-choline, 3 mg gamma-tocopherol, 60 softgels.

Solgar: Phosphatidylserine Complex, 100 mg phosphatidylserine, 100 mg phosphatidylcholine from 500 mg phosphatidylserine complex, 30 tablets.

Phytosterols and Phytostanols

Related Item: Beta-sitosterol.

Description: Phytosterols are compounds found in plants that have a chemical structure similar to cholesterol. Cholesterol is found only in animal products, however. Phytostanols are similar to phytosterols, except they have no double bonds in the sterol ring. In other words, phytostanols are saturated phytosterols.

Uses: Phytosterols and phytostanols have been shown to lower cholesterol. Total cholesterol is reduced by about 10 percent, and

> *Indications:* Cholesterol problems, cardiovascular disease.

LDL cholesterol by about 13 percent. Even better, they seem to have no effect on HDL cholesterol, the good cholesterol.

Phytosterols and phytostanols are very insoluble in water, and dissolve poorly in oil. Esterification of these compounds with long-chain fatty acids increases their solubility in oils and fats. This allows the material to be incorporated into food items such as margarine. But the esters are broken down (hydrolyzed) into the free sterols and stanols in the small intestine before absorption.

The exact mechanism of their cholesterol-lowering action is not known for sure, but it is thought they block the absorption of cholesterol from the diet and the reabsorption of endogenous cholesterol from the GI tract.

Studies so far have shown that the phytosterols and phytostanols seem to be equally effective in lowering cholesterol.

Dosage: The dose of unesterified phytosterols and phytostanols is approximately 1 gram daily. The product should be taken with meals.

Cautions: There is some concern that supplementing with phytosterols and phytostanols may interfere with the absorption of certain nutrients (carotenoids, vitamin E, and lycopene).

Products:

Arkopharma: Basikol Phytosterols, 800 mg phytosterols from soy, corn, and canola oils, 120 g powder.
Twinlab: Cholesterol Success, 900 mg phytosterols (Reducol) per 2 tablets, 120 tablets.

Policosanol

Description: Policosanol is a term used to describe a group of long-chain, aliphatic, saturated alcohols. They are derived from waxes in plants such as sugar cane, yams, and beeswax. The main alcohol in policosanol is octacosanol.

Uses: Both animal and human studies have shown that policosanol is a safe and effective cholesterol-lowering agent. Results

> *Indications:* Cholesterol problems, intermittent claudication.

so far have been impressive, with reductions in LDL cholesterol of 20 to 25 percent. HDL cholesterol was increased. In addition, policosanol seems to reduce platelet aggregation almost as effectively as aspirin, especially at higher dosages.

Some have claimed that policosanol, and its main constituent, octacosanol, can boost energy, athletic performance, and male sexual performance. This is an outgrowth of work done back in the early 1970s by Cureton, using an extract of wheat germ oil. Unfortunately, in over thirty years, no research has been produced to substantiate these early claims.

Dosage: The suggested dose seems to be 5 milligrams, taken once or twice a day with lunch and dinner. It may take several months for the results to appear. Long-term use, at dosages up to 20 milligrams daily, seem to be safe.

Products:

Jarrow: Policosanols, 10 mg, 10 mg policosanols, derived from 36 mg rice bran wax (28%), 100 vegicaps.

Metagenics: Cholarest, 10 mg policosanol from beeswax, 30 softgels.
Pharmanex: Cholestin, 15 mg policosanol from beeswax, 30 softgels.

Polyphenols

Related Items: Red wine, green tea, flavonoids.

Description: Polyphenols is a broad term encompassing over 4,000 individual compounds found in plants. It includes the flavonoids, tannins, proanthocyanidins, isoflavones, and catechins.

Uses: Epidemiolgical studies have shown that both tea consumption and the moderate intake of red wine are inversely related to the risk of heart dis-

> *Indications:* Cardiovascular disease, cholesterol problems, cancer.

ease. Both red wine and tea are rich in polyphenols. While the exact mechanism by which wine or tea consumption could offer protection against atherosclerosis and ischemic heart disease is still under investigation, a large body of literature suggests that the presence of polyphenols in these beverages may account for the protective action.

The polyphenols in wine include phenolic acids, anthocyanins, tannins, caffeic acid, rutin, catechin, myricetin, quercetin, and epicatechin. Proanthocyanidins, polymers or oligomers of catechin units, are the major polyphenols in red wine and grape seeds. Resveratrol is a nonflavonoid polyphenol also found in red wine and grape seeds.

The polyphenols in tea include quercetin, kaempferol, myricetin, catechin, epicatechin, and epigallocatechin (ECG).

The polyphenols in general have potent antioxidant activity. Many studies have shown that they may lower total cholesterol, lower LDL cholesterol, and raise HDL cholesterol. They reduce platelet aggregation and have vasorelaxant effects.

Polyphenols are available in many types of supplements, from green tea and grape seed concentrates, to various flavonoid-rich mixed fruit and vegetable concentrates.

Dosage: Follow the directions on the label.

Products:

Jarrow: Resveratrol Synergy, polyphenols from resveratrol, grapeskin, grape seed, and green tea extracts, plus catechins, anthocyanins, and proanthocyanins, 60 tablets.

Potassium

Description: Potassium is an essential mineral. In conjunction with sodium and chloride, it is involved with regulation of water balance, acidity, blood pressure, and neuromuscular function.

Uses: The largest source of dietary potassium is fruits and vegetables. Many of us eat far too few fruits and vegetables and, at

> *Indications:* Hypertension, cardiovascular disease

the same time, ingest too much sodium and chloride from processed foods. Many believe this is a cause of high blood pressure.

There is evidence that potassium may be useful in the prevention and treatment of hypertension. This may be most pronounced in male African Americans. Potassium may be beneficial in alleviating other cardiovascular problems as well, including the risk of strokes.

Somewhat paradoxically, the amount of potassium in a dietary supplement is limited to 99 milligrams. This is due to concerns over possible side effects, such as stomach irritation. But one banana can contain 500 milligrams of potassium. One-sixth teaspoonful of popular salt substitutes contain 530 milligrams. Prescription potassium products are widely used in dosages ranging from 1.5 to 3.0 grams daily. (Prescription potassium supplements are usually labeled in mEq, or milliequivalents, not milligrams.)

These higher amounts of potassium, when from food, do not cause stomach irritation. And there is much to be said for eating a piece of fruit rather than taking a potassium tablet.

If you suspect that potassium supplementation might be worth considering, you should discuss it with your physician.

Products:

Twinlab: Potassium Capsules, 99 mg potassium from potassium citrate and potassium aspartate, 180 capsules.
Solgar: Potassium Amino Acid Complex, 99 mg potassium as potassium glycinate amino acid complex, 250 tablets.

Pregnenolone

Related Item: DHEA.
Description: Pregnenolone is naturally found in the body, and serves as a precursor for the synthesis of various steroid hormones, including DHEA (dehydroepiandrosterone) and progesterone.

Uses: There are many interesting areas of research on pregnenolone, but it is difficult to justify its use as a nutritional supplement at this time except under medical supervision. It may be shown to have some effect as a memory enhancer, and it may someday be used in treating Alzheimer's disease, cancer, arthritis, and other conditions associated with aging.

Cautions: Pregnenolone should not be used by those with prostate, breast, or uterine cancer. It should not be used by those with seizure disorders.

Products:

Jarrow: Pregnenolone, 50 mg, pharmaceutical grade, 100 capsules.
Country Life: Pregnenolone, 10 mg, 60 capsules.
Allergy Research: Pregnenolone, 150 mg TR, 150 mg pregnenolone in a timed-release lipid matrix, 60 tablets.

Proanthocyanidins

See Grape Seed Extract.

Probiotics

Related Item: Acidophilus.

Description: The term *probiotic* is used to describe live microorganisms that, when ingested, improve the balance of the intestinal microflora, with resultant beneficial health effects. The types of microorganisms commonly used include various lactobacillus species, bifidobacterium species, and yeasts.

Uses: A delicate balance and symbiosis exists between the intestinal microflora and the human host. The beneficial bacteria that reside in the intestinal tract have been shown to exert antimicrobial, immunomodulatory, anticarcinogenic, anti-allergenic, and antidiarrheal activity.

Indications: Diarrhea, candidiasis, immune system, gastrointestinal disorders, allergies (food).

When present in adequate quantities, these beneficial microorganisms reinforce the function of the intestinal mucosa as a barrier against pathogens and toxins. Some probiotic organisms have actually been found to secrete antimicrobial substances. Some have been shown to stimulate general immune system function and inhibit, perhaps indirectly, certain types of tumor formation.

The lining of the intestines should serve as a barrier, preventing the absorption of food-protein antigens. Antigens are protein fragments that can trigger an allergic reaction. Those who suffer from food allergies and sensitivities may have, to varying degrees, a condition called leaky gut, which allows too many antigens to be absorbed. Probiotics enhance the integrity of the intestinal mucosa, preventing the absorption of these allergens.

Probiotics have long been used to combat antibiotic-induced diarrhea, and they may be helpful in other types of intestinal problems as well, including ulcerative colitis and Crohn's disease.

There are many types of bacteria and yeasts now being used in probiotic supplements, including bifidobacteria, lactobacilli, lactococci, saccharomyces, streptococcus thermophilus, and enterococci. There are conflicting claims as to the superiority of one type over another, but each has its own slightly unique properties, and the trend seems to be moving toward mixtures containing synergistic blends. There was also concern over whether certain probiotics were dairy-free or contained dairy products. Some feel this concern may have been overblown. Except for those with a true milk protein allergy (not lactose intolerance, or "sensitivity"), the small amount of dairy residue in a product taken in capsule or partial teaspoon quantities is not always likely to be a problem.

Another problem with probiotic supplements is stability. First, the organisms themselves are delicate, and careful processing and storage are necessary to ensure their continued viability. Newer technology seems to be overcoming the need for refrigerated storage in this regard. Second, the live organisms have to survive the passage through the gastrointestinal tract before reaching the colon. To ensure that a large enough number of live organisms survive, various measures can be taken, including enteric coating and buffering. Some loss is inevitable, and this is why it is important to start with as high a potency product as possible.

Dosage: Follow the directions on the label. To enhance the survival of the probiotic organisms in the acid environment of the stomach and the alkaline environment of the duodenum, some suggest taking them before meals or on an empty stomach. Others suggest taking them with meals. We suggest that, for the first few days, you do both. Then, take them with meals.

Products:

Natren: Healthy Trinity, 5 billion Lactobacillus Acidophilus, 20 billion Bifidobacterium Bifidum, 5 billion Lactobacillus Bulgaricus in a special matrix, 30 capsules. Store below 75°F.
Jarrow: Jarro-dophilus EPS, 4.4 billion total bacilli from 8 different species, enteric coated, 60 vegicaps. No refrigeration required.
Nature's Way: Primadophilus Reuteri, 100 million colony-forming units per capsule, enteric coated, 30 capsules.
Allergy Research: Lactobacillus GG Culturelle, 40 mg Lactobacillus GG delivers 20 billion live/active bacteria, 30 capsules.

Propolis

Description: Propolis is a brownish resinous, glue-like material collected by bees from plant buds and used to seal their hives. It is thought to exert an antimicrobial action, keeping the hives free of germs.

Uses: Propolis has a long history of use in the health food industry, mostly based on its broad antimicrobial and anti-inflammatory action. There is some speculation that propolis, owing to its content of caffeic acid phenethyl ester (CAPE), may have anticancer activity as well.

Indications: **Immune system, arthritis.**

Dosage: Follow the directions on the label.

Products:

Nature's Answer: Propolis, 2,000 mg propolis resin extract, providing 400 mg propolis solids per 2 ml, 1 oz liquid.
Premier One: Bee Propolis, 650 mg bee propolis 2X (1,300 mg propolis) per 2 capsules, 60 capsules.

PSK

See Coriolus Versicolor Extract.

Psyllium Seed

Related Item: Fiber.

Description: Psyllium (*Plantago ovata*) is an annual plant native to India and Iran, but now cultivated in many countries, including southern Europe and the United States. It is also known as plantain and Ispaghula. Both the seed and seed husk are used in supplements.

Uses: Psyllium is recognized by the FDA, along with oats, as being effective in lowering cholesterol and LDL cholesterol. It is also helpful in treating constipation, and may be beneficial to those with diabetes in moderating blood glucose levels.

> *Indications:* Cholesterol problems, constipation, diarrhea, irritable bowel syndrome, weight loss, diabetes.

Dosage: Typical dosage is from 5 to 15 grams daily, before meals or at bedtime.

Cautions: If you are not accustomed to supplementing with dietary fiber, be sure to start out with small doses and gradually increase the amount. Always drink ample quantities of water when taking fiber supplements.

Products:

Yerba Prima: Psyllium Husk Vegicaps, 625 mg psyllium per cap. 4 vegicaps provide 2.2 g fiber, 180 vegicaps.
Yerba Prima: Psyllium Whole Husks, 4.5 g fiber per tablespoon, 12 oz powder.

Pycnogenol®

Related Items: Grape seed extract, OPC, PCO.

Description: Pycnogenol® is a name that originally was used to describe the class of flavonoids called proanthocyanidins or procyanidins. Now, it has been trademarked, and refers to procyanidins derived from the French maritime pine (*Pinus maritima*).

Uses: OPCs represent a type of flavonoid thought to function as a powerful antioxidant, protecting tissues, glands, and organs throughout the body from the deleterious effects of free-radical damage. In addition, they have an ability to strengthen collagen. This explains their value in enhancing the integrity of skin, blood vessels, and connective tissue. They exert an anti-inflammatory action, perhaps by inhibiting the release of pro-inflammatory prostaglandins. There is also compelling evidence that the proanthocyanidins have anticarcinogenic activity.

Products containing OPC flavonoids are considered by many to be the most valuable and inclusive antioxidants available, and should be part of any comprehensive supplement program.

Products:

Country Life: Pycnogenol®, 50 mg, 100% pine bark extract (85–90% total polyphenols), 50 capsules.
Solgar: Pycnogenol®, 100 mg, 100 mg Pycnogenol® extract (95% phenolic components), 30 vegicaps.

Pygeum

Description: Pygeum (*Pygeum africanum*) is an evergreen tree native to Africa. The bark of the tree trunk is the part used medicinally, containing phytosterols, including beta-sitosterol, pentacyclic terpenes, and ferulic esters.

Uses: While saw palmetto seems to be slightly better than pygeum in the treatment of benign prostatic hyperplasia, pygeum

Indications: **Benign prostatic hypertrophy, prostatitis.**

also appears to be effective. It certainly deserves consideration as an alternative to saw palmetto, or as part of a combination therapy approach.

Dosage: The usual dose is 50 to 100 milligrams two times a day.
Products:

Gaia Herbs: Pygeum Africanum Bark, 90 mg *Pygeum africanum* bark extract per 40 drops, 1 oz liquid.
Nature's Herbs: Pygeum Power, 50 mg Pygeum bark extract (13% sterols) per softgel, 60 softgels.

Pyridoxal 5'-Phosphate

Related Item: Vitamin B_6.
Description: Vitamin B_6 is an important vitamin, functioning as a coenzyme in the metabolism of amino acids, glycogen, and structural components of the nervous system, as well as neurotransmitters such as serotonin and dopamine.

Uses: Pyridoxal 5'-phosphate is marketed as a "more absorbable" form of vitamin B$_6$. But vitamin B$_6$ is very readily absorbed, and before pyridoxal 5'-phosphate can be absorbed, it is converted first to pyridoxine. In general, therefore, the regular form of pyridoxine is probably no less effective than the 5'-phosphate.

Cautions: Vitamin B$_6$ is used as a treatment for various peripheral neuropathies. At very high doses—2,000 to 5,000 milligrams daily—over time, it may actually cause sensory neuropathy. It is now agreed that at levels between 200 and 500 milligrams daily, side effects are not likely to occur. During pregnancy, amounts over 100 milligrams daily should be avoided, unless taken under the advice of a health professional.

Products:

Klaire Labs: Pyridoxal 5'-Phosphate, 50 mg per, capsules, 250 kosher gelatin capsules.
Source Naturals: Coenzymated B$_6$, 25 mg B$_6$ from pyridoxal 5'-phosphate (sublingual), 60 tablets.

Pyridoxine

Related Item: Pyridoxal 5'-phosphate.

Description: Vitamin B$_6$ is an important vitamin, functioning as a coenzyme in the metabolism of amino acids, glycogen, and structural components of the nervous system, as well as neurotransmitters (serotonin, dopamine, etc.).

Uses: Supplementation with vitamin B$_6$ is necessary to prevent deficiency, especially in the elderly and the chronically ill. Studies have shown that up to one-third of the healthy elderly population suffers from marginal vitamin B$_6$ deficiency.

Indications: Carpal tunnel syndrome, cardiovascular disease, autism, nausea (morning sickness), depression (oral contraceptives, PMS), premenstrual syndrome, immune system, asthma.

Vitamin B$_6$ is important for immune system function. In the elderly, supplementation with vitamin B$_6$ results in significant improvement in immune system function.

In conjunction with vitamin B$_{12}$ and folic acid, vitamin B$_6$ is important in lowering elevated homocysteine, a risk factor for atherosclerosis.

A COMMENT FROM DR. ABEL

Most orthopedic and hand surgeons feel that symptoms of carpal tunnel syndrome require an operation. But before you consider such invasive therapy, you should recognize that several hundred milligrams of pyridoxine (vitamin B$_6$) may be just what your body needs. Additionally, exercising your flexor and extensor tendons is helpful. This can be done by extending your arm straight and gently pulling your fingers back until discomfort is recognized, holding them there for 10 or 15 seconds. Then, with the elbow straight, move the wrist and fingers down in a similar fashion for another 15 or 20 seconds. Repeat the process twice with each arm and wrist. A combination of exercise and natural therapy may just save you the pain and discomfort, not to mention the cost, of a surgical procedure. Certainly, a surgical procedure is always available for an urgent condition, or one that is unresponsive to natural alternatives.

Vitamin B$_6$ has been shown in several studies to be an effective treatment in some cases of carpal tunnel syndrome. It certainly is something that should be tried before more expensive and invasive treatments are undertaken.

Dosage: The recommended daily value is 2 milligrams. The amount used in nutritional supplements can run up to 75 milligrams per day or more. When treating carpal tunnel syndrome, up to 200 milligrams per day are usually used. When used for premenstrual syndrome, up to 100 milligrams per day are used.

Since vitamin B$_6$ is a water-soluble vitamin, we recommend that it be taken in divided doses, two or three times a day.

There are two forms of vitamin B$_6$ used in supplements, pyridoxine HCl, and pyridoxal 5'-phosphate. Pyridoxine HCl, the regular form of vitamin B$_6$, is very well absorbed, even in high dosages. Any advantage gained by using the pyridoxal 5'-phosphate is problematic.

Cautions: Vitamin B$_6$ is used as a treatment for various peripheral neuropathies. At very high doses—2,000 to 5,000 milligrams daily over time—it may actually cause sensory neuropathy. It is now agreed that at levels between 200 and 500 milligrams daily, side effects are not likely to occur. During pregnancy, amounts over 100 milligrams daily should be avoided, unless under the advice of a health professional.

Products:

Solgar: B₆, 500 mg, vegetarian and kosher, 100 vegicaps.
Twinlab: B₆, 50 mg, 100 capsules.

Pyruvate

Description: Pyruvate is the salt (anionic) form of pyruvic acid, a key metabolite formed when carbohydrates and proteins are converted in the body to energy. Pyruvate itself can be thought of as a biological fuel source.

Uses: Studies have shown that when pyruvate is taken in amounts ranging from 6 to 50 grams a day and combined with a | **Indications: Obesity, weight loss, athletic performance.**

controlled-calorie diet and/or regular exercise, it aids weight loss and improves cholesterol and triglyceride levels. There is no evidence, however, that taking large doses of pyruvate without concomitant calorie restriction and/or a regular exercise program results in significant weight loss.

Dosage: A level of at least 5 or 6 grams daily seems to be required for weight loss. Higher doses may be necessary for enhancing athletic endurance and performance.

Products:

Twinlab: Pyruvate Fuel, 750 mg calcium pyruvate, 60 capsules.
Natrol: Pyruvate 650 mg, 650 mg calcium pyruvate, equal to 528 mg pyruvate, plus 50 mg cayenne pepper, 60 capsules.

Quercetin

Related Items: Bioflavonoids, polyphenols.

Description: Quercetin is a flavonol type of flavonoid, a type of polyphenol. It is found in relatively high levels in onions, green tea, red wine, and apples.

Uses: Quercetin is a strong antioxidant, with anti-inflammatory, anti-allergy, antiviral, immunomodulatory, anticancer, and gastroprotective activity. It enjoys a | **Indications: Cardiovascular disease, prostatitis, allergies, asthma, cataracts.**

well-earned reputation as one of the premier antioxidant flavonoid compounds. It may be especially valuable to diabetics, preventing the nerve, eye, and kidney damage common to the condition. It may help fight allergies owing to an antihistamine-type action. And it may even offer some protection against breast cancer owing to its possible antiestrogenic activity.

Dosage: The usual dosage ranges from 200 to 1,200 milligrams daily.

Products:

Jarrow: Quercetin 500 mg, from eucalyptus, 200 capsules.

Red Yeast Rice

Description: Red yeast rice is the fermentation product obtained when certain strains of yeast (*Monascus purpureus*) grow on rice. It has been used for hundreds of years in China as a food and medicine. It has been shown to contain a compound (HMG-CoA reductase inhibitor) that inhibits the production of cholesterol in the liver. The drug lovastatin (Mevacor) contains the same material. This has caused the FDA to challenge the legal status of red yeast rice. They claim it should be regulated as a drug, not a food.

Uses: Red yeast rice has been shown to lower cholesterol and triglycerides. Its action, in certain respects, was superior to the drug lovastatin, and may indicate that

> *Indications:* Cholesterol problems.

there are other active ingredients in red yeast rice that contribute to its action. But the product may no longer be available as a supplement owing to ongoing regulatory problems.

Dosage: At the time this was written, the continued availability of this product is uncertain.

Cautions: If available, all of the warnings and cautions appropriate to the use of lovastatin-type drugs would apply to this product.

Products:

Solaray: Red Yeast Rice, 600 mg, 45 capsules. Only product currently available at the time this was written.

Reishi

Related Item: Medicinal mushroom.

Description: Reishi mushrooms grow on decaying logs and stumps in the coastal regions of China. The red variety is most often used, and is cultivated throughout the Orient and North America.

Uses: Certain mushrooms have been shown to have immunomodulatory activity, as well as possible antitumor, antimicrobial, lipid-lowering and glucose-regulating actions. The components thought to be responsible for this are polysaccharide complexes found in the cell walls of the organism. The active constituent is beta-D-glucan, or beta-glucans.

> *Indications:* Immune system, hypertension, diabetes.

Reishi, in addition, contains triterpenoids (ganoderic acids), which may lower blood pressure and LDL cholesterol. Reishi may be of some benefit to those with diabetes as well.

Dosage: Reishi is available in powder, tea, and tincture form. Follow the directions on the label.

Products:

Nature's Herbs: Reishi Power, 60 mg Reishi mushroom extract, providing 4% triterpenoids and 12.5% polysaccharides, and 540 mg Reishi mushroom powder, 60 capsules.
Maitake Products: Super Reishi, 500 mg reishi fruit body, 300 mg reishi 14:1 extract, plus ginger, maitake D fraction, vitamin C, and bioperine per 4 vegetable tablets, 120 tablets.
Nature's Answer: Reishi Alcohol Free, 1,000 mg reishi fruiting body fluid extract per ml, 1 oz liquid.

Resveratrol

Description: Resveratrol is a nonflavonoid polyphenol found in grape skin and red wine. It can also be found in the dried roots and stems of the plant *Polygonum cuspidatum*.

Uses: Resveratrol has been shown to be an antioxidant with cardioprotective action. It is thought to be of value as an anti-atherosclerotic agent, and may

> *Indications:* Cardiovascular disease, cholesterol problems, immune system.

also have immune-stimulating and anticancer activity.

Dosage: Follow the directions on the label.
Products:

Natrol: Resveratrol, 50 mg, 12 mg total resveratrol from 50 mg
Polygonum cuspidatum root extract, 60 capsules.
Source Naturals: Resveratrol, 10 mg resveratrol from 500 mg
Polygonum cuspidatum (8% total resveratrols), 60 tablets.
Seagate Gold: Grape Seed Extract, 250 mg, 150 mg red grape
seed extract, 100 mg red grape skin extract. 90 capsules. Note that
this product contains not only an extract of the grape skin, but also
an extract of grape seed. (See Grape Seed Extract.)

Riboflavin

Description: Riboflavin (vitamin B$_2$) plays a key role in energy production and the generation of antioxidants such as glutathione.

Uses: Recent research indicates that high-dose supplementation with riboflavin may prevent migraine headaches. It may also protect against esophageal cancer, malaria, and cataracts.

Indications: Migraine headaches, nutritional support (elderly), canker sores.

Dosage: The recommended daily allowance is 1.7 milligrams, but supplements normally contain from 25 to 50 milligrams. For treatment of migraine headaches, doses as high as 400 milligrams daily may be used. This should be done under the supervision of a health professional.

Cautions: Riboflavin has a greenish-yellow fluorescent color. Excess riboflavin is excreted in the urine and imparts this color to the urine. This is of no consequence.

Products:

Twinlab: B$_2$, 100 mg, 100 mg riboflavin from riboflavin 5'-phosphate and riboflavin, 100 capsules.
Nature's Plus: Vitamin B$_2$, 250 mg SR 60 tablets. Base provides for gradual release over a prolonged period.

Rose Hip Vitamin C

Related Items: Vitamin C.
Description: Rose hips is the fruit of the rose plant. It is a very rich source of vitamin C.

Uses: A concentrate or extract of rose hips can be used in supplements as a source of "natural" vitamin C. Although "natural" vitamin C is no different from "synthetic" vitamin C, there are other substances in rose hips (flavonoids, carotenoids, other vitamins, minerals) that offer additional benefit.

Just as it is desirable to take vitamin C with bioflavonoids rather than vitamin C alone, it may be of some benefit to take vitamin C either from rose hips or with rose hip concentrate.

Be careful not to be misled about what is actually in the product. If it is a high-potency vitamin C supplement, it is unlikely to be providing vitamin C only from rose hips. Instead, it is more likely a mixture of rose hip–derived vitamin C and synthetic vitamin C.

Read the label carefully. Products that used to be labeled "Rose Hip C, 500 mg" some years ago now call themselves "Vitamin C 500 mg with Rose Hips." The content of the product did not change, but the wording on the label did! If a product is labeled in such a way to imply that it contains 500 or 1,000 milligrams of Vitamin C "from rose hips," we suggest you move on to another brand.

Products:

Solgar: Vitamin C, 1,000 with Rose Hips, 62.5 mg rose hips fruit, 1,000 mg L-ascorbic acid, 100 tablets.

Rosemary Leaf

Description: Rosemary (*Rosmarinus officinalis*) is a small, fragrant evergreen shrub native to the Mediterranean but now found cultivated throughout the world. Rosemary contains phenolic acids, phenolic diterpenoid bitter substances, triterpenoid acids, flavonoids, volatile oils, and tannins.

Uses: Rosemary has been used medicinally since the time of the Greeks. In Europe, it has been used as a tonic, stimulant, and carminative to treat dyspepsia (indigestion), headaches, and nervous tension. A carminative is an agent that helps to expel gas, relieving colic and cramping. It is used as a spasmolytic, to relieve intestinal cramping, and as a choleretic, promoting bile secretion by the liver.

> *Indications:* Indigestion, gastrointestinal disorders, candidiasis, immune system, headaches.

The volatile oils in rosemary are thought to have powerful antibacterial action. There is some evidence that certain of the components in rosemary have anticancer activity as well.

Dosage: One or two capsules of standardized extract, two or three times daily. Or up to 10 milliliters of the tincture, two or three times daily.

Products:

Gaia Herbs: Rosemary Leaf, 1 oz liquid.
Arkopharma: Rosemary, 300 mg, 300 mg rosemary flower head powder (1.5% essential oil), 100 capsules.
Natrol: RoseOx, 250 mg, 250 mg rosemary leaf powdered extract, 30 capsules.

Royal Jelly

Description: Royal jelly is the substance secreted by nurse worker bees that stimulates the growth and development of the queen bee. Without this substance, the queen bee would apparently be no different from a worker bee, living for only seven or eight weeks rather than five to seven years.

Uses: While royal jelly has not yet been shown to increase the life span of humans tenfold, as it does for the queen bee, it does seem to

Indications: **Cholesterol problems.**

have some beneficial effects as a supplement. Studies have shown that royal jelly may have cholesterol-lowering activity. There is also some evidence that it may have some antibacterial, immune system stimulating, and anti-inflammatory action.

Dosage: The usual dose is from 50 to 100 milligrams daily.

Cautions: Those with allergies and sensitivities should exert caution.

Products:

Premier One: Royal Jelly 1000, 286 mg royal jelly 3.5X, equivalent to 1,000 mg royal jelly, 60 capsules.

Rutin

Related Items: Bioflavonoids, quercetin.
Description: Rutin is a flavonoid, commonly present in the "citrus

bioflavonoid" type of supplements. Rutin is the rhamnoglucoside of quercetin; when hydrolyzed, it yields quercetin, rhamnose, and glucose.

Uses: The powerful antioxidant action of the flavonoids protects the membranes of both the red blood cells and the cells lining the capillary walls. This prevents those cells, the endothelial cells, from becoming brittle and damaged. This condition, sometimes called capillary fragility, can lead to poor circulation, easy bruising, varicose veins, spider veins, and hemorrhoids. When fluid leaks from fragile capillaries, swelling and inflammation result.

Historically, the flavonoids are associated with vitamin-P activity. *Vitamin P* was a term originally applied by Albert Szent-Gyorgyi, who discovered vitamin C, because of his observation that this group of compounds reduced capillary permeability. We now feel that the most important biochemical, or therapeutic, action of the flavonoids as a group is their powerful antioxidant activity. Some have referred to them as biological response modifiers due to their anti-inflammatory, antiviral, anticarcinogenic, and anti-allergy properties.

Products:

Solgar: Rutin, 500 mg, 500 mg rutin from *Dimorphandra mollis* fruit (Brazilian tree), 250 tablets.

S-Adenosyl-L-Methionine

See SAMe.

SAMe

Description: S-adenosyl-L-methionine (SAMe) is a substance naturally present in the body. It plays a crucial role in the biochemical reactions involving transmethylation. SAMe is a "methyl donor." Thus, SAMe is involved in the biosynthesis of DNA, RNA, phospholipids, proteins, melatonin, epinephrine, creatine, and other proteins.

Uses: In Europe, SAMe is categorized as a drug, and is recommended for the treatment of depression, liver disorders, osteoarthritis, and fibromyalgia. In the United States, it is being used to support emotional well-being and en-

Indications: Depression, arthritis (osteo), fibromyalgia, liver disorders.

hance mood, in addition to treating mild to moderate depression. It is also used to treat joint problems and osteoarthritis. It may be useful in certain liver disorders as well.

Unlike traditional antidepressants, SAMe has few side effects, and a more rapid onset of action—only one or two weeks.

SAMe is generally unstable, and various measures are used to overcome this problem. Various modified forms are available, as is the use of an enteric coating. Even the enteric-coated forms are subject to deterioration from moisture and temperature, so it is important that moisture-resistant packaging is used and careful storage requirements are adhered to.

Many suggest taking SAMe with additional vitamin B_6, B_{12}, folic acid, and perhaps trimethylglycine, to assist in controlling the levels of homocysteine, the end product of SAMe metabolism.

Dosage: For joint problems and osteoarthritis, the dosage ranges between 400 and 1,200 milligrams daily. For depression, from 800 to 1,600 milligrams can be used. Always take the product on an empty stomach (one hour before or two hours after meals).

Read the label carefully to determine if you are getting 200 milligrams of SAMe or SAMe tosylate disulfate.

Cautions: There is some question as to whether SAMe is beneficial or detrimental to those with Parkinson's disease.

Products:

Jarrow: SAMe 200 mg Enteric Coated, 200 mg SAMe from 400 mg SAMe tosylate disulfate, 60 tablets. Take on an empty stomach.

Saw Palmetto

Description: Saw palmetto (*Serenoa repens*) is a small palm tree native to southeastern North America. The fruits, or berries, were used as a staple food and medicine by the Seminole inhabitants of Florida before European colonization.

Uses: Saw palmetto, particularly the fat-soluble (lipophilic) extract, has been shown, very convincingly, to be as good or

> *Indications:* Benign prostatic hypertrophy.

better in treating benign prostatic hyperplasia than the popular prescription medication (finasteride). At the very least, saw palmetto is as effective as the drugs, but with significantly lower incidence of side effects.

The role of saw palmetto in preventing prostate cancer is still being investigated. Most recent evidence now indicates that, contrary to early thinking, saw palmetto actually results in a reduction of the enlargement of the prostate. Also, it is reported that saw palmetto does not interfere with PSA measurements.

Dosage: Typically, 160 milligrams of the lipophilic extract, twice daily. One 320-milligram capsule daily may work as well. Allow four to six weeks for effects to fully manifest themselves.

Products:

Nature's Way: ProstActive, 320 mg saw palmetto berry extract (12:1), 30 softgels.
Nature's Herbs: Saw Palmetto, 600 mg saw palmetto berry powder, 100 capsules.
Nature's Answer: Saw Palmetto Berry, 2,000 mg saw palmetto berry fluid extract per 2 ml (56 drops), 2 oz liquid.

Sea Cucumber

Related Items: Cartilage, shark cartilage, bovine cartilage, green-lipped mussel.

Description: A source of mucopolysaccharides thought to be helpful in reducing the pain and inflammation of arthritis and sports injuries.

Indications: Arthritis, sports injuries.

Products:

Solgar: Sea Cucumber, 500 mg blend of sea cucumber and sea plant, 30 vegicaps.
Nutraceutical Research: Marine Care, 500 mg sea cucumber, 60 capsules.

Selenium

Related Items: Selenium yeast, selenomethionine.

Description: Selenium is an essential trace element. It is a component of the enzyme glutathione peroxidase, a powerful antioxidant.

Uses: Low levels of selenium have been linked to increased risk of cancer, cardiovascular disease, and inflammatory disorders.

> *Indications:* Cancer, cardiovascular disease, immune system, HIV, cataracts.

Selenium is a powerful antioxidant, working in conjunction with vitamin E to protect against oxidative, free radical damage. Selenium is important for proper immune system function, and may play a role in detoxification and male fertility.

In certain areas, the soil is low in selenium, resulting in widespread selenium deficiency. Plants (crops) can be low in selenium even though they look normal.

The importance of selenium in reducing the incidence of certain cancers (prostate, lung, colorectal, and skin) is well documented and impressive. There is strong epidemiological evidence of a similar role for selenium in reducing the risk of cardiovascular disease.

There is some evidence that selenium levels are also inversely related to cataract formation. Glutathione peroxidase, a major antioxidant enzyme in the eye, is selenium dependent.

In the light of the overwhelming evidence supporting the benefit of ensuring an optimal level of selenium intake, it is difficult to understand why anyone interested in living a long and healthy life would not supplement with this trace mineral.

Dosage: The currently accepted range of selenium in supplements is between 50 and 200 micrograms daily, with doses up to 400 micrograms being used by those with cancer, heart disease, or otherwise at risk to conditions influenced by selenium. The tolerable upper limit is 400 micrograms. Adverse effects are rarely seen at dosages below 900 micrograms daily.

There are three types of selenium supplements available. There is a selenium-enriched brewer's-type yeast that is an excellent source of selenium. Another "organic" form is selenomethionine. The active form of selenium in the body (and in the yeast supplement) is actually this same selenomethionine compound. It is an excellent source. For those who prefer not to ingest yeast, selenomethionine is fine. For those who do not like the natural sulfur odor of the selenomethinine, the yeast form is fine. In fact, studies show that the inorganic forms of selenium, sodium selenite and sodium selenate, while not as good as the organic forms, are sufficiently well absorbed to be used without concern for availability.

For most individuals, the 200 micrograms of selenium contained in a balanced daily multivitamin-multimineral supplement will be all that are needed. Usually, a comprehensive antioxidant blend will contain additional selenium and vitamin E. So the combination of a balanced multivitamin and an antioxidant blend may provide ample amounts of selenium.

Products:

Twinlab: Sodium Selenite, 250 mcg selenium from sodium selenite, yeast-free, 100 capsules.

Selenium Yeast

Related Item: Selenium.

Description: Selenium-enriched yeast has been grown in a selenium-rich media so that it incorporates higher than normal levels of selenium. On enzymatic hydrolysis, the selenomethionine complex is released, which is then readily absorbed from the small intestine.

Uses: Low levels of selenium have been linked to increased risk of cancer, cardiovascular disease, and inflammatory disorders. Selenium is a powerful antioxidant, working in conjunction with vitamin E to protect against oxidative, free-radical damage. Selenium is important for proper immune system function and may play a role in detoxification and male fertility.

The importance of selenium in reducing the incidence of certain cancers (prostate, lung, colorectal, and skin is well documented and impressive. There is strong epidemiological evidence of a similar role for selenium in reducing the risk of cardiovascular disease.

Some evidence exists that selenium levels are also inversely related to cataract formation. Glutathione peroxidase, a major antioxidant enzyme in the eye, is selenium-dependent.

This form of supplemental selenium is very well utilized by the body.

Cautions: For those with yeast sensitivities, the selenomethionine form or the inorganic forms of selenium can be used.

Products:

Country Life: Selenium, 100 mcg, 100 mcg selenium as high-selenium yeast, 100 tablets.
Solgar: Selenium 200 mcg, 200 mcg selenium as primary grown yeast, 100 tablets.

Selenomethionine

Related Item: Selenium.

Description: L-selenomethionine is a compound containing selenium and an amino acid, methionine. This form of selenium is readily absorbed from the small intestine.

Uses: Low levels of selenium have been linked to increased risk of cancer, cardiovascular disease, and inflammatory disorders. Selenium is a powerful antioxidant, working in conjunction with vitamin E to protect against oxidative, free-radical damage. Selenium is important for proper immune system function and may play a role in detoxification and male fertility.

The importance of selenium in reducing the incidence of certain cancers (prostate, lung, colorectal, and skin) is well documented and impressive. There is strong epidemiological evidence of a similar role for selenium in reducing the risk of cardiovascular disease.

Some evidence exists that selenium levels are also inversely related to cataract formation. Glutathione peroxidase, a major antioxidant enzyme in the eye, is selenium-dependent.

This form of supplemental selenium is very well utilized by the body.

Cautions: Methionine is a sulfur-containing amino acid, and may have a slight sulfurous odor. This is normal.

Products:

Solgar: Seleno-6, 100 mcg, vegetarian and kosher, 250 tablets.
Klaire Labs: Seleno Met, 200 mcg, 100 capsules.

Shark Cartilage

Related Items: Cartilage, bovine cartilage.

Description: In general terms, cartilage is composed of collagen and proteoglycans, which in turn contain glycosaminoglycans (GAGs) or mucopolysaccharides, which in turn contain chondroitin sulfate, which in turn contains glucosamine. There is considerable argument and debate in the nutritional-supplement industry over which of the forms of cartilage—shark cartilage, bovine cartilage, glucosamine sulfate, chondroitin sulfate, or another mucopolysaccharide-rich substance such as green-lipped mussel extract or sea cucumber—is most effective. There is no clear answer, as there is some degree of support for each argument, and there is clinical evidence supporting the efficacy for each supplement.

Uses: The primary use for these supplements, in general, is to rebuild damaged connective tissue and joints, reduce inflammation, and relieve the pain associated with osteoarthritis and sports injuries.

Cartilage supplements, however, especially shark cartilage, have historically been used for a different purpose—as a treatment for certain forms of cancer. The basis for the use of cartilage in treating cancer was that it was thought to inhibit the formation of new blood vessels (angiogenesis). In spite of early enthusiasm in this area, follow-up research in support of this use has not been forthcoming.

It is difficult to assign a specific use for shark-cartilage supplements today. Rich in the minerals and protein building blocks of bone and connective tissue, they certainly could be part of any supplement regimen for arthritis or osteoporisis. But as a primary treatment for a condition such as arthritis, one would have to wonder if glucosamine sulfate and/or chondroitin sulfate should take precedence. For cancer, the advice of a qualified health professional should be sought out, to determine whether or not cartilage treatment is appropriate.

Dosage: For cancer, extremely large doses were utilized. For arthritis, in support of other supplements, up to 2 grams a day are sufficient.

Products:

Seagate: Shark Cartilage, 650 mg, 100 capsules.
Lane Labs: Benefin Caplets, 750 mg shark cartilage per caplet, 270 caplets.

Shark Liver Oil

See Alkylglycerol.

Shiitake Mushroom

Related Item: Medicinal mushroom.

Description: Originally native to Japan, China, and other Asian countries, shiitake mushroom *(Lentinus edodes)* is now widely cultivated throughout the world. It normally grows on fallen broadleaf trees.

Uses: Certain mushrooms have been shown to have immunomodulatory activity, as well as possible antitumor, antimicrobial, lipid-lowering, and glucose-regulating actions. The components thought

> *Indications:* Immune system, HIV, liver disorders, cancer (prostate).

to be responsible for this are polysaccharide complexes found in the cell walls of the organism. The active constituent is beta-D-glucan, or beta-glucans.

Shiitake contains a unique polysaccharide called lentinan. A preparation of the powdered mycelium is called lentinus edodes mycelium extract, or LEM. A purified version is available in Japan as a treatment for cancer.

There are many interesting studies supporting the efficacy of shiitake mushroom extracts, including one that showed that the recurrence rate of genital warts was reduced significantly in those who took a lentinan supplement.

Dosage: Shiitake is available as a food, and as a concentrate. The dose of the concentrate is 1 to 3 grams, two or three times daily.

Products:

Nature's Answer: Shiitake Alcohol Free, 2,000 mg shiitake fruiting body fluid Extract per 2 ml, 1 oz liquid.
Nature's Herbs: Shiitake Mushroom, 600 mg shiitake mushroom powder per capsule, 100 capsules.

Siberian Ginseng

Related Item: Ginseng.

Description: Siberian ginseng (*Eleutherococcus senticosus*) is technically not a ginseng, and it is not from Siberia. It is a separate species, also known as Eleuthero or, in China, as Ci Wu Jia.

Uses: The German Commission E approves Siberian ginseng as a tonic in times of fatigue and debility, declining capacity for work or concentration, and during convalescence.

> *Indications:* Athletic performance, energy (low), chronic fatigue syndrome, stress, immune system, cancer (breast), cold and flu, diabetes.

There have been, according to some reports, over 1,000 scientific studies on Siberian ginseng. Most of them were in Russia, and many do not meet today's rigid standards. But the general consensus regarding its value has to be compelling, especially when taken in context of its persistent popularity.

The term *adaptogen* was coined by Soviet researchers to describe Siberian ginseng's ability to increase nonspecific resistance, help modulate stress, and improve performance under stressful conditions.

Siberian ginseng has been shown to indeed demonstrate the qualities originally designated as adaptogenic. Its use seems to improve endurance, memory, and stamina. It has immunomodulating and immunostimulatory action. There is some evidence that it has hypoglycemic activity, platelet aggregation–inhibiting action, and antiproliferative effects on leukemia cells. It may protect the liver from toxins, and has been shown to protect against the effects of radiation. Some interesting research on eye conditions shows that it helps patients with glaucoma, eye burns, and even myopia. In another study, it improved color distinction in people with normal color vision.

Siberian ginseng may help alleviate the side effects and enhance recovery in people undergoing chemotherapy and radiation therapy for cancer.

Dosage: Powdered root and rhizomes, 2 or 3 grams per day. Standardized powdered extracts are available, and 300 to 450 milligrams daily are a common dose. Liquid extracts and tinctures are available as well, and are effective. Follow the dosage recommendations on the label.

Cautions: Commission E cautions against using Siberian ginseng if you have high blood pressure. No one seems to understand why they say this, except that two old Russian studies made that recommendation. However, research indicates that, if anything, Siberian ginseng lowers blood pressure. Other studies have shown that it raises low blood pressure and lowers elevated blood pressure.

Products:

Nature's Answer: Siberian Ginseng Root Alcohol Free, 2,000 mg Siberian ginseng root fluid extract per 2 ml, 2 oz liquid.
Solgar: Siberian Ginseng Root Extract, 150 mg Siberian ginseng root extract (0.8% eleuthrosides), and 300 mg Siberian ginseng root powder, 180 vegicaps.

Silicon

Related Items: Horsetail, orthosilicic acid.

Description: Silicon is the most abundant mineral on earth, and it is now recognized as an essential mineral in humans.

Uses: Silicon appears to be involved in maintaining the integrity of the skin, ligaments, tendon, bone, hair, and nails.

Indications: Hair, skin, and nails, osteoporosis.

Silicon seems to be required for collagen and glycosaminoglycan formation. Claims that silicon may be helpful in preventing atherosclerosis are no doubt related to this function.

The exact role played by silicon is yet to be determined, and evidence for its effectiveness is lacking, but anecdotal support abounds. We have seen impressive improvement in nail and hair strength and growth after silicon supplementation. In Europe, the combination of silicon and herbs such as devil's claw is a popular and effective treatment for arthritis.

Dosage: There is no established dose. Amounts ranging from 2 to 20 milligrams have be used.

Products:

Natureworks: Silica Gel Liquid, 420 mg silica from quartz (silicon dioxide), 17 oz liquid.
Solgar: Oceanic Silica, 25 mg elemental silicon from red algae powder, 100 vegicaps.

Soy Isoflavones

Related Items: Soy protein, ipriflavone.

Description: Soy isoflavones are phytoestrogens, plant-derived non-steroidal compounds that resemble estrogen and demonstrate weak estrogenic and weak anti-estrogenic effects. The three main isoflavones in soy are genistein (50%), diadzein (40%), and glycitein (10%).

Uses: Soy isoflavones may help to prevent, and treat, various types of heart disease and cancer. Studies have shown benefit in breast, lung, and prostate cancer,

Indications: Cardiovascular disease, cholesterol problems, cancer, osteoporosis, menopause.

as well as leukemia. Numerous studies have shown that soy isoflavones can lower cholesterol levels. (*See* Soy Protein.)

Soy isoflavones, perhaps due to their weak estrogenic activity, seem to alleviate many of the symptoms of menopause, including hot flashes, and may be very valuable in preventing osteoporosis. (*See* Ipriflavone.)

Studies have shown that long-term soy protein consumption does not affect normal hormone levels in postmenopausal women.

Dosage: The optimal dose is still being determined, but between 50 and 125 milligrams of soy isoflavones are commonly employed.

Products:

Twinlab: Mega Soy, 200 mg soy bean extract (40% isoflavones, 80 mg), providing 40 mg genistin, 31 mg diadzin, and 8 mg glycetin, 60 capsules.
Jarrow: Isoflavone 50, 50 mg isoflavonoid complex providing 25 mg genistein, 18 mg diadzein, and 7 mg glycetein, 60 capsules.
Solgar: Super Concentrated Isoflavones, 38 mg total isoflavones from soy isoflavone extract, 120 tablets.

Soy Protein

Related Item: Soy isoflavones.

Description: Soy protein is marketed as soy protein isolate and contains approximately 90 percent protein. Soy protein is a complete protein, but its biological value is not as high as casein, whey, or egg. When fortified with methionine, its biological value can be enhanced to the equivalent of casein. Soy protein is not only a source of dietary amino acids, but also a source of isoflavones, saponins, and bioactive peptides.

Uses: Diets high in soy protein and low in animal protein lead to a decrease in levels of total cholesterol, LDL cholesterol, and triglycerides. The evidence of this

Indications: Nutritional support, cholesterol problems, cardiovascular disease.

is so convincing that the FDA now allows the following label claim: "Diets low in saturated fat and cholesterol that include 25 grams of soy protein a day may reduce the risk of heart disease."

This beneficial effect on cholesterol and triglycerides seems to be due to a synergistic action of the soy protein, soy isoflavones, and perhaps saponins.

Soy protein isolate can be used as a source of additional dietary protein, necessary for tissue synthesis and repair.

There are other possible benefits associated with the isoflavones in soy protein (*See* Soy Isoflavones).

Products:

Jarrow: Iso-Rich Soy, 25 g protein, 56 mg isoflavones per dose, vanilla flavor, 15.8 oz (449 g).
Nature's Life: Protein 95, 25 grams protein, 69 mg total isoflavones per scoop, vanilla flavor, 1 lb (450 g).

Spirulina

Related Items: Chlorella, green foods, wheat grass, barley grass, chlorophyll, blue green algae.

Description: Spirulina is a type of unicellular blue green algae, or bacteria, that, in spite of the enthusiastic marketing claims to the contrary, can be grouped along with similar supplements as a green food.

All green-food supplements are relatively rich in protein, chlorophyll, gamma-linolenic acid (GLA), and carotenoids.

Uses: Green-food concentrates of this type are claimed to have anticancer activity, modulate immune system function, lower cholesterol, treat gastrointestinal problems, and function, generally, as detoxification agents.

> *Indications:* Immune system, liver disorders, allergies, cholesterol problems, detoxification.

While convincing proof of all of these actions may be lacking, there is certainly no reason not to include one of the green-food concentrates in a comprehensive supplement program. They are all rich in phytonutrients, antioxidants, and varying amounts of trace nutrients. The problem with these supplements is that exaggerated marketing claims often accompany the products, and consumers may overestimate their value. As a general rule, they should be considered adjuncts to other supplements, not replacements or alternatives to them.

Cautions: Green-food supplements may be rich in vitamin K, so caution should be exercised if you are taking anticoagulant medication.

Products:

Nutrex Hawaii: Spirulina Pacifica, 3 g of protein, plus carotenoids and SOD per teaspoon (5 g), 16 oz powder.
Solgar: Spirulina, 750 mg, 2 g of protein, plus 14,000 IU beta-carotene per 4 tablets, 250 tablets.

Squalene

See Alkylglycerol.

St. John's Wort

Description: St. John's wort is a perennial herb native to Europe, North Africa, and western Asia. Medicinally, the dried aboveground parts are used.

Uses: St. John's wort is used as a treatment for mild to moderate depression. This is supported by a long history of usage and numer-

Indications: Depression, anxiety, seasonal affective disorder.

ous clinical studies. Conventional medicine and the regulatory agencies are reluctant to acknowledge its efficacy, demanding more scientifically exacting research, but their caution may be inappropriate.

It was originally thought that hypericin was the active ingredient in St. John's wort; however, there is now some question as to whether that is indeed the case.

Dose: The usual dose for mild to moderate depression is 500 to 1,000 milligrams of the extract per day.

Cautions: St. John's wort is reported to increase the skin's sensitivity to sunlight. Fair-skinned people should exert caution. People with manic-depressive illness (bipolar disorder) should not take St. John's wort unless advised otherwise by a physician.

There is also some concern that St. John's wort may affect the metabolism of certain prescription drugs. It seems that St. John's wort speeds up the liver's detoxification functions. In certain respects, this is beneficial. But it may result in an increased rate of drug metabolism, shortening the life of certain medications. The net result is that certain conventional medications may be less effective when taken in conjunction with St. John's wort. Some examples include contraceptives, HIV medications, and cyclosporine. If you are taking prescription medications, make sure your physician knows that you are also taking St. John's wort.

Products:

Nature's Answer: St. John's Wort, 1,000 mg St. John's wort fluid extract per ml, 1 oz liquid.
Nature's Way: Perika St. John's Wort Extract, 300 mg St. John's wort Extract (WS5572), providing 0.3% hyperformin, 60 tablets.

Sterols

Related Items: Plant sterols, phytosterols, beta-sitosterol, stanols.

Description: Sterols are components of plants, with a structure similar to cholesterol. They are very poorly absorbed from the digestive tract (small intestine).

Uses: Sterols have been shown to lower elevated cholesterol levels. This may be due to inhibition of cholesterol absorption. For this purpose, sterol supplements should be taken with meals.

Sterols have also been shown to be an effective treatment for BPH (benign prostatic hypertrophy). In addition, there is some evidence that sterols can normalize immune system function. Specific conditions that this might benefit include viral infections, rheumatoid arthritis, allergies, cancer, autoimmune diseases.

Products:

Essential Phytosterolins: Moducare, 20 mg plant sterols, 0.2 mg plant sterolins, 90 vegicaps.

Stinging Nettle

Description: Stinging nettle (*Urtica dioica*) is a perennial herb that grows wild throughout the world's temperate zones. The name comes from the hairs that burn or sting. There are two types of stinging nettle supplements. One type is derived from the root, and the other is derived from the herb and leaf, or the aboveground parts.

Uses: The root is used primarily as a treatment for benign prostatic hyperplasia and prostatitis. The leaf is used as a treatment for arthritis and respiratory allergies and can also function as a diuretic.

> *Indications:* Root: Benign prostatic hypertrophy, prostatitis. Leaf and herb: Arthritis, allergies, kidney stones.

Dosage: When treating BPH, 120 milligrams of a concentrated root extract can be taken twice a day. For arthritis, or allergies, take one or two capsules of the leaf concentrate twice a day, or as directed.

Products:

Nature's Answer: Nettle Leaf, 2,000 mg nettle leaf fluid extract per 2 ml, 2 oz liquid.
Solgar: Stinging Nettle Leaf Extract, 275 mg nettle leaf extract,

standardized to 0.1% (3 mg) silicic acid, and 200 mg stinging nettle leaf powder, 60 vegicaps.

Eclectic Institute: Urtica Dioica, 250 mg, 250 mg freeze dried stinging nettle root, 90 capsules.

Gaia Herbs: Nettle Root, 25 mg organically grown stinging nettle root extract per 30 drops, 2 oz liquid.

Taurine

Description: Taurine is a nonprotein amino acid. It is formed in the body as an end product of the metabolism of L-cysteine. It is found in high levels in the brain, retina, and muscle tissue, including heart muscle. Taurine is considered an essential amino acid for infants, and may be necessary for normal retina and brain development.

Uses: Taurine is an antioxidant, and seems to play a role in bile acid production. Taurine has been shown to be of value in treating congestive heart failure,

> *Indications:* Congestive heart failure, cystic fibrosis, epilepsy, liver disorders.

arrhythmias, and possibly hypertension. It has also been shown to be of benefit in cystic fibrosis, reducing the degree of fat malabsorption. There is also a possible role for taurine in treating epileptic seizures.

Dosage: The dose can range from 500 to 6,000 milligrams per day.

Products:

Jarrow: Taurine 1000 mg, pharmaceutical grade, 100 capsules.

Solgar: Taurine, 500 mg, vegetarian and kosher, 250 vegicaps.

Tea Tree Oil

Description: Tea tree oil (*Melaleuca alternifolia*) is derived from the leaves of the tree, a tall evergreen that grows in Australia and Asia. The oil contains numerous terpenoids, with terpinen-4-ol used as a standardization marker, required in concentrations not less than 30 percent of the oil. Another compound, cineole, should not be present at levels over 15 percent.

Uses: Tea tree oil seems to be an effective antifungal and antibacterial agent. It has been

> *Indications:* Fungal infections (topical).

shown to be effective for conditions such as athlete's foot, acne, toe nail fungus, and thrush.

Dosage: The full-strength oil (70 percent to 100 percent) can be applied to the affected area twice a day. For acne, a diluted oil is used (around 10 percent). Tea tree oil is available in several premixed forms for various uses (mouthwash, douche, and so forth), and the directions on the container should be followed carefully.

Cautions: Use caution if treating a large area. Test a small amount for sensitivity first. Do not take tea tree oil internally.

Products:

Desert Essence: Tea Tree Oil, 100%, 2 oz liquid.
Thursday Plantation: Tea Tree Oil, 100%, minimum 36% terpinen-4-ol, 50 ml.

Theanine

Related Item: Green tea extract.

Description: L-theanine is an amino acid found in green tea. It is a derivative of L-glutamic acid, and is thought to be what gives green tea its characteristic flavor.

Uses: Interest in theanine has resulted from research showing that it seems to enhance the activity of some anticancer drugs while protecting noncancerous cells from their side effects. When used in conjunction with chemotherapeutic drugs, it may exert a synergistic and protective action.

Indications: Cancer, anxiety.

Theanine also seems to have a mood-modulating, relaxing effect that may indicate some value in treating stress and anxiety.

Products:

Jarrow: Theanine, 100 mg, 60 capsules.

Thiamine

Description: Thiamine (vitamin B_1) plays a role in the metabolism of carbohydrates and other nutrients, providing energy to all cells in the body. It is directly involved with nerve cell function. A deficiency of Vitamin B_1 results in the condition known as beriberi. The early stage of beriberi causes fatigue, irritation, poor memory, sleep disturbances, precordial pain, anorexia, abdominal discomfort, and constipation. Later, severe peripheral neurologic symptoms appear, initially in the lower legs. The condition was first characterized when it became popular to "polish" rice, that is, remove the outer husk. This resulted in loss of thiamine, and beriberi resulted.

Uses: Marginal thiamine deficiency may be more common than many realize, especially among the elderly and those with chronic illness. Heavy alcohol consumption is known to cause thiamine deficiency as well. In fact, there

> *Indications:* Alzheimer's disease, diabetes, fibromyalgia, chronic fatigue syndrome, nutritional support (elderly), multiple sclerosis.

was a movement in the past to fortify alcholic beverages with thiamine to prevent the condition called Wernicke's encephalopathy.

Because of thiamine's role in carbohydrate metabolism and nerve cell function, supplementation is often recommended for those with diabetes.

Thiamine works in concert with the other B vitamins, and except in special circumstances, a B-complex mixture of B vitamins is the preferred means of supplementation.

Dosage: The recommended daily allowance is as little as 1.5 milligrams, but supplements commonly provide from 25 to 75 milligrams daily. For those wanting higher doses, we suggest taking a fifty-milligram dose twice daily, rather than one 100-milligram dose.

Thiamine is usually present in supplements as the hydrochloride or mononitrate. Both forms are stable and well absorbed, although the higher the dose, the lower the percentage absorbed. A fat-soluble form of thiamine, allithiamine is available, and may be better absorbed at high doses. Normally, there would seem to be little need for that.

Products:

Twinlab: B₁, 500 mg, thiamine mononitrate, 100 capsules.
Solgar: B₁, 50 mg, thiamine hydrochloride, 100 tablets.
Ecological Formulas: Allithiamine, 50 mg thiamine tetrahydro furfuryl disulfide per capsule, 60 capsules.

Thioctic Acid

See Lipoic Acid.

TMG

Related Item: Betaine.

Description: TMG (trimethlglycine) is also known as betaine. It is closely related to choline. It functions biochemically as a methyl donor. It is also involved in the synthesis of the essential amino acid methionine from homocysteine.

Choline has four methyl groups. When choline reacts chemically and donates one of those methyl groups to another molecule, it forms betaine (trimethylglycine). When betaine donates one of its methyl groups, it forms DMG (dimethylglycine).

Uses: In enhancing the conversion of homocysteine to methionine, which requires folic acid, vitamin B_6, and vitamin B_{12}, betaine may lower the risk of heart

> *Indications:* Cholesterol problems, liver disorders, cardiovascular disease.

disease. Betaine and choline may be involved in the prevention of fatty liver, neurotransmitter function, and the metabolism of fat. Agents that facilitate the liver's ability to process fats are called lipotropic agents.

The body manufactures choline from methionine, with the aid of folic acid and vitamin B_{12} as coenzymes.

Another form of betaine often seen in supplement form is betaine hydrochloride. This form is usually used as a source of hydrochloric acid, for digestive problems, rather than as a source of betaine.

Products:

Jarrow: TMG-500, anhydrous betaine, 120 tablets.
Jarrow: TMG Crystals, anhydrous betaine, one teaspoon equals 2.6 g, 50 g.
Source Naturals: TMG, 750 mg, 120 tablets.

Tocotrienols

Related Item: Vitamin E.

Description: Vitamin E is composed of two types of compounds, tocopherols and tocotrienols. Chemically, they differ in the structure of the side chain, with the tocotrienols having three double bonds and the tocopherols a saturated side chain.

Uses: Tocotrienols have similar activity, in general, to vitamin E. There is some evidence, how-

> *Indications:* Cholesterol problems, cancer (breast).

ever, that the tocotrienols are actually more effective in lowering cholesterol than vitamin E. Tocotrienols have hypocholesterolemic, antiatherogenic, and antithrombotic activity.

Some studies have also shown that tocotrienols may be of value in treating breast cancer.

Tocotrienols are available alone, and in combination with mixed tocopherols. For general supplementation, we recommend using a mixed tocopherol vitamin E supplement that includes tocotrienols. For indications, *see* Vitamin E.

For those with cardiovascular disease or who are at risk of breast cancer, additional tocotrienols may be desirable.

Dosage: The usual dose ranges from 100 to 400 milligrams daily.

Cautions: Those taking blood-thinning medication should be aware that vitamin E may also exert some blood-thinning action. Their prothrombin times should be monitored, and the amount of medication (Coumadin) should be adjusted accordingly.

Products:

Yasoo Health: Vitamin E Factor Tocotrienols, 60 mg gamma tocotrienol, 68 mg total tocotrienols (rice source), and 39 mg vitamin E, 60 softgels.
Solgar: Tocotrienol Complex, 25 mg gamma tocotrienol, 100 IU vitamin E, 60 softgels.

Trametes Versicolor

See Coriolus Versicolor.

Trimethylglycine

See TMG.

Tryptophan

Related Item: 5-HTP.

Description: Tryptophan is an essential amino acid. It is a precursor to serotonin synthesis in the body.

Uses: As a precursor to serotonin, tryptophan may induce sleep, as well as influence mood. It has been recommended for mild depression and as an appetite suppressant. Increasing serotonin intake results in increased melatonin, the natural hormone that regulates the body's sleep cycle.

Cautions: Several years ago, a contaminated batch of tryptophan, manufactured in Japan, was thought to have caused eosinophilia-myalgia. The FDA removed tryptophan from the market, and has refused to rescind that ban, even though the problem may no longer exist.

Turmeric

See Curcumin.

Tyrosine

Description: L-tyrosine is an amino acid. In most instances, the body can synthesize enough tyrosine to fill its needs. Tyrosine is made from phenylalanine, and for those with phenylketonuria, it is an essential amino acid. Tyrosine is a precursor for the synthesis of the catecholamines epinephrine, norepinephrine, and dopamine, as well as the thyroid hormones thyroxine and triiodothyronine.

Uses: Supplemental L-tyrosine has been used as an antidepressant owing to its role as a precursor to the neurotransmitters norepinephrine and dopamine. Research in support of this function has not been overly convincing, with mixed results.

Indications: **Depression.**

Dosage: The typical dose is from 500 to 2,000 milligrams daily, but tyrosine supplementation should best be under the direction of a health professional.

Products:

Solgar: Tyrosine, 500 mg, vegetarian and kosher, 250 vegicaps.

Uva Ursi

Description: Uva ursi *(Arctostaphylos uva ursi)* is an evergeen perennial shrub found in colder, northern climates. It is also known as bearberry, perhaps because bears like to eat its red berries. The active ingredient is thought to be arbutin, a hydroquinone derivative.

Uses: Uva ursi exerts an astringent and antiseptic action in the urinary tract.

> **Indications:** Urinary tract infections.

It is used as a urinary antiinflammatory agent, for the treatment of cystitis, and a treatment for mild infections of the urinary tract.

Dosage: For standardized extracts (20% arbutin), use 700 to 1,000 milligrams, three times a day. A tea can be made by steeping about 3 grams of uva ursi in a cup of boiling water. Take this three or four times daily.

For maximum effect, uva ursi should be used when the urine is alkaline. An alkaline pH can be encouraged by eating a diet rich in dairy products, vegetables, fruits, and potatoes. Or those who do not have high blood pressure (sodium restriction) can take baking soda (sodium bicarbonate).

Cautions: Treatment of a urinary tract infection is a medical problem, and should be done under the supervision of a health professional. Use of uva ursi or baking soda should not be required for more than two weeks.

Products:

Nature's Herbs: Uva Ursi, 500 mg uva ursi leaf, 100 capsules.
Nature's Answer: Uva Ursi, 2,000 mg uva ursi leaf fluid extract in 2 ml, 2 oz liquid.
Nature's Way: Uva Ursi Standardized Extract, 665 mg uva ursi leaf extract (20% arbutin), 300 mg uva ursi leaf per 2 capsules, 60 capsules.

Valerian Root

Description: Valerian root, as the name implies, consists of the underground part of the plant *Valeriana officinalis.* The components have been identified, but those actually responsible for its sedative activity remain undetermined.

Uses: Valerian root has sedative and sleep-promoting action.

> **Indications:** Insomnia.

It is used alone, as a tea, tincture, tablet, or capsule, and in combination with other sedative herbs (hops, lemon balm, passion flower, etc.). The Commission E has officially recognized valerian for restlessness and sleeping disorders based on nervous conditions. Valerian is also reported to be of value in relieving pain and reducing muscle spasms.

Dosage: Valerian is available in a wide variety of dosage forms. Follow the directions on the container.

Products:

Solaray: Valerian Root, 470 mg, 100 capsules.
Nature's Way: Valerian Nightime, 320 mg valerian root extract (0.2% valerenic acid), 160 mg lemon balm leaf extract, odor-free, 100 tablets.
Nature's Answer: Valerian Root, 1,000 mg valerian root fluid extract per ml, 2 oz liquid.

Vanadium

Related Item: Vanadyl sulfate.

Description: Vanadium is a trace mineral that has been shown to be essential in animals, but not yet for humans.

Uses: Vanadium is of interest because it seems to mimic the action of insulin and, in large dosages, may improve glucose control in diabetics. The amounts used in preliminary studies are sufficiently high to raise serious concerns about toxicity. Since no actual deficiency state has been induced in humans, we do not know what the recommended daily intake will be. Estimates are in the range of only 10 to 50 micrograms per day.

Cautions: At this time, the higher doses used by some, including bodybuilders, are not recommended.

Vanadyl Sulfate

Related Item: Vanadium.

Description: Vanadyl sulfate is a form of vanadium used in dietary supplements.

Uses: Vanadium, even as vanadyl sulfate, is very poorly absorbed. It may eventually be shown to be of value to diabetics in controlling blood glucose, but additional research is necessary. For one thing, a dose that is effective while not toxic remains to be determined.

Dosages vary over a wide range (50 to 10,000 micrograms), but the safety of long-term use remains to be determined. Therefore, we suggest using higher doses only when recommended by a health professional.

Products:

Country Life: Vanadyl Sulfate, 5,000 mcg vanadyl sulfate, 90 capsules.

Vinpocetine

Description: Vinpocetine is a derivative of an alkaloid derived from a plant in the periwinkle family (*Vinca minor*).

Uses: Vinpocetine has been used to enhance mental function. It may be helpful in treating or preventing dementia, but additional research is needed. It seems

> **Indications:** Age-related cognitive decline, stroke, mental function, tinnitus.

to enhance memory and learning. It has also been shown to be of benefit in the treatment of stroke, perhaps owing to its powerful cerebral vasodilating and blood-thinning activity.

In many respects, its actions and roles seem similar to those associated with ginkgo biloba.

Cautions: Vinpocetine may add to the effect of anticoagulant medications such as Coumadin (warfarin).

Products:

Jarrow: Vinpocetine, 5 mg, extracted from the periwinkle plant, 100 capsules.

Vitamin A

Related Item: Carotenoids.

Description: Vitamin A is a fat-soluble vitamin. It is actually a group of substances of similar structure. The prominent component is retinol. The term *retinoids* refers to retinol, its metabolites (retinoic acid), and related compounds.

Uses: Vitamin A is essential to embryonic cell differentiation and growth. It is required for vision and the maintenance of the retina and other parts of the eye. It is involved in immune system function,

> **Indications:** Immune system, night blindness, vision problems, skin disorders, cancer, cystic fibrosis, bronchitis, macular degeneration.

and may have certain anticancer roles in the body. It has also been shown to be useful in preventing various skin disorders, and is required for optimal integrity of the mucous membranes. Adequate vitamin A status is necessary for normal reproductive function.

A COMMENT FROM DR. ABEL

Vitamin A is an essential nutrient and is produced in the liver from its precursor, beta-carotene. It can be found naturally in plants or fish oil, and is also available in synthetic forms. Cod liver oil, which also contains vitamin D and essential fats, is an excellent source. Vitamin A is necessary for normal growth, color vision, reproduction, immune function, to avoid dry eye, and is an important fat-soluble antioxidant. Beta-carotene is the best-known representative of the carotenoid family, a group of approximately 600 compounds that are commonly found in fruits and vegetables. In addition to beta-carotene, a precursor to vitamin A, lutein, zeaxanthin, and lycopene are other important carotenoids. Vitamin A was recognized as an essential nutrient when discovered in 1909, but it took another twenty years before it was chemically recognized for its value. Fat-deficient animals develop an inability to grow, weakened immunity, and poor eyesight. Red, inflamed eyes can be quickly reversed by adding cod liver oil to the diet. Some physicians warn about frequent intake of high levels of vitamin A, especially since an article indicated the association of high levels with osteoporotic hip fractures in women (*JAMA*, 2002). However, an eleven-year survey could find only ten cases of vitamin A toxicity in the United States; and those people consumed well over 30,000 IU daily for many years (*Am J Clin Nutr* 1989; 49: 358–71). It was felt that an administration of the precursor beta-carotene was safer, since the body will not produce more vitamin A than is necessary.

Too much vitamin A can lead to toxicity, but too little vitamin A can be equally detrimental. Women who might become pregnant, for example, have been warned, quite rightly, to avoid too much vitamin A, as it may lead to an increased incidence of birth defects. They have been warned to keep their daily intake of vitamin A below 5,000 IU daily. Some actually warn them to avoid vitamin A altogether, and take only carotenoids. This leads to confusion, with some women thinking that they cannot even take more than 5,000 IU of carotenoids. What they forget, unfortunately, is that too little vitamin A causes birth defects as well! Just as it is often a mistake to think that if a little of something is good for you, a larger amount is even better, it is also a mistake to think that if too much of something is bad for you, none at all is even better!

Everyone needs vitamin A, and that includes pregnant and soon-to-be pregnant women. Dosages up to 5,000 IU of preformed vitamin A daily are appropriate for pregnant women. Carotenoids, the substances that can serve as dietary precursors of vitamin A, can be taken in higher amounts. (*See* Carotenoids.) Most supplements contain 15,000 to 25,000 IU of carotenoids.

There are some multivitamin formulations that contain no preformed vitamin A at all. Instead, they rely only on carotenoids to provide the equivalent of 5,000 to 10,000 IU of vitamin A. This may be a mistake. We prefer to have at least part of the vitamin A requirement met by preformed vitamin A.

Note: Vitamin A can be obtained either from preformed vitamin A (vitamin A palmitate, vitamin A acetate, fish oil) or from the dietary precursor to vitamin A, carotenoids (beta-carotene, mixed carotenoids). Both forms are labeled in terms of their vitamin A activity. On labels, the units of activity are IUs, or International Units.

This can lead to confusion, as vitamin A, in high doses, can be toxic while carotenoids are not. If a label states: 8,000 IU of vitamin A (4,000 IU vitamin A palmitate, 4,000 IU natural beta-carotene), this means only 4,000 of the 8,000 IU of vitamin A activity actually comes from preformed vitamin A. It means, as well, that this product can be used by a woman who might become pregnant.

Even though taking higher doses of carotenoids has not been shown to be dangerous, many physicians recommend limiting the total intake of carotenes during pregnancy to under 8,000 to 10,000 IU daily as well. Others feel that higher levels of carotenes are not a problem. Carotenes themselves are safe in high quantities. Bear in mind that one medium-size carrot has 8,000 IU of beta-carotene! The body converts only the amount of carotene to vitamin A that it needs. Taking higher doses of carotene does not mean you are getting more vitamin A. Beyond their role as precursors to vitamin A, carotenes are powerful antioxidants and it is a mistake to reduce your intake of natural carotenoids for fear of vitamin A toxicity.

Dosage: The recommended daily intake of preformed vitamin A is 3,000 to 5,000 IU. Supplements often contain up to 10,000 IU daily, but there is little justification for more than 5,000 IU of that to be supplied by preformed vitamin A. Vitamin A as carotenoids or beta-carotene can be taken in substantially higher amounts.

Vitamin A is present in supplements in two forms: vitamin A palmitate (retinyl palmitate) and vitamin A acetate (retinyl acetate). Both forms are well absorbed. Emulsified and "micellized" forms of vitamin A are available as well, but as the regular form is well absorbed, the advantages claimed for these liquid forms is questionable.

Cautions: Preformed vitamin A (vitamin A acetate, vitamin A palmitate, retinol) can be toxic (hypervitaminosis A) at high levels. Natural carotenes have not been shown to be toxic at high doses. Women who might become pregnant should limit their intake of preformed vitamin A to no more than 5,000 to 8,000 IU daily.

Products:

Twinlab: Allergy A Caps, 10,000 IU vitamin A from retinyl acetate, dry, fish-free, water-dispersed for easier digestion, 100 capsules.
Carlson: Vitamin A, 25,000 IU emulsified, 25,000 IU vitamin A from fish liver oil, 100 softgels.

Vitamin B$_1$

See Thiamine.

Vitamin B$_2$

See Riboflavin.

Vitamin B$_3$

See Niacin.

Vitamin B$_5$

See Pantothenic Acid.

Vitamin B$_6$

See Pyridoxine.

Vitamin B$_{12}$

Related Items: Cobalamin, methylcobalamin.

Description: Vitamin B$_{12}$ is one of the B vitamins. It contains cobalt as might be surmised from its other name, cobalamin. It is one of the most complex of all of the vitamins, and resembles hemoglobin and chlorophyl in structure. It is needed for the proper functioning of all cells, especially those of the nervous system, bone marrow, and gastrointestinal tract. Vitamin B$_{12}$ is required for red blood cell formation, and it works closely with folic acid to form methionine, influencing homocysteine levels.

Uses: Vitamin B$_{12}$ deficiency is associated with pernicious anemia, gastric surgery, chronic illness, and old age. People who are strict vegetarians are very likely to be deficient in vitamin B$_{12}$. People with *H. pylori* infections, HIV, and parasitic infections are often deficient.

> *Indications:* Anemia (pernicious), malabsorption conditions, chronic fatigue syndrome, gastrointestinal disorders, cardiovascular disease, nutritional support (elderly), tinnitus.

For optimal absorption of vitamin B$_{12}$, a substance called intrinsic factor, found in the lining of the stomach, is required. When insufficient levels of intrinsic factor are present, pernicious anemia results.

Unlike the other water-soluble B vitamins, vitamin B$_{12}$ is stored in the body, and it may take some time for the overt symptoms of a deficiency to manifest themselves—sometimes up to five years of low intake or impaired absorption.

Vitamin B$_{12}$ is not found in plants. This is why strict vegetarians, or vegans, are at risk of B$_{12}$ deficiency. Some have claimed that products like spirulina and blue green algae contain vitamin B$_{12}$, but this does not seem to be the case. They contain similar compounds, but these substances do not exhibit vitamin B$_{12}$ activity.

A deficiency manifests itself through impaired nerve and mental function, anemia, and disorders of the lining of the mouth, tongue, and bowels. Often, the symptoms resemble Alzheimer's disease.

Some nutritionists feel that the elderly should all be given vitamin B$_{12}$ on a preventive basis.

Contrary to previous dogma, oral vitamin B_{12} can be an effective supplementation route. Injectable B_{12} is not the only option. It turns out that a small amount of vitamin B_{12} will be absorbed regardless of intrinsic factor status. The higher the dose of oral vitamin B_{12}, the lower the percentage that gets absorbed. But some does. And what has been found is that when a high enough dose is given, sometimes in the 500- to 1,000-microgram range, enough vitamin B_{12} is absorbed to satisfy the body's requirements, and correct a deficiency.

There are several forms of vitamin B_{12} available as supplements. The regular form, also called cyanocobalamin or cobalamin, is available in tablets, capsules, and lozenges. Cyanocobalamin is stable and effective. Another similar form is hydroxocobalamin. Some studies indicate that the hydroxocobalamin form is better retained by the body.

These forms of vitamin B_{12} are converted in the body to one of two active (coenzyme) forms, methylcobalamin and adenosylcobalamin (*see* Dibencozide). Both are also available in supplements. Each of the coenzyme forms of B_{12}, however, participate in different enzyme systems, and we question whether taking one or the other alone is more advantageous than taking a high-potency cobalamin supplement.

The use of sublingual lozenges, or nuggets, as a way of enhancing the absorption of oral vitamin B_{12} has been popularized over the years. Unfortunately, there is little evidence that it works. Vitamin B_{12} is a very large molecule, and one would not logically expect it to be readily absorbed sublingually. Instead, as the lozenge dissolves, the B_{12} is swallowed, and absorbed the same way as are the other forms. There is no harm in taking vitamin B_{12} in lozenge form, but there may be no advantage in doing so.

Dosage: The recommended daily intake is from 2.4 to 6 micrograms, but oral supplementation is usually given in doses from 100 up to 5,000 micrograms. Vitamin B_{12} is nontoxic and safe at high doses.

Products:

Twinlab: B_{12} Dots, 500 mcg, 250 lozenges.
Solgar: B_{12} Nuggets, 1,000 mcg, 250 tablets.
Solgar: B_{12} Megasorb Nuggets, 5,000 mcg, 5,000 mcg cobalamin and 100 mcg dibencozide, 60 tablets.

Vitamin C

Related Items: Buffered vitamin C; magnesium ascorbate; calcium ascorbate; ascorbyl palmitate; ester-C.

Description: Vitamin C (ascorbic acid) is a water-soluble vitamin with numerous functions. To be most precise, it is the L-form, L-ascorbic acid, that possess vitamin activity. A powerful antioxidant, vitamin C protects against oxidative damage throughout the body. It also enhances the activity of other antioxidant vitamins. Vitamin C is needed in the formation of collagen, the main protein essential to the integrity of connective tissue, cartilage, bone matrix, tooth dentin, skin, and tendons

---

A COMMENT FROM DR. ABEL

Not only does ascorbic acid (vitamin C) help build collagen and capillaries, but it has the ability to provide extra electrons to all of your cells. Since vitamin C is water soluble, it can travel throughout your body and provide reinforcements for your cell membrane antioxidants (SOD, glutathione, and vitamin E). All of these antioxidants work in concert in order to deal with the scavenger free radicals that are constantly around. Vitamin C also helps build such tissues as your cornea and your heart valves, and you never know if you are getting enough. Too much vitamin C (3,000, 5,000, or 10,000 milligrams for some people) can cause diarrhea. If this occurs, simply reduce the dose.

Uses: There are several different forms of vitamin C. Some, like the D-ascorbic acid, or erythorbic acid, which is often added to foods as an antioxidant, actually have little vitamin C activity.

> *Indications:* Cancer, cataracts, cold and flu, cholesterol problems, cardiovascular disease, hypertension, *Helicobacter pylori*, asthma, stress.

Other forms of vitamin C that can be found in nutritional supplements are: buffered vitamin C, vitamin C with bioflavonoids, effervescent vitamin C, acerola vitamin C, rose hip vitamin C, Ester-C, and ascorbyl palmitate.

Infections, cold, and flu: Vitamin C has been shown to be effective in treating various viral infections, including, according to many complementary physicians, chronic fatigue syndrome, hepatitis, herpes, and AIDS. While vitamin C's ability to protect against, or cure, the common cold remains somewhat controversial, there seems to be no question that it reduces the severity of the symptoms and the duration.

Heart disease: Vitamin C protects against heart disease by preventing the oxidation of LDL cholesterol, which can then turn into atherosclerotic plaque.

Stress: Vitamin C is involved in adrenal cortical hormone production and function. During periods of emotional, psychological, or physiologic stress, levels of these hormones are increased, and urinary excretion of vitamin C is increased. During periods of stress, therefore, supplementation with vitamin C may be helpful.

Cancer: There is evidence that vitamin C can prevent certain cancers, such as gastric, breast, and cervical cancers, perhaps owing to its protective antioxidant action, for example, blocking the creation of nitrosamine from nitrates. Many complementary physicians utilize vitamin C as part of their cancer treatment protocols; it is thought to lengthen survival time and improve quality of life.

Bruising, capillary fragility, hemorrhoids, varicose veins: Vitamin C, especially when administered with bioflavanoids, is recommended for these problems owing to its role in strengthening and tonifying the vessel wall.

Glaucoma, cataracts, vision disorders: Vitamin C is one of the antioxidants that protects the eye from free radical oxidative damage; high doses of vitamin C have been shown in several studies to reduce elevated intraocular pressure.

There are many additional conditions that may benefit from vitamin C supplementation: gout, gallstones, asthma, allergies, bronchitis, gingivitis, periodontal disease, wound healing, autism, cold sores, diabetes, gastritis, immune function, iron-deficiency anemia, lead toxicity, among others.

Dosage: The recommended daily allowance for vitamin C is from 75 to 90 milligrams for nonsmokers, and 110 to 125 milligrams for smokers. The amounts typically found in supplements will provide between 500 and 1,000 milligrams daily, although some claim that 200 milligrams are enough to ensure maximum tissue levels. Many take much higher amounts. Some, for example, take 4 to 5 grams daily to ameliorate the symptoms of a cold. Some of the research studies have used doses in the 5-gram daily range. Daily intakes up to 2 or 3 grams a day are generally considered benign. Too high a dose will result in diarrhea.

Cautions: The only consistent adverse effect of high dose vitamin C is gastric upset or diarrhea. Because the normal catabolism of vitamin C leads to oxalate, there is concern that high doses of vitamin C could increase the risk of kidney stones. Clinically, this does not seem to be the case, but those with a history of oxalate stone formation should consult with their physician before taking doses over 1 gram.

Products:

Solgar: Vitamin C, 1,000 mg, L-ascorbic acid, 100 vegicaps.
Allergy Research: Pure Vitamin C, 2,000 mg ascorbic acid (beet source) per half teaspoon, 120 g powder.

Vitamin C with Bioflavonoids

Related Item: Vitamin C.

Description: Vitamin C is often presented in supplements with bioflavonoids. The most common flavonoids used in these products are citrus bioflavonoids, although a wide variety of mixtures can be employed.

Uses: There is a persistent belief that vitamin C and bioflavonoids work synergistically together. While both vitamin C and the various flavonoids have many actions totally independent of each other, they also share many functions. They are both powerful antioxidants. They often occur together in nature. The flavonoids have historically been thought to strengthen blood capillaries, along with vitamin C.

Vitamin C is good, flavonoids are good, they are found together in food, and it makes sense to take them together in supplements as well.

Products:

Solgar: Hy-Bio, 500 mg vitamin C, 500 mg citrus bioflavonoids, 50 mg rutin and 50 mg rose hips fruit, 250 tablets. Note: One of the highest level of bioflavonoids in a combination product.
Twinlab: C-Plus Citrus Bioflavonoids, 1,000 mg vitamin C, 650 mg citrus bioflavonoids, 50 mg rutin per 2 capsules, 250 capsules.

Vitamin D

Description: Vitamin D can be considered both a vitamin and a hormone. There are two forms of vitamin D found in food, vitamin D_2

(ergocalciferol) and vitamin D_3 (cholecalciferol). Our body can produce vitamin D through the action of sunlight on the skin.

Ergocalciferol (D_2) is derived from plants, and cholecalciferol (D_3) is derived from animal sources. For those who prefer a nonanimal source, D_2 supplements are available.

Uses: A deficiency of vitamin D results in rickets (children) or osteomalacia (adults). It is caused by an inability to incorporate calcium in bone. This was once a

> *Indications:* Osteoporosis, Crohn's disease, cystic fibrosis, osteomalacia.

common problem, but now usually seen only in elderly people who fail to get adequate exposure to sunlight.

While vitamin D is usually associated with the absorption of calcium and bone status, it also seems to have a role in the prevention of breast and colon cancer. It may also have some influence on the prevention of diabetes, multiple sclerosis, and general immune system function.

Dosage: For those who are frequently exposed to sunlight, supplemental vitamin D may be unnecessary. For most, however, 400 IU per day are recommended. Those who at risk, such as the elderly and those not exposed to sunlight, should be taking 800 IU daily.

Products:

Solgar: Vitamin D, 400 IU, 400 IU vitamin D_3 (cholecalciferol) and 1,000 IU vitamin A from fish liver oil, 100 softgels.
Twinlab: Allergy D Caps, 400 IU, fish-free, water-dispersed vitamin D_3, 100 capsules.

Vitamin E

Related Items: Tocopherol, tocotrienol, dry vitamin E, mixed tocopherols.

Description: Vitamin E is a collective term for a family of substances that includes four tocopherols (alpha, beta, gamma and delta) and four tocotrienols (alpha, beta, gamma, and delta). Vitamin E is a fat-soluble vitamin and a powerful antioxidant. In the case of vitamin E, there is a difference in activity between natural and synthetic forms. New evidence indicated that the natural form may actually be twice as active as the synthetic form.

Uses: Vitamin E is an important antioxidant. Because it is fat-soluble, it exerts its protective effect very efficiently at the cell membrane (which contains a high proportion of fat) level. Vitamin E is now recognized, even by mainstream medicine, as protective against cardiovascular disease

> **Indications:** Anti-aging, cardiovascular disease, immune system, cancer, asthma, arthritis, cataracts, Alzheimer's disease, skin conditions (topical), tardive dyskinesia, diabetes.

and some forms of cancer. It may also be of some benefit to those with rheumatoid arthritis, asthma, neurological diseases, cataracts, diabetes, and premenstrual syndrome. It can protect against environmental toxins and enhances immune system function.

For historical and regulatory purposes, the potency of vitamin E is related to one form, alpha tocopherol. But each form of vitamin E has value, and some are more beneficial than others depending on the function. Alpha tocotrienol, for example, may have higher antitumor activity than alpha tocopherol, even though the latter has higher "vitamin E" activity.

Here are the choices available to you for vitamin E supplements:

- *Natural or synthetic.* The natural forms of vitamin E can be identified by the prefix "d-" (d-alpha tocopheryl acetate) and the synthetic form has the prefix "dl-" (dl-alpha tocopheryl acetate). The natural form is generally twice as potent as the synthetic form.
- *Esterified or unesterified.* When the form of vitamin E ends in "- ol," it is the unesterified, free form (tocopherol), and when it ends in "-yl" it is the esterified form, either an acetate ester or a succinate ester (tocopheryl acetate). The esterified forms are more stable.
- *Alpha tocopherol only or the mixture of all of the tocopherols.* Mixed tocopherols consist of a mixture of all four tocopherols (alpha, beta, gamma, and delta). They can also contain the four tocotrienols. The labeled potency, in IU, only refers to alpha tocopherol, but each of the eight isomers has activity, and some have different actions.
- *Tocopherols or tocotrienols.* As already mentioned, there are four tocopherols and four tocotrienols in the vitamin E family of compounds. The tocotrienols have different activity, and may be uniquely beneficial in treating cardiovascular disease and certain types of cancer.

Here is our recommendation: Natural vitamin E (the d- form) is superior to the synthetic form (the dl- form). The esterified form, the acetate or succinate, is preferred as a supplement because it is more stable. The mixed tocopherol form, however, while not esterified, is superior because it contains the three other isomers of vitamin E, and a mixed tocopherol with tocotrienols is even better.

So we suggest a mixed tocopherol and tocotrienol complex as the best form of vitamin E supplement.

Dosage: The current situation regarding the labeling of alpha tocopherol activity is very confusing. Forget it. Instead, an appropriate dose of natural vitamin E supplements should be from 100 to 400 IU daily. If using the synthetic form, it should be 200 to 800 IU daily. Doses up to 800 IU of natural vitamin E are acceptable when indicated. Even though vitamin E is a fat-soluble vitamin, it has an excellent safety record.

Cautions: Those taking blood-thinning medication should be aware that vitamin E may also exert some blood-thinning action. Their prothrombin times should be monitored, and the amount of medication (Coumadin) should be adjusted accordingly.

Products:

Yasoo Health: Vitamin E Factor 400/400, 400 IU vitamin E as d-alpha tocopherol, 400 mg beta, gamma, and delta tocopherols, 31 mg gamma tocotrienol, 5 mg alpha, beta, and delta tocotrienols, 60 softgels.
Solgar: E 400 Mixed Tocopherols, 400 IU vitamin E as d-alpha tocopherol, plus beta, gamma, and delta tocopherols, 250 softgels.
Solgar: E 400 Dry, 400 IU vitamin E as d-alpha tocopheryl succinate, 250 vegicaps.
Carlson: E Gems 400 IU, 400 IU vitamin E as d-alpha tocopheryl acetate, 200 softgels.
Allergy Research: Vitamin E, 400 IU, synthetic vitamin E, dl-alpha tocopheryl acetate (hypoallergenic), 120 softgels.

Vitamin K

Description: Vitamin K is essential for proper blood clotting. The "K" is derived from the German word *Koagulation*, which means clotting. Vitamin K is available in three forms. The natural form, Vitamin K_1 (phylloquinone or phytonadione), found in green leafy vegetables, is the preferred type, as it seems to have the broadest activity.

Uses: A deficiency of vitamin K is rare, but can occur in those who do not eat vegetables, are on long-term anticoagulant and/or

> *Indications:* Nutritional support, osteoporosis, malabsorption conditions.

antibiotic therapy, or suffer from various types of malabsorption conditions or liver disease.

There is some interest in the role of vitamin K in osteoporosis. It is involved in bone formation, and evidence is accumulating that those who might be low in vitamin K have increased osteoporosis.

Dosage: For general supplementation, usually as part of a broad-spectrum multivitamin product, amounts of vitamin K between 50 and 100 micrograms are recommended. The recommended daily value is 80 micrograms.

The preferable form of vitamin K in supplements is vitamin K_1 (or phylloquinone). It is also present in oil-soluble chlorophyll supplements.

Cautions: Those taking anticoagulant medications (warfarin, Coumadin) should avoid supplementation, especially at doses over the daily value (80 micrograms), without notifying their physician.

Products:

Solgar: Vitamin K, 100 mcg, phytonadione, 250 tablets.
Orjene: Vitamin K Cream, 2% phytonadione cream, 60 grams.

Vitex

See Chaste Tree Berry.

Western Larch

See Larch, Western.

Wheat Grass

Related Items: Spirulina, green foods, chlorella, chlorophyll, blue green algae.

Description: As with all green-food supplements, wheat grass concentrate is relatively rich in protein, chlorophyll, and carotenoids. Marketing claims to the contrary, there is little documented therapeutic difference among these products.

Uses: Green food concentrates of this type are claimed to have anti-cancer activity, modulate immune system function, lower cholesterol, treat gastrointestinal problems, and function, generally, as detoxification agents.

While convincing proof of all these actions may be lacking, there is certainly no reason not to include one of the green food concentrates in a comprehensive supplement program. They are all rich in phytonutrients, antioxidants, and varying amounts of trace nutrients. The problem with these supplements is that exaggerated marketing claims often accompany the products, and consumers may overestimate their value. As a general rule, they should be considered adjuncts to other supplements, not replacements or alternatives to them.

Cautions: Green food supplements may be rich in vitamin K, so caution should be exercised if you are taking anticoagulant medication.

Products:

Pines: Wheat Grass Powder, 2 teaspoons equal one large serving of green leafy vegetable, 10 oz powder.

Whey Protein

Description: There are two main types of protein in milk. The most plentiful type is casein, which is easily precipitated (curds) in making cheese. The soluble protein fraction, whey, has a higher biological value and remains after the curd (casein) is removed.

As the water, fat, and lactose are removed, a whey protein concentrate is obtained. Such concentrates can contain up to 80 percent whey protein, with the balance consisting mostly of lactose. Further removal of the remaining lactose results in highly purified, high-protein whey isolates.

Uses: Whey protein can be used for two purposes. As a protein, a source of amino acids that are the building blocks for almost

Indications: Nutritional support, immune system.

all parts of the body, whey is one of the highest-quality sources available. The higher the quality of protein, the less amount one needs to fulfill the body's requirements. Whey is relatively bland in flavor, and easily tolerated, making it an ideal protein supplement for those who need general nutritional support, and those who need additional protein for bodybuilding and athletic purposes.

The other use for whey protein revolves around its possible immunomodulating and antimicrobial activity. This is related to certain specific components of whey, such as lactoferrin, various immunoglobulins, bovine serum albumin, etc.

These compounds are thought to exert their beneficial actions in different ways. The lactoferrin, for example, binds iron. Iron is a nutrient essential to microbial growth. So by depriving pathogenic bacteria of the iron they need for growth, lactoferrin-containing whey protein may exert antimicrobial activity. Whey contains precursor components to glutathione, and by increasing glutathione levels, whey may affect immune function. The immunoglobulins in whey function as antibodies. When immunoglobulins are made in our body, in response to various antigens, it is called active immunity. When the immunoglobulins are obtained from an external source, as from whey protein, it is called passive immunity.

There are three types of whey protein isolates now being marketed:

1. Ion-exchange.
2. Microfiltration or ultrafiltration.
3. Cross-flow microfiltration.

The proponents of each type claim theirs is superior to the others.

Arguing that one is better than the other, as an immunomodulating agent, because it contains more glutathione precursors, seems pointless. One type yields more lactoferrin, but less serum albumin. The other yields more serum albumin and less lactoferrin. If it is the lactoferrin that is so important, why not take a lactoferrin supplement? If it is the glutathione precursors that are so important, why not just take a glutathione supplement?

As a source of high-quality protein, the isolation process is of no consequence. The same is probably true for whey's other purposes as well. The heightened interest in whey's possible anticancer and immune-enhancing action is exciting, but preliminary.

Products:

Bioplex Nutrition: Pure Whey Protein Isolate, 22.2 g whey protein isolate, providing 20 g protein, no fat or carbohydrate, 5570 mg.

BCAAs (branched chain amino acids) per scoop, 2 lb powder (908 g). Note: This product positioned as a post-workout supplement. **Jarrow: Whey Protein,** 23 g whey protein, providing 18 g protein, 4600 mg BCAAs per scoop, and 51% beta lactoglobulin, 20% alpha lactalbumin, 10% immunoglobulin, 2 lb powder (908 g). Note: This product positioned as post-workout and immune-enhancing supplement.

Willow Bark

Description: The bark of young willow tree branches is the source of this herbal supplement. The bark contains natural salicylates, which account for its anti-inflammatory, fever-reducing, and analgesic activity. Salicin is the primary salicylate present. These natural salicylates, first isolated from the plant meadowsweet, are the precursors to the drug acetylsalicylic acid, commonly known as aspirin.

Uses: Willow bark (*Salix alba*) is used as an analgesic, anti-inflammatory, and antipyretic (fever-reducing) agent. Natural

> *Indications:* Pain, arthritis, sports injuries, bursitis.

salicylic acid is thought to produce fewer side effects than synthetic acetylsalicylic acid (aspirin).

Like aspirin, the salicin in willow bark is thought to exert its analgesic action by blocking prostaglandin synthesis.

Dosage: Typically, an amount of herbal extract is used that is equivalent to between 60 and 120 milligrams of total salicin daily. Follow the directions on the label. Willow bark is available as dry extract (capsules), as well as tinctures and teas.

Cautions: Some caution that willow bark preparations should not be used by small children with the flu (Reye's syndrome), but this may not be a valid concern. The salicylates in willow are not metabolized in the same way as aspirin (acetylsalicylic acid). Follow your doctor's advice.

Products:

Nature's Answer: White Willow Bark, 200 mg white willow bark extract (15% salicin), 200 mg white willow bark powder, 60 vegicaps.
Nature's Answer: White Willow Bark Alcohol Free, 2,000 mg white willow bark fluid extract per 2 ml, 1 oz liquid.

Yohimbe Bark

Description: Yohimbe (*Pausinystalia yohimbe*) is a tall evergreen forest tree, native to Africa. Its main constituent is an indole alkaloid, yohimbine, and most of the research has been on yohimbine rather than yohimbe bark.

Uses: The bark has been used traditionally in western Africa as an aphrodisiac, especially for male erectile problems. There is

> *Indications:* Sexual performance.

evidence that yohimbine is effective in some cases of impotence, but isolated yohimbine is very drug-like, with side effects and contraindications to match. There is a lack of positive research on the crude bark. There is also some question as to the integrity of some of the yohimbe bark products on the store shelves, many of which have been found to contain little if any yohimbine.

Dosage: Follow directions on the bottle.

Cautions: Yohimbine can cause nervousness, tremor, sleeplessness, anxiety, increased blood pressure, rapid heartbeat, dizziness, nausea, and vomiting. Do not use yohimbe in the presence of liver and kidney disease, peptic ulcer, or inflammation of the prostate. If taking antidepressant medication, do not take yohimbe unless under the supervision of a physician.

Products:

Twinlab: Yohimbe Fuel, 400 mg yohimbe bark extract (8% yohimbine alkaloids), 100 capsules.
Country Life: Yohimbe Power 1000, 1,000 mg yohimbe bark (4% yohimbine alkaloids, 90 capsules.

Zeaxanthin

Related Items: Carotenoids, lutein.

Description: Zeaxanthin is one of the xanthophyll carotenoids. Lutein is another. The carotenoids, or carotenes, are the red, orange, and yellow plant pigments that protect against oxidative damage during photosynthesis. There are more than 600 carotenoids in nature.

Uses: The macula of the eye contains very high concentrations of lutein and zeaxanthin. These carotenoids protect the macula

> *Indications:* Cataracts, macular degeneration.

from the harmful effects of ultraviolet light. Studies have shown that older people with the highest intake of carotenoids have the lowest rate of age-related macula degeneration. The lutein and zeaxanthin in supplements are often made from marigolds.

Zinc

Related Item: Zinc lozenges.

Description: Zinc is an essential mineral. It is involved in the function of hundreds of different enzymes throughout the body. It is required for the proper function of many of the important hormones, and is involved in growth and energy production. While severe zinc deficiency is rare in developed countries, mild to moderate deficiency is common, especially among the elderly. The average American diet, for example, does not provide the recommended daily level of zinc.

Uses: Zinc is important for proper immune system function. Several studies have shown that zinc, in the form of a lozenge, reduces the duration of the common cold in adults.

Indications: Alzheimer's disease, benign prostatic hypertrophy, cancer (prostate), cold and flu, fertility (male), immune system, macular degeneration, night blindness, sexual performance, wound healing.

Zinc is essential for growth, and seems to play a role in promoting or accelerating wound healing.

Preliminary research indicates zinc may be protective against prostate cancer. It has long been used by those with benign prostatic hypertrophy, and is also thought to be involved in male fertility, prostate, and sexual function.

Zinc is involved in maintaining optimal vision, taste, and smell. Poor night vision, for example, is one sign of zinc deficiency, as is loss of taste.

Zinc has also been used as a treatment for acne. Not all studies have shown zinc to be effective, but this may be due to the type of zinc used.

Zinc's benefit to those with vision problems, including macular degeneration, continues to garner support. Studies that include zinc along with other antioxidants have supported its role for this condition.

There is also some evidence that a zinc deficiency contributes to Alzheimer's disease. As already mentioned, moderate zinc deficiency is common among the elderly. Some research has shown that zinc supplementation in those who already have Alzheimer's disease results in improvement.

Dosage: The general range of zinc dosage is between 15 to 30 milligrams. When zinc is used therapeutically, amounts up to 60 milligrams daily are commonly recommended by health professionals. The amount of zinc in lozenges intended for treating the common cold ranges from 13 to 25 milligrams. These lozenges can be taken every 2 hours, but should be limited to two or three days only.

Too much zinc, over an extended period of time, can result in depressed copper levels. This is because zinc competes with copper for absorption. As little as 2 milligrams of copper daily, an amount in most multivitamin supplements, may be all that is needed to prevent this problem.

There are many different forms of zinc available in supplements. Some, like zinc oxide, are generally considered to be poorly absorbed, and supplements containing this form of zinc should be avoided. Zinc sulfate may be slightly better than oxide, but it is not as good as other forms of zinc, and should also be avoided. Zinc gluconate, zinc citrate, zinc chelate (amino acid), zinc picolinate, and similar organic compounds of zinc are the preferred forms. For zinc lozenges, so far the best results have been obtained with zinc gluconate.

If there are differences between the forms of zinc recommended above, the differences seem to be small, while the improvement over the inorganic oxide and sulfate form seems to be what is important.

Cautions: If taking high levels of zinc for an extended period of time, be sure to include at least 2 milligrams of copper in your supplement program.

Products:

Ethical Nutrients: Zinc Status Liquid, 2.4 mg zinc sulfate per 10 ml, 4 oz. After placing 10 ml in the mouth, a lack of taste or a delayed taste perception suggests a possible zinc insufficiency.

Zinc Chelate

Related Item: Zinc.

Description: Zinc chelate, or zinc amino acid chelate, or zinc glycinate are forms of zinc intended for use in dietary supplements. Zinc is complexed with organic compounds, usually amino acids, to form a chelate that is more readily absorbed by the body than inorganic forms of zinc such as the sulfate and oxide.

Uses: Zinc is important for proper immune system function. It is essential for growth and seems to play a role in promoting or accelerating wound healing.

Preliminary research indicates zinc may be protective against prostate cancer. It has long been used by those with benign prostatic hypertrophy and is also thought to be involved in male fertility, and prostate and sexual function.

Zinc is involved in maintaining optimal vision, taste, and smell. Poor night vision, for example, is one sign of zinc deficiency, as is loss of taste. Zinc's benefit to those with vision problems, including macular degeneration, continues to garner support. Studies that include zinc along with other antioxidants have supported its role for this condition.

Zinc has also been used as a treatment for acne. Some evidence also exists that a zinc deficiency contributes to Alzheimer's disease. It is well known that moderate zinc deficiency is common among the elderly. Some research has shown that zinc supplementation in those who already have Alzheimer's disease results in improvement.

Products:

Solgar: Chelated Zinc, 22 mg zinc glycinate, 250 tablets.
Natrol: OptiZinc 30, mg, zinc monomethionine, 120 capsules.

Zinc Gluconate

Related Item: Zinc.

Description: Zinc gluconate is a form of zinc used in nutritional supplements. A gluconate is a mineral-glucose compound that is absorbed better than inorganic zinc salts such as zinc oxide or zinc sulfate.

Uses: Zinc is important for proper immune system function. It is essential for growth and seems to play a role in promoting or accelerating wound healing.

Preliminary research indicates zinc may be protective against prostate cancer. It has long been used by those with benign prostatic hypertrophy and is also thought to be involved in male fertility, and prostate and sexual function.

Zinc is involved in maintaining optimal vision, taste, and smell. Poor night vision, for example, is one sign of zinc deficiency, as is loss of taste. Zinc's benefit to those with vision problems, including macular degeneration, continues to garner support. Studies that include zinc along with other antioxidants have supported its role for this condition.

Zinc has also been used as a treatment for acne. Some evidence also exists that a zinc deficiency contributes to Alzheimer's disease. It is well known that moderate zinc deficiency is common among the elderly. Some research has shown that zinc supplementation in those who already have Alzheimer's disease results in improvement.

Products:

Solgar: Zinc "50," 50 mg zinc gluconate, 100 tablets.
Twinlab: Zinc Caps, 50 mg, zinc gluconate and zinc picolinate, 180 capsules.

Zinc Lozenges

Related Item: Zinc.

Description: Zinc lozenges are supplements containing zinc, usually as zinc gluconate, gluconate/glycinate, or acetate, intended to be dissolved in the mouth.

Uses: Zinc lozenges are specifically intended for use as a treatment for the common cold. Several studies have shown that zinc lozenges are indeed effective in this regard, especially if the form of zinc mentioned above is used. The product may exert a direct antiviral action in the throat.

The use of the term *homeopathic* in conjuction with this type of product seems to be more of a marketing gimmick than anything else. Homeopathic remedies for the cold or flu are fine, and often effective. But zinc lozenges, with zinc levels between 13 and 25 milligrams, are not homeopathic preparations.

Dosage: One lozenge, dissolved in the mouth, every two hours, for two or three days.

Cautions: Zinc lozenges are not intended for long-term use. With the intended purpose of limiting the duration and severity of the common cold, there should be no reason to continue taking zinc lozenges for more than two or three days, at most.

Products:

Country Life: Zinc Lozenges Lemon Flavor, 23 mg zinc gluconate and citrate, and 100 mg vitamin C, 120 lozenges.
Twinlab: Zinc Lozenges Cherry Flavor, 23 mg zinc gluconate, and 30 mg Vitamin C, 75 lozenges.

Zinc Picolinate

Related Item: Zinc.

Description: Zinc picolinate is a form of zinc used in nutritional supplements. It is a complex formed by reacting picolinic acid, a natural metabolite found in breast milk, related to the B-vitamin niacin, with zinc. Zinc picolinate is absorbed better than inorganic zinc salts such as zinc oxide or sulfate.

Uses: Zinc is important for proper immune system function. Zinc is essential for growth and seems to play a role in promoting or accelerating wound healing.

Preliminary research indicates zinc may be protective against prostate cancer. It has long been used by those with benign prostatic hypertrophy and is also thought to be involved in male fertility, and prostate and sexual function.

Zinc is involved in maintaining optimal vision, taste, and smell. Poor night vision, for example, is one sign of zinc deficiency, as is loss of taste. Zinc's benefit to those with vision problems, including macular degeneration, continues to garner support. Studies that include zinc along with other antioxidants have supported its role for this condition.

Zinc has also been used as a treatment for acne. Some evidence also exists that a zinc deficiency contributes to Alzheimer's disease. It is well known that moderate zinc deficiency is common among the elderly. Some research has shown that zinc supplementation in those who already have Alzheimer's disease results in improvement.

Products:

Solgar: Zinc Picolinate, 22 mg, vegetarian and kosher, 100 tablets.
NOW Foods: Zinc Picolinate, 50 mg, 120 capsules.

THERAPEUTIC CROSS-REFERENCE

The following cross-reference is intended to help you pick out the appropriate supplements to use for a certain purpose, such as treating a disorder. To use the cross-reference, first find the purpose in the list, then read across for the suggested supplements. For more information on the supplements, look them up alphabetically in Chapter 5 (individual nutrients and herbs) and Chapter 6 (combination supplements).

Age-related cognitive decline. *See* Ginkgo biloba; Phosphatidylserine; Vinpocetine.

Allergies. *See* Grape seed extract; Hesperidin; Quercetin; Spirulina; Stinging nettle leaf.

Allergies, food. *See* Probiotics.

Alzheimer's disease. *See* Acetyl-L-carnitine; CDP-choline; Choline; Folic acid; Ginkgo biloba; Huperzine A; Lecithin; Phosphatidylcholine; Phosphatidylserine; Thiamine (vitamin B_1); Vitamin E; Zinc.

Anemia, iron deficiency. *See* Iron.

Anemia, pernicious. *See* Vitamin B_{12}.

Angina, hypertension. *See* CoQ$_{10}$.

Anti-aging. *See* 7-keto DHEA; Acetyl-L-carnitine; Carnosine; Cordyceps; DHEA; Ginseng; Grape seed extract; Huperzine A; Lipoic acid; Vitamin E.

Anxiety. *See* 5-HTP; Inositol; Kava kava; St. John's wort; Theanine.

Appetite, loss of. *See* Devil's claw; Fenugreek.

Arthritis. *See* Alkylglycerol; Ashwagandha; Boron; Boswellia; Bovine cartilage; Bromelain; Cartilage; Cat's claw; Cetyl myristoleate (CMO); Chondroitin; Curcumin; Devil's claw; Flaxseed oil; Ginger; Glucosamine; Grape seed extract; Green tea extract; Green-lipped mussel extract; Propolis; Sea cucumber; Stinging nettle leaf.

Arthritis, osteo. *See* Manganese; Niacinamide (vitamin B_3).

Arthritis, rheumatoid. *See* Borage oil; Evening primrose oil; Fish oil; Pantothenic acid (vitamin B_5).

Asthma. *See* Beta-carotene; Boswellia; Bromelain; Coleus forskohlii; Cordyceps; Ginkgo biloba; Magnesium; Pyridoxine (vitamin B_6); Quercetin; Vitamin C; Vitamin E.

Asthma, sulfite sensitivity. *See* Molybdenum.

Athletic performance. *See* Arginine; Carnitine; Conjugated linoleic acid (CLA); Cordyceps; Creatine; Ginseng; Glutamine; HMB (beta-Hydroxy beta-MethylButyrate); Ornithine, Ornithine alpha-ketoglutarate (OKG); Pyruvate; Siberian ginseng.

Autism. *See* Pyridoxine (vitamin B_6).

Benign prostatic hypertrophy. *See* Beta-sitosterol; Flower pollen; Genistein; Pygeum; Saw palmetto; Stinging nettle root; Zinc.

Bronchitis. *See* N-acetyl cysteine (NAC); Vitamin A.

Burns. *See* Aloe vera gel.

Bursitis. *See* Willow bark.

Cancer. *See* Alkylglycerol; Astragalus; Beta-1,3-glucan; Beta-carotene; Bovine cartilage; Broccoli extract; Cartilage; Cat's claw; Chlorophyll; Conjugated linoleic acid (CLA); Cordyceps; Coriolus versicolor extract (PSK); Curcumin; Folic acid; Garlic; Ginseng; Glutathione; Grape seed extract; Green foods; Green tea extract; Lycopene; Maitake mushroom; Molybdenum; Polyphenols; Selenium; Soy isoflavones; Theanine; Vitamin A; Vitamin C.

Cancer, breast. *See* Genistein; Indole-3-carbinol; Siberian ginseng; Tocotrienols.

Cancer, cervical. *See* Indole-3-carbinol.

Cancer, colon. *See* Calcium; Fiber; FOS (fructo-oligosaccharides).

Cancer, prostate. *See* Genistein; Green tea extract; Lycopene; Modified citrus pectin; Shiitake mushroom; Zinc.

Candidiasis. *See* Barberry; Caprylic acid; Probiotics; Rosemary leaf.

Canker Sores. *See* Deglycyrrhizinated licorice (DGL); Goldenseal; Oregon grape; Riboflavin (vitamin B_2).

Cardiovascular disease. *See* Acetyl-L-carnitine; Arginine; Beta-carotene; Betaine; Bilberry; Black currant seed oil; Carnitine; CDP-choline; Coleus forskohlii; Conjugated linoleic acid (CLA); Copper; CoQ_{10}; Creatine; Curcumin; Fiber; Fish oil; Folic acid; Garlic; Grape seed extract; Green tea extract; Hawthorn; Hesperidin; Lycopene; Magnesium; N-acetyl cysteine (NAC); Pantethine; Phytosterols and phytostanols; Polyphenols; Potassium; Pyridoxine (vitamin B_6); Quercetin; Resveratrol; Selenium; Soy isoflavones; Soy protein; Vitamin B_{12}; Vitamin C; Vitamin E.

Carpal tunnel syndrome. *See* Pyridoxine (vitamin B_6).

Cataracts. *See* Beta-carotene; Bilberry; Curcumin; Glutathione; Grape seed extract; Lutein; Pantethine; Quercetin; Selenium; Vitamin C; Zeaxanthin.

Cholesterol problems. *See* Artichoke leaf; Ascorbyl palmitate; Beta-1,3-glucan; Beta-sitosterol; Betaine; Carnitine; Chitosan; Choline; Chromium; Chromium picolinate; Chromium polynicotinate; Fenugreek; Fiber; Flaxseed oil; Garlic; Genistein; Guggul; Hawthorn; Hesperidin; Lecithin; Lycopene; Niacin (nicotinic acid, vitamin B_3); Niacin, no-flush; Pantethine; Pectin; Phosphatidylcholine; Phytosterols and phytostanols; Polyphenols; Psyllium seed; Red yeast rice; Resveratrol; Royal jelly; Soy isoflavones; Soy protein; Spirulina; Tocotrienols; Vitamin C.

Chronic fatigue syndrome. *See* Cordyceps; DHEA; Ginseng; Magnesium; Siberian ginseng; Thiamine (vitamin B_1); Vitamin B_{12}.

Chronic venous insufficiency. *See* Butcher's broom; Grape seed extract; Horse chestnut.

Cirrhosis, liver. *See* Milk Thistle.

Cold and flu. *See* Astragalus; Echinacea; Elderberry; Ephedra (ma huang); Ginseng; Siberian ginseng; Vitamin C; Zinc.

Cold sores. *See* Lysine.

Congestive heart failure. *See* Taurine.

Constipation. *See* Aloe vera; FOS (fructo-oligosaccharides); Psyllium seed.

Crohn's disease. *See* Boswellia; Cat's claw; Fish oil; Vitamin D.

Cystic fibrosis. *See* Taurine; Vitamin A; Vitamin D.

Depression. *See* 5-HTP; DL-Phenylalanine (DLPA); Inositol; Phosphatidylserine; SAMe; St. John's wort; Tyrosine.

Depression, from oral contraceptives or PMS. *See* Pyridoxine (vitamin B_6).

Detoxification. *See* Chlorophyll; Glutathione; Green foods; N-acetyl cysteine (NAC); Pantethine; Spirulina.

Diabetes. *See* Aloe vera gel juice; Bilberry; Biotin (vitamin H); Carnitine; Chromium; Chromium picolinate; Chromium polynicotinate; Conjugated linoleic acid (CLA); Evening primrose oil; Fenugreek; Ginseng; Glutathione; Gymnema sylvestre; Inositol; Lipoic acid; Magnesium; Niacinamide (vitamin B_3); Psyllium seed; Siberian ginseng; Reishi; Thiamine (vitamin B_1); Vitamin E.

Diabetic neuropathy. *See* Black currant seed oil; Lipoic acid.

Diarrhea. *See* Bromelain; Colostrum; Fiber; FOS (fructo-oligosaccharides); Probiotics; Psyllium seed.

Digestive aid. *See* Bromelain; Curcumin; Peppermint oil.

Down syndrome. *See* Acetyl-L-carnitine.

Eczema. *See* Borage oil; Evening primrose oil.

Energy. *See* 7-keto DHEA.

Energy, low. *See* Carnitine; Cordyceps; Ginseng; Siberian ginseng.

Epilepsy. *See* Taurine.

Erectile dysfunction. *See* Arginine; Ginkgo biloba; Ginseng.

Fertility, male. *See* Arginine; Ginseng; Zinc.

Fibrocystic breast disease. *See* Chaste tree berry; Evening primrose oil; Iodine.

Fibromyalgia. *See* 5-HTP; Cetyl myristoleate (CMO); SAMe; Thiamine (vitamin B_1).

Fungal infections, topical. *See* Oregano oil; Tea tree oil.

Gastroesophageal Reflux Disease (GERD). *See* Deglycyrrhizinated licorice (DGL).

Gastrointestinal disorders. *See* Aloe vera gel juice; FOS (fructo-oligosaccharides); Ginger; Glutamine; Goldenseal; Oregon grape; Probiotics; Rosemary leaf; Vitamin B_{12}.

Glaucoma. *See* Coleus forskohlii; Lipoic acid.

Goiter. *See* Iodine.

Hair, Skin, and Nails. *See* Horsetail; Orthosilicic acid; Silicon.

Headaches. *See* 5-HTP; Rosemary leaf.

Healing. *See* Glutamine.

Helicobacter pylori. *See* Vitamin C.

Hemorrhoids. *See* Bilberry; Butcher's broom; Grape seed extract; Hesperidin; Horse chestnut.

Hepatitis. *See* Astragalus; Choline; Milk thistle; N-acetyl cysteine (NAC); Phosphatidylcholine.

Herpes simplex virus. *See* Lysine.

HIV. *See* Alkylglycerol; Beta-carotene; Cat's claw; Glutathione; Maitake mushroom; Selenium; Shiitake mushroom.

Hypertension. *See* Calcium; Fish oil; Garlic; Hawthorn; Magnesium; Olive leaf extract; Potassium; Reishi.

Hypoglycemia. *See* Chromium; Chromium picolinate; Chromium polynicotinate.

Hypothyroidism. *See* Iodine.

Immune system. *See* Alkylglycerol; Ashwagandha; Astragalus; Barberry; Beta-1,3-glucan; beta-carotene; Cat's claw; Chlorophyll; Colostrum; Coriolus versicolor extract (PSK); Curcumin; Echinacea; Elderberry; FOS (fructo-oligosaccharides); Garlic; Ginseng; Glutamine; Green foods; Larch, western; Maitake mushroom; N-acetyl cysteine (NAC); Olive leaf extract; Oregon grape; Probiotics; Propolis; Pyridoxine (vitamin B_6); Reishi; Resveratrol; Rosemary leaf; Selenium; Shiitake mushroom; Siberian ginseng; Spirulina; Vitamin A; Vitamin E; Whey protein; Zinc.

Indigestion. *See* Artichoke leaf; Bromelain; Devil's claw; Rosemary leaf.

Infertility. *See* Acetyl-L-carnitine; Chaste tree berry

Infertility, male. *See* Glutathione.

Insomnia. *See* 5-HTP; Kava kava; Melatonin; Valerian root.

Intermittent claudication. *See* Ginkgo biloba; Niacin (nicotinic acid, vitamin B_3); Niacin, no-flush.

Irritable bowel syndrome. *See* Artichoke leaf; Boswellia; Cat's claw; Fiber; FOS (fructo-oligosaccharides); Peppermint oil; Psyllium seed.

Jet lag. *See* Melatonin.

Kidney stones. *See* Chlorophyll; Cranberry; Stinging nettle leaf.

Leg cramps. *See* Horse chestnut.

Leukoplakia. *See* Beta-carotene.

Liver disorders. *See* Artichoke leaf; Astragalus; Betaine; Choline; Inositol; Lecithin; N-acetyl cysteine (NAC); Phosphatidyl-choline; SAMe; Shiitake mushroom; Spirulina; Taurine.

Low immune system. *See* 7-keto DHEA.

Lung disease. *See* N-acetyl cysteine (NAC).

Macular degeneration. *See* Beta-carotene; Bilberry; Ginkgo biloba; Grape seed extract; Lutein; Vitamin A; Zeaxanthin; Zinc.

Malabsorption conditions. *See* Vitamin B_{12}; Vitamin K.

Manic depression. *See* Choline; Phosphatidylcholine.

Menopause. *See* Black cohosh; Chaste tree berry; genistein; Soy isoflavones.

Menstrual irregularities. *See* Chaste tree berry.

Mental function. *See* Choline; Huperzine A; Phosphatidyl-choline; Vinpocetine.

Migraine headaches. *See* 5-HTP; Feverfew; Magnesium; Riboflavin (vitamin B_2).

Multiple sclerosis. *See* Thiamine (vitamin B_1).

Muscle spasm. *See* Kava kava.

Nausea. *See* Ginger.

Nausea, morning sickness. *See* Pyridoxine (vitamin B_6).

Nervousness. *See* Kava kava.

Neuropathies. *See* Acetyl-L-carnitine.

Night blindness. *See* Beta-carotene; Grape seed extract; Vitamin A; Zinc.

Nutritional support. *See* Copper; Glutamine; Green foods; MCT (Medium Chain Triglycerides); Soy protein; Vitamin K; Whey protein.

Nutritional support, for the elderly. *See* riboflavin (vitamin B_2); Thiamine (vitamin B_1); Vitamin B_{12}.

Obesity. *See* 5-HTP; 7-Keto DHEA; Ephedra (ma huang); Garcinia cambogia; Green tea extract; Pyruvate.

Obsessive-compulsive disorder. *See* Inositol.

Odor. *See* Chlorophyll.

Osteomalacia. *See* Vitamin D.

Osteoporosis. *See* Black cohosh; Boron; Calcium; Ipriflavone; Magnesium; Manganese; Orthosilicic acid; Silicon; Vitamin D; Vitamin K.

Pain. *See* DL-Phenylalanine (DLPA); Kava kava; Willow bark.

Parasites. *See* Garlic; Goldenseal; Oregon grape.

Parkinson's disease. *See* CDP-choline; Choline; Phosphatidyl-choline; Phosphatidylserine.

Periodontal disease. *See* CoQ_{10}; Cranberry.

Pregnancy. *See* Folic acid.

Premenstrual syndrome. *See* Black cohosh; Chaste tree berry; Evening primrose oil; Pyridoxine (vitamin B_6).

Prostatitis. *See* Flower pollen; Pygeum; Quercetin; Stinging nettle root.

Psoriasis. *See* Alkylglycerol; Aloe vera gel; Barberry; Coleus forskohlii; Fish oil; Oregon grape.

Raynaud's phenomenon. *See* Niacin (nicotinic acid, vitamin B_3); Niacin, no-flush.

Retinopathy. *See* Bilberry; Ginkgo biloba; Grape seed extract.

Seasonal affective disorder. *See* 5-HTP; St. John's wort.

Sexual performance. *See* 7-Keto DHEA; DHEA; Yohimbe bark; Zinc.

Shingles. *See* Lysine.

Sinusitis. *See* Bromelain; Ephedra (ma huang).

Skin conditions, topical. *See* Ascorbyl palmitate; Vitamin E.

Skin disorders. *See* Biotin (Vitamin H); Borage oil; Evening primrose oil; Oregon grape; Pantothenic acid (vitamin B_5); Vitamin A.

Sports injuries. *See* Boswellia; Bromelain; Chondroitin; Devil's claw; Glucosamine; Grape seed extract; Sea cucumber; Willow bark.

Stress. *See* 7-Keto DHEA; Ashwagandha; Astragalus; Kava kava; Pantothenic acid (vitamin B_5); Siberian ginseng; Vitamin C.

Stroke. *See* Garlic; Vinpocetine.

Tardive dyskinesia. *See* Choline; Phosphatidylcholine.

Tinnitus. *See* Ginkgo biloba; Vinpocetine; Vitamin B_{12}.

Triglycerides, high. *See* Carnitine; Chromium; Chromium picolinate; Chromium polynicotinate; DHA (docosahexaenoic acid); Fish oil; Flaxseed oil; Garlic.

Ulcer, peptic. *See* Carnosine; Deglycyrrhizinated licorice (DGL).

Ulcerative colitis. *See* Boswellia; Fish oil.

Urinary tract infections. *See* Barberry; Cranberry; Horsetail; Uva ursi.

Varicose veins. *See* Bilberry; Butcher's broom; Grape seed extract; Hesperidin; Horse chestnut.

Ventricular arrhythmias. *See* Barberry.

Vertigo. *See* Ginkgo biloba.

Vision problems. *See* Grape seed extract; Vitamin A.

Weight loss. *See* 7-Keto DHEA; Carnitine; Chitosan; Chromium; Chromium picolinate; Chromium polynicotinate; Colostrum; Conjugated linoleic acid (CLA); Ephedra (ma huang); Garcinia cambogia; Green tea extract; Psyllium seed; Pyruvate.

Wound healing. *See* Aloe vera gel; Arginine; Ornithine, Ornithine alpha-ketoglutarate (OKG); Zinc.

CHAPTER SIX

Combination Remedies

As shown in Chapter 5, for any given health problem there may be numerous vitamins, herbs, and mineral supplements that may be appropriate. We have emphasized that the foundation for every program should be a broad-spectrum multivitamin and multimineral supplement, including the recommended amount of calcium and magnesium. Then, any additional supplements that might be appropriate, based on each individual's unique health situation, should be added.

For some people, this can result in quite a large number of additional supplements. This can be expensive and confusing. To make it easier, you may find it more convenient to select one or more combination supplements that are designed specifically for your health problems.

For example, let's say you have arthritis. How would you set up your supplement program? Well, you could start with a two-per-day multivitamin such as Solgar's VM2000. You add a calcium-magnesium supplement. And you take a broad-spectrum antioxidant blend. For the arthritis, you can add glucosamine and chondroitin. Maybe you want to also take MSM. And the herb devil's claw to reduce the inflammation. To help with the pain, you also want to take some white willow bark and DLPA. What about SAMe?

Where does it end? You have already added six additional products to the multivitamin, calcium-magnesium, and antioxidant blend. That's nine separate products already.

Is there an easier way? Yes, you can select a combination product, one that contains a blend of ingredients designed for the problems you are concerned with. You may be able to find a comprehensive arthritis supplement, for example, that contains most of the individual nutrients you need. Instead of taking nine separate products, you may need to take only four or five.

And if you have more than one health problem, arthritis *and* high cholesterol, for example, the advantage of relying on combination products becomes even greater.

In this chapter, we will introduce you to a representative selection of combination products, with some commentary that will enable you to better decide which are right for you. We could not include all of the products, or categories, of course. If you do not see products suitable for your particular health problem, talk to your nutritional pharmacist, or check our website, www.bestsupplementsforyourhealth.com, for additional listings.

Antioxidant Flavonoid Formulas

Description: There are many antioxidants available for use in nutritional supplements. Some of the most powerful ones are those found in plants, generally categorized as flavonoids. Many of these powerful phytonutrients are available as individual supplements, for example, grape seed extract, Pycnogenol, and quercetin. Each is slightly different, however, and a combination product may provide the most benefit.

Ingredients: See the listings for each individual component in Chapter 5.

Sample Products:

- *Advanced Proanthocyanidin Complex* (Solgar). Every two vegicaps contain the following:

Pycnogenol (as pine bark extract)	12.5 g
Grape Seed Extract (24 mg [95%] oligomeric proanthocyanidins)	25 mg
Green Tea Extract (leaf)	10 mg
Red Wine Extract	10 mg

Standardized Ginkgo Biloba Extract (leaf) (1 mg [24%] ginkgoflavoglycosides)	5 mg
Standardized Billberry Extract (berry) (1 mg [25%] anthocyanosides)	5 mg
Citrus Bioflavonoids	5 mg
Hesperidin	5 mg
Rutin (Dimorphandra mollis) (fruit)	5 mg
Quercetin	5 mg

- *Antioxidant Supreme* (Nature's Answer) is a combination of vitamin C (Ester-C), vitamin E, and selenium along with the antioxidant-rich herbal extracts of curcumin, green tea, tomato, pine bark, and grapeseed.

Antioxidant Formulas

Description: Most of the degenerative diseases encountered as we age are mediated, at least in part, through oxidative damage. Oxidation is a two-edged sword. It is involved in many of the biochemical reactions necessary for life, including energy production. But when it gets out of control, it causes cellular damage. Aging itself is due to oxidative damage. Cancer, atherosclerosis, arthritis, cataracts, Parkinson's disease—these conditions result from the damage caused by free radicals, molecules with an unbalanced structure that attack other molecules. Antioxidants are the substances in our body that function to block these dangerous free radicals.

Ingredients: The antioxidant vitamins include vitamin C, beta-carotene, and vitamin E. Selenium and zinc are antioxidant minerals. Some of the strongest antioxidants are the phytonutrients such as the polyphenols and flavonoid compounds, which are found in fruits and vegetables.

Sample Products: Antioxidant nutrients are best taken in combination. They work synergistically, often serving to regenerate each other. This is a situation where using a combination product is definitely functional as well as convenient.

One of most basic types of antioxidant combination formulas can be thought of as the "ACE" group, because it contains the three basic antioxidant vitamins, A, C, and E. Two examples of enhanced versions of this type are as follows:

- *ACES+Zn* (Carlson) contains vitamins A, C, and E, along with zinc and selenium.
- *ImmunACE* (Nature's Plus) is a product that contains vitamins A, C, and E as well as folate, iron, zinc, selenium, and L-cysteine. The vitamin A is in the form of beta-carotene.

Another version of the above is the following formula from Solgar. As you see, it contains the same basic antioxidants as do those above (A, C, E, zinc, and selenium), but it also contains glutathione and the glutathione precursor, cysteine, as well as the carotenoid antioxidants and lutein.

- *Antioxidant Factors* (Solgar). Every tablet contains the following:

Vitamin A (as 100% natural beta-carotene from D.salina) 11,000 IU	
Vitamin C (as L-ascorbic acid)	600 mg
Vitamin E (as D-alpha tocopheryl succinate)	250 IU
Zinc (as zinc aspartate)	22 mg
Selenium (as L-selenomethionine)	75 mcg
L-Cysteine (as L-cysteine HCl)	100 mg
L-Glutathione	25 mg
Carotenoid mix (alpha-carotene, lutein, zeaxanthin, cryptoxanthin)	125 mcg

There are now more comprehensive formulas available containing additional antioxidant nutrients such as alpha-lipoic acid, CoQ_{10}, tocotrienols, NAC (n-acetyl-cysteine), taurine, and glutathione. In addition, they may have significant levels of phyto-antioxidants such as proanthocyanidins, grape seed extract, pine bark extract, polyphenols, and other flavonoids. In fact, these phytochemical antioxidants are so important, we have created a separate category of "Antioxidant Flavonoid Formulas" (see page 304).

Examples of broader-spectrum, complete antioxidant blends are as follows:

- *Lipoxidant Complex* (Willner Chemists). This is a comprehensive blend of water-soluble and fat-soluble antioxidant nutrients and phytonutrients. Every two capsules contain the following:

NAC (N-acetyl-cysteine)	100 mg
Alpha-Lipoic Acid	30 mg
Vitamin C (mineral ascorbates)	200 mg
Vitamin E (D-alpha tocopheryl succinate)	100 mg
Tocotrienol Complex (alpha, delta, gamma tocotrienols)	30 mg
Coenzyme Q_{10}	15 mg
Beta-Carotene/Natural Carotenoid Blend (D.salina)	10,000 IU
Fruit Polyphenols (40% oligophenolics from apricot, apple, prune, pomegranate, cherry)	50 mg
Zinc (fully reacted glycinate chelate)	15 mg
Copper (fully reacted glycinate chelate)	1 mg
Selenium (l-selenomethionine)	50 mcg

- *Advanced Antioxidant Formula* (Solgar). A comprehensive formula, with SOD inducers and proanthocyanidins. Every two vegicaps contain the following:

Vitamin A (as palmitate 2500 IU, 75% [7500 IU] as natural beta-carotene	10,000 IU
Vitamin C (as calcium ascorbate)	500 mg
Vitamin E (as d-alpha tocopheryl succinate)	200 IU
Calcium (as calcium ascorbate)	60 mg
Zinc (as zinc glycinate)	10 mg
Selenium (as L-selenomethionine)	50 mcg
Copper (as copper lysinate)	1 mg
Manganese (as manganese glycinate)	4 mg
L-Cysteine HCl	100 mg
Taurine	50 mg
L-Glutathione	25 mg
Coenzyme Pyridoxal-5-Phosphate	6 mg
Coenzyme Riboflavin-5-Phosphate	6 mg
Carotenoid mix (alpha-carotene, lutein, zeaxanthin, cryptoxanthin)	86 mcg

Proanthocyanidin Complex Blend, Green Tea Extract, Red Wine Extract, Pycnogenol	50 mg
Food and Herbal Blend Ginkgo Biloba Extract (leaf), Spirulina, Gotu Kola Extract (aerial), Milk Thistle Extract (aerial)	70 mg

- *Radical Fighters* (Twinlab). This is a nice formula, but it contains relatively high levels of the various B vitamins, which may make it an inappropriate choice if you are already taking other multivitamins. On the other hand, it has some nice features, such as ascorbyl palmitate, the fat-soluble form of Vitamin C.
- *Antioxidant Free Radical Formula* (Solgar). This is another antioxidant combination from Solgar, and illustrates how many options are available. This product has a wide range of phytonutrient antioxidant extracts along with the carotenoids, tocotrienols, and alpha-lipoic acid. Every two vegicaps contain the following:

Vitamin A (100% as natural beta-carotene from D. salina, carrot)	5,000 IU
Vitamin C (as calcium, potassium, magnesium, and zinc ascorbates)	200 mg
Vitamin E (as D-alpha tocopheryl succinate)	100 IU
Zinc (as zinc glycinate)	10 mg
Selenium (as L-selenomethionine)	25 mcg
Copper (as copper glycinate)	1 mg
Lycopene (from tomato)	1 mg
Lutein (from marigold flower)	1 mg
Zeaxanthin (from marigold flower)	50 mcg
Carotenoid Blend (phytoene, phytofluene, and zeta-carotene)	80 mcg
Gamma Tocopherol	50 mcg
Tocotrienols (as alpha, beta, gamma, and delta)	15 mg
Alpha-Lipoic Acid	30 mg
N-Acetyl-L-Cysteine (NAC)	100 mg
Standardized Fruit Polyphenols (phenolics 10 mg [40%] as apple, cherry, prune, apricot/nectarine, pomegranate)	25 mg

Grape Seed Extract (phenolics 14 mg [95%])	15 mg
Pine Bark Extract (phenolics 9 mg [60%])	15 mg
Standardized Ginkgo Biloba Extract (leaf)(ginkgoflavo-glycosides 4 mg [24%], terpene lactones 1 mg [6%])	15 mg
Standardized Turmeric Extract (root) (curcuminoids 14 mg [95%])	15 mg
Standardized Bilberry Extract (berry) (anthocyanosides 4 mg [25%])	15 mg
Standardized Green Tea Extract (leaf) (polyphenols 8 mg [50%])	15 mg

Arthritis Formulas—Osteoarthritis

Description: Osteoarthritis is a normal consequence of the aging process. The lining of the joints deteriorate, leading to pain and decreased mobility. Osteoarthritis is sometimes referred to as "wear and tear" arthritis to differentiate it from rheumatoid arthritis.

Ingredients: The treatment of osteoarthritis is as much directed to the healing and regeneration of the joint tissue as it is to reducing the inflammation and pain associated with the condition. Glucosamine sulfate, chondroitin sulfate, and other mucopolysaccharide-rich substances (cartilage, green-lipped mussel, sea cucumber, etc.) are very effective. MSM can be used as well. SAMe may be helpful. Secondarily, supplements that reduce inflammation can help, and could include the omega-3 oils, black currant oil, borage oil, and herbs such as devil's claw, boswellia, turmeric, and ginger. White willow bark and DLPA might be helpful as analgesic agents. There is some research supporting the use of niacinamide, not niacin, in treating osteoarthritis.

Sample Products: There are many excellent combination products suitable for treating osteoarthritis, including the following:

- *FlexAnew* (Natrol). This product contains a natural COX-2 inhibitor, to reduce inflammation and pain, along with glucosamine and chondroitin. Every two tablets contain the following:

Calcium (as calcium carbonate)	330 mg
Glucosamine Sulfate	750 mg

Chondroitin Sulfate	300 mg
Nexrutine (Phellodendron amurense)	250 mg

There is a companion product to FlexAnew called Remedief that is designed for the temporary relief of pain. It contains analgesic and anti-inflammatory herbs (boswellia and white willow bark), Nexrutine™, the natural COX-2 inhibitor, and kava kava root extract, which adds a skeletal muscle relaxant action as well.

- *Joint Formula* (Willner Chemists) is a unique blend of glucosamine sulfate, chondroitin sulfate, manganese, and vitamin C with anti-inflammatory herbs such as devil's claw, turmeric, and boswellin. The product contains proline, an amino acid needed for connective tissue repair, and niacinamide, which has been utilized extensively in arthritis treatment based on the work of Drs. William Kaufman and Abram Hoffer. Bromelain, a proteolytic enzyme, enhances the anti-inflammatory action and horsetail, a source of organic silica, has been shown to work synergistically with devil's claw as an antiarthritic treatment. Every two capsules of Joint Formula contain the following:

Vitamin C	50 mg
Niacinamide	75 mg
Manganese Gluconate	2 mg
Glucosamine Sulfate	500 mg
Chondroitin Sulfate	150 mg
DLPA (dl-phenylalanine)	100 mg
Turmeric Extract (95%)	100 mg
Devil's Claw Extract (4:1)	100 mg
L-Proline	100 mg
Horsetail Extract (2%)	50 mg
Boswellin Extract (60%)	50 mg
Grape Seed Extract	45 mg
Grape Skin Extract	30 mg
Bromelain (2400 GDU)	25 mg

• *Joint Modulators* (Solgar). This product is somewhat similar to Joint Formula. Both products contain DLPA, which provides some analgesic action. Every two tablets of Joint Modulators contain the following:

Vitamin C (as L-ascorbic acid)	100 mg
Niacin (as niacinamide)	100 mg
Manganese (as manganese glycinate)	4 mg
Iron	0.5 mg
Glucosamine Sulfate (from shellfish)	1 g
Bovine Cartilage	500 mg
DLPA (as DL-phenylalanine)	400 mg
Standardized Turmeric Extract (root) (curcuminoids 190 mg[95%])	200 mg
Ulva Seaweed	200 mg
L-Proline	200 mg
Grape Seed Extract (phenolics 50 mg [50%])	100 mg

• *MaxiLife Joint Protector* (Twinlab). Every six capsules contain the following:

Glucosamine Sulfate	1,500 mg
Chondroitin Sulfate A (CSA)	100 mg
Zinc (from chelated zinc picolinate)	15 mg
Vitamin C	1,000 mg
Vitamin D_3	400 IU
Natural Vitamin E	800 IU
Selenium (from selenomethionine)	200 mcg
Turmeric (Curcuma longa) Extract (standardized for 95% curcumin)	1,300 mg
Boswellia Serrata Extract (standardized for 60–65% boswellic acids)	25 mg
Quercetin	25 mg
Bromelain	25 mg

Arthritis Formulas—Rheumatoid Arthritis

Description: Rheumatoid arthritis is a chronic inflammatory disease, usually affecting the joints throughout the body. It is an autoimmune disease, a condition in which the body's own immune system mistakenly attacks its own tissue. The cause of this condition has yet to be determined.

Ingredients: Because rheumatoid arthritis is an inflammatory disease, the main treatment approach is to reduce inflammation. Thus, anti-inflammatory nutrients such as borage oil, fish oil (EPA-DHA), and vitamin E are indicated. The same can be said for anti-inflammatory and antioxidant herbs such as devil's claw, turmeric, boswellin, and ginger.

A COMMENT FROM DR. ABEL

The Chinese have long recognized that the joints and ligaments are essential to the body's mobility. Chinese medicine and martial arts encourage hydration and protect movement. The inflammation of joints is commonly known as arthritis. The two major kinds of arthritis are osteoarthritis (degenerative arthritis or degenerative joint diseases) and rheumatoid arthritis. Osteoarthritis includes the wear and tear of the joint cartilage. It is due to the constant pressure, over years, on the weight-bearing joints and stiffness of their supporting tendons. Selective exercise and supplements can be very helpful in improving osteoarthritic joint pain. Remember that joint pains may be the body's cries for water, and reflect discomfort in the ligaments and tendons. This discomfort, which is often interpreted as arthritis, may actually be due to tendonitis or bursitis. People may actually have one leg longer than the other, which, over time, causes chronic back and neck aches. Rheumatoid arthritis is a category of inflammatory rather than degenerative joint disease, and result from infection or autoimmune disease. The infection may present elsewhere in the body, and follow a common cold that creates antibodies that attack not only the cold virus but also the joint capsules. This leaves the individual with an inflamed joint that may act up later in life. Many patients with rheumatoid arthritis may find that dairy products and nightshade plants (white potatoes, tomatoes, cucumber, and eggplant) aggravate the condition. There are several supplements such as the essential fatty acids, glucosamine and chondroitin sulfate, and SAMe that may be effective in minimizing joint pain. Even probiotics, the good bacteria that can replenish your colon's bacteria, are helpful in reducing joint pain. One study showed a 50 percent reduction in joint pain in people who took probiotic supplements. This is related to the fact that at any one time, 50 percent of our inflammatory lymphocytes are in our bowels and can be affected by what we eat and our normal bowel flora. Once again, this shows that our body is a harmonious whole, which must be treated not in parts, but together.

Sample Products:

- *Joint Rescue* (Twinlab). Joint Rescue combines anti-inflammatory essential fatty acids and herbal extracts with vitamin E and glucosamine/chondroitin. Every three softgels contain the following:

Vitamin E (from d-alpha tocopherols)	400 IU
Glucosamine HCl and Glucosamine Sulfate	750 mg
Chondroitin Sulfate	50 mg
Turmeric Powder Extract (standardized for 95% curcumin)	650 mg
Boswellin (Boswellia serrata extract) (standardized for 65% boswellic acids)	13 mg
Ginger Root Extract	50 mg
EPA	750 mg
DHA	750 mg
Borage Oil	100 mg

There are a number of new products that consist of herbal COX-2 inhibitors that should be effective anti-inflammatory supplements for use by those with rheumatoid arthritis:

- *FlexAnew* (Natrol). Two tablets of FlexAnew contain glucosamine sulfate, 750 milligrams, chondroitin sulfate, 300 milligrams, Nexrutine™, 250 milligrams, and calcium, 330 milligrams. Nexrutine™ is a plant extract derived from *Phellodendron amurense* bark. This extract has been scientifically shown to inhibit the COX-2 enzyme that is found naturally in our body. The COX-2 enzyme is involved with how we feel and experience pain. For maximum benefit, the active constituents in the extract need to be absorbed into the body. If taken with a meal, food may interfere with the absorption of Nexrutine™. Furthermore, animal data and human clinical experience suggest that taking this plant extract on an empty stomach is well tolerated.

- *Zyflamend* (New Chapter) is another blend, containing various plant-derived COX-2 inhibitors. It is a mixture of ten herbs, including turmeric and ginger, that are known for either their COX-2-inhibiting action or their anti-inflammatory effect.

Brain and Mental Support Formulas

Description: Mental deterioration can be related to aging, leading to memory impairment and Alzheimer's disease. But other, short term cognitive problems can be related to optimal brain function as well.

Ingredients: There are a wide variety of vitamins, herbs, and nutritional supplements that can impact mental function and perhaps retard age-related cognitive decline. The herb gingko biloba has been considered valuable in this regard in Europe for many years, and recently published studies in this country have confirmed this. Other herbs, such as huperzine A, may help as well. Antioxidants seem to be important, including vitamins C and E. Other vitamins, such as B_6 and B_{12}, have been found to be present at lower levels in elderly patients with cognitive problems. And the various neurotransmitter precursors, phosphatidylserine, phosphatidylcholine, acetyl-L-carnitine, seem to be especially useful in enhancing brain function.

Sample Products:

- *Brain Modulators* (Solgar) is a nice blend of several key vitamins, folic acid and B_{12}, and the neurotransmitter precursor substances phosphatidylcholine, acetyl-L-carnitine, and phosphatidylserine. In addition, it contains ginkgo biloba, as well as a decent amount of DHA, the essential fatty acid shown to be directly involved in brain and nervous system growth and development. Every three tablets of Brain Modulators contain the following:

Folic Acid	200 mcg
Vitamin B_{12} (as cobalamin)	200 mcg
Phosphatidylcholine	500 mg
Acetyl-L-Carnitine	300 mg
Phosphatidylserine	160 mg
Docosahexaenoic Acid [DHA]	120 mg
Standardized Ginkgo Biloba Extract *leaf) (ginkgoflavo-glycosides 19 mg [24%], terpene lactones 5 mg [6%])	80 mg

- *MaxiLife Brain Protector* (Twinlab) differs slightly from the above formula. For one thing, it contains CoQ_{10} and vitamin E. In comparing the two, however, be aware that this product is per six capsules, and the Solgar product above is per three tablets. Every six capsules of MaxiLife contain the following:

Choline	1,000 mg
Phosphatidylserine Complex	250 mg
Phosphatidylserine	50 mg
Phosphatidylcholine	50 mg
Phosphatidylethanolamine	30 mg
Phosphatidylinositol	15 mg
Acetyl-L-Carnitine	1,000 mg
Ginkgo Biloba Extract (standardized for 24% flavonoid glycoside)	120 mg
Vitamin B_5	100 mg
Vitamin B_{12}	1,000 mcg
Folic Acid	800 mcg
Vitamin B_6	25 mg
Natural Vitamin E	400 IU
CoQ_{10}	30 mg

- *Memory Complex* (Natrol) employs a different approach, with an emphasis on herbs, containing vinpocetine, huperzine, and ginkgo biloba, rather than high levels of acetyl-L-carnitine, and phosphatidylserine. Lecithin, of course, is a source of phosphatidylcholine. Every two tablets of Memory Complex contain the following:

Thiamin (as thiamin HCl) (vitamin B$_1$)	1.5 mg
Niacin (as niacinamide)	20 mg
Vitamin B$_6$ (as Pyridoxine)	2 mg
Folate (folic acid)	400 mcg
Vitamin B$_{12}$ (cyanocobalamin)	6 mcg
Calcium (as Di-calcium phosphate)	130 mg
Vinpocetine (from periwinkle seed extract)	10 mg
Huperzine (from Huperzia serrate extract)	100 mcg
Ginkgo Biloba Leaf Extract (25% ginkgo flavone-glycosides, 6% triterpenes)	120 mg
Phosphatidyl Serine Complex	15 mg
Lecithin	100 mg

- *Brain Function* (Willner Chemists) is perhaps most similar to the approach taken by Solgar, in that it contains a blend of neurotransmitter precursors, along with DHA and ginkgo biloba. For those taking CoQ$_{10}$, herbs such as huperzine, and vitamins separately, this product would be ideal. Every three tablets of Brain Fuction contain the following:

DHA (Neuromins—Algae & Fish Oil)	50 mg
Phosphatidylserine (Leci-PS)	50 mg
Neurocholine (choline, phosphatidylcholine, CDP choline)	300 mg
Acetyl-L-Carnitine	150 mg
Standardized Ginkgo Biloba Root Ext. (24% ginkgo flavoneglycosides/6% terpene lactones)	30 mg
Vitamin B$_{12}$ (cobalamin)	100 mcg

Additional products to consider:

- *Neuro Optimizer* (Jarrow Formulas) is an excellent neuroprotective and cognition-enhancing product. The only thing missing is ginkgo biloba. Every four capsules of Neuro Optimizer contain the following:

Cytidine 5'-diphoscholine (CDP choline)	300 mg
Phosphatidyl Serine (PS)	100 mg
Acetyl L-Carnitine	500 mg
L-Glutamine	500 mg
Alpha Lipoic Acid	50 mg
Taurine	500 mg
Phosphatidylcholine	135 mg

- *Memory Formula* (Country Life) contains huperzine and vinpocetine, making this combination ideal for those trying to enhance memory.
- *Brainstorm Alcohol Free Liquid Extract* (Nature's Answer) is designed to promote mental clarity. It contains gotu kola, ginkgo biloba, periwinkle, plus other herbs.

Calming and Relaxing Formulas

Description: Mild to moderate anxiety, nervousness, and depression can often be alleviated through the use of nutritional supplements and herbs. It is important to consult with a physician, however, as depression, if serious, should be handled by a qualified health professional.

Ingredients: Many herbs have been shown to have calming, relaxing, and even antidepressant actions, including kava, passion flower, hops, lemon balm, valerian, and St. John's wort. Inositol has been shown to be helpful, along with niacinamide and magnesium.

Sample Products:

- *Brain Calmplex* (Willner Chemists) is a comprehensive blend of calming herbs, neurotransmitter modulators, and glucose regulators. Trimethylglycine is a methyl donor, and a precursor to the formation of SAMe, a natural antidepressant. Chromium is included to ensure that blood sugar levels remain in the normal range, which is essential for normal brain function. Every three tablets of Brain Calmplex contain the following:

DHA (Neuromins®—Algae & Fish Oil)	50 mg
Phosphatidylserine (Leci-PS®)	50 mg
Inositol (myo-inositol)	400 mg
Trimethylglycine	200 mg
St. John Wort Standard Extract (0.3% kavalactones)	200 mg
Kava Kava Standard Root Ext. (30% kavalactones)	100 mg
Chromium (nicotinate/glycinate chelate)	100 mcg

- *Mood Modulators* (Solgar) is a variation on Brain Calmplex in that it contains less DHA, but adds schisandra and rhodiola in place of kava kava. It also contains preformed SAMe. Every three vegicaps of Mood Modulators contain the following:

Chromium (as chromium nicotinoglycinate)	25 mcg
Standardized St. John's Wort Extract (aerial) (hypericin 0.45 mg [0.3%])	150 mg
SAMe (from 30 mg S-adenosyl-L-methionine sulfate)	16 mg
Trimethylglycine [TMG] (from beets)	250 mg
Phosphatidylserine	75 mg
Docosahexaenoic Acid [DHA] (from algae)	5 mg
Inositol (as myo-inositol)	500 mg
Standardized Rhodiola Extract (root) (salidrozid 0.75 mg [1%], polyphehnols 30 mg [40%])	75 mg
Standardized Schisandra Extract (fruit)(schisandrins 0.75 mg [1%])	75 mg

Additional products to consider:

- *Tense-Ease* (Nature's Answer) is an alcohol-free liquid combination of hawthorn berry, linden flower, wood betony, and hops strobile. The label says it promotes "stressless moments."
- *Serenity with Kava Kava* (Gaia Herbs) is a liquid-filled vegetarian capsule containing skullcap, passion flower, kava kava, chamomile flowers, and four more relaxant herbs. This is an excellent relaxing formula.

Candida Yeast Formulas

Description: Chronic candidiasis is a situation that results when *Candida albicans,* a common yeast, or fungus, proliferates in the gastrointestinal tract, causing symptoms that include fatigue, immune system problems, allergies and sensitivities, digestive disturbances, and depression. The condition is considered rare by conventional medicine, but common by alternative practitioners. Since candida is ubiquitous, a compromised immune system must be at least part of the explanation of why certain individuals have this problem, and others do not.

Ingredients: Certain immune-stimulating nutrients and herbs seem to have specific antifungal activity, and these are usually included in products intended for the treatment of chronic candidiasis. It must be kept in mind, however, that the underlying treatment of the condition must also target generally enhanced immune function and optimal health.

Sample Products:

- *Yeast Fighters* (Twinlab) is probably one of the most successful products available for general use in treating this problem. The probiotics and fiber blend help to strengthen the gastrointestinal tract integrity. Caprylic acid is thought to exert specific antifungal activity. Garlic also has antimicrobial activity. Every five capsules of Yeast Fighters contain the following:

High Potency Freeze Dried Lacto-bacillus acidophilus (milk free) (supplying 2.5 billion viable cells)	1,000 mg
Concentrated Odorless Garlic Extract Powder (equivalent to 1,500 mg of fresh garlic)	100 mg
Natural Caprylic Acid	100 mg
Biotin	900 mcg
Fiber Blend (psyllium seed husks, guar gum, apple pectin). In a concentrated specially prepared herbal tea extract base of pau d'arco, onion, black walnut, echinacea, and golden seal root.	3,000 mg

- *Yeast-Cleanse*™ (Solaray) is another comprehensive formula. It contains grapefruit seed extract, pau d'arco, and tea tree oil, which are not found in the above product. Yeast-Cleanse™ contains, per 6 capsules: calcium (as calcium caprylate), 162 mg; magnesium (as magnesium caprylate), 82 mg; zinc (as zinc caprylate), 7 mg; caprylic acid, 2.16 g; pau d'arco (Ipe Roxo) (inner bark), 240 mg; grapefruit seed extract *(Citrus paradisi)*, 240 mg; GP garlic *(Allium sativum)* (bulb), supplying 10,000 mcg/g (2,400 mcg) Allicin Releasing Potential, 240 mg; licorice root (*Glycyrrhiza glabra*), 240 mg; tea tree oil, 180 mg.

Carbohydrate Control Formulas

Description: There are two types of carbohydrate metabolism problems, hyperglycemia, or diabetes, and hypoglycemia. In many respects, from a nutritional supplement standpoint, they are similar. In diabetes, the body does not properly metabolize carbohydrate, resulting in elevated glucose levels in the blood. Normally, in response to elevated blood glucose, the body secretes insulin, which in turn results in the lowering of the blood glucose levels. Those who have Type 1, or childhood diabetes, do not secrete adequate amounts of insulin. Those who have Type 2, or adult-onset diabetes, may secrete enough insulin, but the body does not properly respond to it. In the presence of too much insulin, blood glucose levels can fall too low, resulting in hypoglycemia. It is crucial to maintain blood glucose levels within the normal range.

A COMMENT FROM DR. ABEL

It is well recognized that people living in industrial societies are overfed and undernourished. There is a startling increase in obesity and consequent diabetes, even in younger people. The following are some basic tips to avoid or help manage diabetes:

(1) Reduce simple sugars while keeping a small amount of complex carbohydrates in your diet. (2) Include polyunsaturated fats, especially omega-3 fatty acids, in your diet while minimizing the trans fats and hydrogenated oils. Research indicates a higher incidence of diabetes among individuals who consume more saturated fats. (3) Use stevia, a naturally sweet herb from Paraguay, instead of artificial sweeteners or processed sugar. (4) Build stronger blood vessels with vitamin C, 1,000 to 2,000 milligrams per day, and the important bioflavonoid quercetin, 1,000 milligrams per day. (5) The eye is the only place to observe blood vessels; when leakage from the blood vessels is noted, it can be treated promptly. Therefore, an annual dilated eye exam is mandatory for diabetics. (6) Lower cho-

lesterol as well as maintain blood sugar with an appropriate diet. Two good choices are the American Diabetic Association's restricted calorie diet and the Atkins low-carbohydrate diet. By reducing carbohydrates, less insulin is secreted and fats will not be absorbed. Consequently, fat in the diet will pass right through, and individuals will burn their own body fat. (7) Take a comprehensive multivitamin daily. It should include zinc and selenium. (8) Magnesium levels are lower in diabetics. Therefore, 500 milligrams of magnesium should be taken daily, with the exception of those with kidney disease. (9) Chromium picolinate (200 micrograms) and alpha-lipoic acid (250 milligrams twice daily) will make circulating levels of insulin more effective. (10) Exercise regularly. (11) Keep all of your health-care providers informed of your medications and supplements.

Ingredients: Several herbs have been shown to be helpful in controlling carbohydrate metabolism, including fenugreek, gymnema, and various other fiber-rich herbs. Alpha-lipoic acid has been shown to be important to those with diabetes, along with the trace mineral chromium. Normally, only 200 micrograms of chromium are needed, but for those with diabetes, 400 to 600 micrograms or more may be required. There seems to be a strong association between magnesium deficiency and diabetes. Fiber supplements (psyllium, glucomannan, etc.) help by slowing gastric emptying, and moderating the absorption of sugar. Certain nutrients, such as vitamin E and alpha-lipoic acid, may be included because they help to prevent some of the side effects of diabetes.

Sample Products:

- *Glucose Modulators* (Solgar) is a comprehensive blend of the important carbohydrate-regulating minerals, chromium, magnesium, and zinc, along with several key herbal extracts. Every two tablets contain the following:

Niacin	10 mg
Vitamin B$_6$ (as pyridoxine HCl)	5 mg
Magnesium (as magnesium oxide)	200 mg
Zinc (as zinc citrate)	5 mg
Chromium (as chromium picolinate)	200 mg

Insulin Powder	300 mg
Standardized Gymnema Sylvestre Extract (leaf) (gymnemic acid 75 mg [75%])	100 mg
Standardized Momordica Charantis Extract (fruit) (min. bitter principles 2.5 mg [2.5])	100 mg
Standardized Milk Thistle Extract (aerial, seed) (silymarin 120 mg [80%])	30 mg
Fenugreek Extract (4:1) (seed)	30 mcg
Green Tea Extract [leaf] (polyphenois 7.5 mg [25%])	30 mg
Alpha-Lipoic Acid	30 mg
Vanadium (as vanadyl sulfate)	500 mg

- *Glycemic Factors* (Country Life) relies on different herbs, but is otherwise similar to the above formula. Every tablet contains the following:

Vitamin B$_6$ (as pyridoxine alpha-ketoglutarate)	12.5 mg
Vitamin B$_{12}$ (as cyanoccobalamin)	50 mcg
Folic Acid	200 mcg
Calcium (as calcium carbonate)	60 mg
Magnesium (as magnesium aspartate)	50 mg
Zinc (as zinc monomethionine)	2.5 mg
Copper (as copper lysinate)	0.5 mg
Manganese (as manganese citrate)	1.5 mg
Chromium (as chromium polynicotinate)	200 mcg
Potassium (as potassium aspartate)	49.5 mg
Gymnema Sylvester (leaf) (from 6.3 mg of 40:1 extract)	250 mg
Fenugreek (seed) (from 37.5 mg of 4:1 extract)	150 mg
Bitter Melon Extract 4:1 (Momordica charantia) (fruit)	100 mg
PAK (pyridoxine alpha-ketoglutarate)	12.5 mg
Vanadyl Sulfate	2.5 mg

- *Glucose Tolerance with ChromeMate*™ (Allergy Research Group). This combination of nutrients supports the body in regulating blood sugar levels. It contains ChromeMate®, a patented chromium complex. Chromium is an essential mineral known to be involved in blood sugar regulation. Galactomannan (*Cyamopsis tetragonoloba*), also known as guar gum, is a soluble fiber, and plays a role in blood sugar regulation. Hypoallergenic.

Each capsule contains: chromium (as ChromeMate®, chromium nicotinate), 250 mcg; niacin, 50 mg; vitamin B_6 (as pyridoxine hydrochloride), 20 mg; L-glutathione, 2.5 mg; galactomannan (as guar gum, *Cyamopsis tetragonoloba*), 450 mg.

Cardiovascular Formulas—Blood Pressure

Description: High blood pressure, or hypertension, is a major risk factor for heart attack or stroke. The heart "beat" is the muscular contraction that pushes blood through the arteries. The amount of resistance to that pulse of blood flow is the "blood pressure." In most instances, doctors do not know why the pressure is elevated, and this is called essential, or idiopathic hypertension. There are many possible causes. If the arteries are partially blocked by plaque buildup, or if they are hard and inelastic, for example, the resistance to blood flow can be increased. Hypertension is a serious problem, and should be treated under a doctor's supervision. Many doctors, however, are quick to prescribe medication. Medication, according to much research, should not be the treatment of choice if at all possible. Discuss with your doctor the possibility of nondrug treatments, including nutritional and herbal supplements.

A COMMENT FROM DR. ABEL

High blood pressure is related to many dietary and lifestyle imbalances. Some of these are high-sodium/low-potassium diet, obesity, and a high-sugar/low-fiber diet, high saturated fats/low essential fats. Some researchers have found that diets low in calcium, magnesium, and vitamin C are also prone to high blood pressure. Reversing these trends is a first step in the management, and therefore appropriate supplementation under medical supervision is advisable.

Ingredients: Numerous studies have shown that CoQ_{10} is effective in lowering high blood pressure. Omega-3 oils are effective as well.

Additional calcium helps, as does fiber supplementation, taurine, and perhaps the amino acid arginine, which is needed by the body to make nitric oxide. Nitric oxide causes blood vessels to dilate, and a dilated blood vessel will cause less resistance to the flow of blood. Several herbs, including hawthorn, garlic, European mistletoe, and olive leaf have been shown to lower elevated blood pressure as well.

Sample Products:

- *Cardiovascular Support* (Solgar). Every three tablets contain the following:

Calcium	175 mg
Magnesium (as magnesium glycinate, magnesium oxide)	200 mg
Taurine	800 mg
Trimethylglycine [TMG] (from beets)	800 mg
Soy Isoflavone Concentrate (seed)	400 mg
L-Carnitine	300 mg
Standardized Hawthorn Extract (leaf/flower) (vitexin 2 mg [1.8%])	125 mg
Cayenne Powder (fruit)	100 mg
Coenzyme Q_{10} (as ubiquinone)	60 mg
Grape Seed Extract (phenolics 48 mg [95%])	50 mg

- *CardioNutriv (Heart Tonic) Liquid Extract* (Nature's Answer) is a blend of hawthorn, linden, and cayenne that can be used adjunctively.
- *Circu-Pressure* (Country Life). Ingredients such as coleus forskholli, hawthorn, and ginger, plus magnesium and potassium, make this product a good choice for lowering blood pressure.

Cardiovascular Formulas—Cholesterol

Description: An elevated cholesterol level is one of the key risk factors for heart disease. A serum cholesterol level of under 180 is considered optimal. But perhaps more important than total cholesterol is the ratio of "bad" cholesterol (LDL) to "good" cholesterol (HDL). Some think, for example, that it is the oxidation of LDL cholesterol that actually leads to clot formation.

A short time ago, the importance of triglycerides was downplayed, but this is now acknowledged to be a risk factor as well.

Ingredients: The goal in treating elevated cholesterol is to lower total cholesterol, lower LDL cholesterol, and/or raise HDL cholesterol. This can be accomplished with a number of different supplements, including niacin (vitamin B_3), gum guggul, phytosterols, phytostanols, policosanols, soluble fiber (psyllium, oat bran, guar gum, pectin), and omega-3 oils. What is important to realize is that to achieve a sufficient reduction without using drugs, a combination of natural remedies is usually required.

Sample Products:

- *Cholesterol Modulators* (Solgar) is an excellent combination. It contains "no flush" niacin, but probably not at a level high enough to be effective on its own. Instead, the combination of gum guggul, soy isoflavones, beta-glucan-rich oat bran fiber, and garlic synergistically work to lower cholesterol and raise HDL. Every three tablets of Cholesterol Modulators contain the following:

Niacin (as inositol hexanicotinate)	171 mg
Standardized Gugulipid Extract (resin) (guggulsterones 15 mg [2.5%])	600 mg
Phosphatidycholine	400 mg
Soy Isoflavone Concentrate (seed)	400 mg
Ultra Oat Bran Fiber	400 mg
Organic Garlic (clove)	300 mg
Hong Qu (as fermented red yeast)	300 mg
Pantethine	160 mg
Tocotrienols	60 mg
Grape Seed Extract (phenolics 25 [50%])	50 mg
Inositol (as inositol hexanicotinate)	29 mg

- *Cholestame* (Jarrow) tackles high cholesterol using policosanol, phytosterols, artichoke leaf, and pantethine. It also provides antioxidants such as grape seed extract and lutein.
- *Nutri Chol-Less* (Country Life) is an effective cholesterol-lower-

ing formula providing a mixture of no-flush niacin, pantethine, and guggulsterones, along with garlic, hawthorn berry, fenugreek, and vanadyl sulfate.

Cardiovascular Formulas—Homocysteine

Description: An elevated homocysteine level appears to be a significant and independent risk factor for heart disease. Homocysteine is a metabolic end product of methionine breakdown.

Ingredients: Homocysteine levels can be reduced by supplementing with folic acid, vitamin B_{12}, and vitamin B_6. In addition, methyl donors such as trimethylglycine (betaine) and choline have also been shown to lower homocysteine levels.

Sample Products:

- *Homocysteine Modulators* (Solgar). Every two vegicaps contain the following:

Vitamin B_6 (as pyridoxine HCl)	50 mg
Folic Acid	400 mcg
Vitamin B_{12} (as cobalamin)	500 mcg
Trimethylglycine [TMG] (from beets)	1 g
Pyridoxal-5-Phosphate	6 mg
Dibencozide	6 mg

Cardiovascular Formulas—Multivitamin

Description: Wouldn't it be nice, you might ask, if there was a multivitamin formula specifically designed for those with heart problems? A multivitamin that had higher levels of magnesium? A multivitamin that contained CoQ_{10}, tocotrienols, red wine concentrate, L-carnitine, taurine, garlic, high folic acid levels, trimethylglycine, and alpha-lipoic acid in addition to the regular vitamins and minerals normally found in regular supplements? Well, such products are available. And for those looking for convenience and simplicity, this may be an attractive option.

Ingredients: Magnesium, CoQ_{10}, tocotrienols, red wine concentrate, L-carnitine, taurine, garlic, high folic acid levels, trimethylglycine, and alpha-lipoic acid are all beneficial to those with various types of cardiovascular problems.

Sample Products:

- *MaxiLife Cardio Protector* (Twinlab) is a comprehensive multi-vitamin-multimineral supplement for those with heart disease. It provides 600 milligrams of magnesium, but only twenty-five milligrams of calcium. This is fine, if supplemented with a regular calcium or calcium/magnesium supplement. Many with heart disease benefit from a higher ratio of magnesium to calcium, but this does not necessarily mean that the need for calcium's bone building and other functions no longer exists. Unless advised otherwise, then, if you continue to take a regular calcium-magnesium supplement, the extra magnesium in this product will alter the ratio, without depriving you of calcium.

MaxLife Cardio Protector contains full homocysteine support nutrients, as well as other cardiovascular-specific items such as red wine concentrate, CoQ_{10}, tocotrienols, carnitine, taurine, and alpha-lipoic acid. It is an excellent supplement for those with heart disease who want to minimze the number of products they use. Every six capsules contain the following:

Beta-Carotene (pro vitamin A activity)	25,000 IU
Vitamin D$_3$	400 IU
Vitamin C	1,000 mg
Red Wine Concentrate (standardized for 30% polyphenols and flavonoids)	50 mg
Natural Vitamin E	800 IU
Tocotrienol Concentrate (standardized for 15% tocotrienols)	50 mg
CoQ$_{10}$ (coenzyme Q$_{10}$)	60 mg
L-Carnitine	250 mg
Taurine	500 mg
Alpha-Lipoic Acid	50 mg
Garlic (from odor-controlled garlic powder)	100 mg
Vitamin B$_1$ (thiamine)	25 mg

Vitamin B$_2$ (riboflavin)	25 mg
Vitamin B$_6$ (pyridoxine)	50 mg
Vitamin B$_{12}$ cobalamin	500 mcg
Trimethylglycine (betaine)	100 mg
Folic Acid	800 mcg
Niacinamide	50 mg
Pantothenic Acid	100 mg
Biotin	300 mcg
PABA (para-aminobenzoic acid)	25 mg
Choline Bitartrate	25 mg
Inositol	50 mg
Calcium (from calcium citrate and carbonate)	25 mg
Magnesium (magnesium aspartate and oxide)	600 mg
Potassium (from potassium aspartate and citrate)	100 mg
Zinc (from zinc picolinate)	30 mg
Copper (from coated copper gluconate)	2 mg
Manganese (from managanese gluconate)	1 mg
Iodine (from potassium iodide)	150 mcg
Selenium (from selenomethionine)	200 mcg
Chromium (from ChromeMate® chromium nicotinate)	400 mcg
Molybdenum (from natural molybdic acid)	150 mcg

Children's Formulas

Description: It is important to provide multivitamin supplements to children. The challenge, of course, is to make them palatable without turning them into candy.

Ingredients: Some children's vitamin products contain only a limited number of nutrients. We prefer formulas that have a broad spectrum of vitamins and minerals.

Sample Products:

- *Kid's Companion Multiple* (Natrol) is an excellent children's multi, containing over thirty vitamins, minerals, and other nutrients. It is a natural grape-berry flavored chewable wafer, sweetened with fructose.

• *Animal Friends* (Twinlab) is also an excellent product. It is not quite as robust as the Natrol's product, providing only 25 milligrams of calcium and 12 milligrams of magnesium to Natrol's 100 milligrams and 50 milligrams, respectively. But the Natrol product is based on a two-per-day dose, while the Twinlab product is one per day. It is also fruit flavored, and in animal shapes, which may make it more acceptable to some small children.

Detoxification Formulas

Description: We are exposed to toxins of many types, in many ways. We breathe in airborne toxins from industrial and automotive pollution. Pollutants—pesticide residues, heavy metals, and microbial toxins—are in our food and water. The metabolic breakdown products of drugs and other proteins can be toxic to the body. Our body has ways to neutralize and eliminate these toxins, with the liver being the main tool charged with this task. When liver function is compromised, or the integrity of the intestinal wall is compromised, the body's normal detoxification process may become inadequate. Some feel that the mere magnitude of environmental toxins we are now exposed to, compared to what was experienced by our ancestors, is a contributory factor to many of the chronic diseases now on the increase.

A COMMENT FROM DR. ABEL

The kidneys, in addition to the liver, excrete toxins from the body. The kidney cleans out water-soluble chemicals and waste, and the liver excretes fat-soluble materials. Blood goes through the renal arteries into the capillaries, and then passes through a cluster of tubules called glomeruli. It is these renal tubules where critical nutrients are absorbed and other molecules are excreted. For instance, we need to retain potassium while excreting sodium, and our kidneys help us do that. Through this process, they help control our blood pressure. Certain medications, such as diuretics, used for congestive heart failure and high blood pressure, may alter the kidney's efficiency. Dehydration, increased alcohol consumption, a high-protein diet, a high-saturated-fat/low-fiber diet, too much vitamin D-enriched food (more than 600 IU per day) are dietary imbalances that can cause kidney stones. If kidney function is reduced, there may be metabolic imbalances, including fluid retention, weight gain, bleeding, and loss of water-soluble antioxidants.

Ingredients: The purpose of detoxification is to aid the body in eliminating excess toxins. We do this by enhancing liver function, with herbs such as milk thistle and artichoke leaf. We cleanse the bowel with mild laxative herbs such as senna and cascara. We use antioxidants such as vitamin C and glutathione. We drink extra water and increase fiber levels to improve elimination of waste. We encourage bile flow, using lipotropic agents and choleretic herbs.

Sample Products:

- *Detox* Capsules (Natrol) contains zinc, garlic, dandelion, yellow dock, sarsaparilla, burdock, cascara sagrada, goldenseal, licorice, parsley, milk thistle, NAC, and aloe vera gel.
- *Detoxicates* Capsules (Twinlab) is a mixture of vitamin B_1, L-cysteine, vitamin C, and glutathione specifically indicated for smokers and drinkers.
- *Detox Formula* Capsules (Nature's Answer) contains prickly ash bark extract (4:1), dandelion root, burdock root, psyllium husk, green tea, and bilberry fruit.
- *Daily Detox* (Gaia Herbs) contains corydalis, yellow dock, black alder, mayapple, and figwort. This product designed for internal cleansing of the liver and gall bladder.
- *Colon Cleanse* Powder and Tea (Health Plus) is a psyllium husk powder designed as a bulk cleanse. *Super Colon Cleanse* (Health Plus) adds senna, buckthorn, and cascara sagrada to the psyllium for those folks who need a bit more stimulation to help them cleanse properly.
- *Liver Cleanse* (Health Plus) contains artichoke extract, beet leaf, black radish, dandelion root, milk thistle, B vitamins, turmeric extract, and astaxanthin, the powerful carotenoid antioxidant.
- *Heart Cleanse, Blood Cleanse, Kidney Cleanse, Joint Cleanse, Prostate Cleanse* and *Adrenal Cleanse* (Health Plus) are additional detoxification products designed, obviously, for specific types of health problems.

Digestive Enzyme Formulas

Description: Digestive enzymes are needed to break down food—proteases digest protein, lipases digest fat, and amylases digest carbohydrates. Different enzymes are secreted by the body at different times during the digestive processes, and each is designed to work optimally in that area. For example, pepsin works in an acid environment—with the hydrochloric acid in the stomach—to digest protein. Pancreatic enzymes, on the other hand, are designed to work in the more alkaline environment of the duodenum. Supplementation with digestive enzymes can be indicated for indigestion, pancreatic insufficiency, celiac disease, Crohn's disease, GERD, and people with food allergies.

Ingredients: Digestive enzymes can be derived from animal sources (pancreatin, pepsin), plant sources (papain, bromelain), or fungal sources. Each has its unique advantages and disadvantages. The plant enzymes only digest protein. The animal proteins work only within a specific pH range, but they work very well. Pancreatin digests proteins, carbohydrates, and fat. The fungal enzymes work over a very broad pH range, and are preferred by those who do not want to take animal products. Enzymes should be labeled in terms of potency units, not milligrams. Products that label the potency of enzymes in milligrams only, with no indication of units of activity (for example, 4X, or 200 GDU/gm), should not be purchased.

Sample Products:

- *Digestive Aid Tablets* (Solgar) and the following product, *Super Enzyme Capsules*, from Twinlab, are typical digestive enzyme combinations. Both suffer from the above labeling defect. According to the label, every Digestive Aid Tablet contains the following:

Pancreatin (4x USP) (derived from 130 mg quadruple-strength concentrate)	500 mg
Ox bile extract	130 mg
Pepsin	100 mg
Betaine HCl	65 mg
Diastase (as Aspergillus oryzae)	65 mg
Papain	32 mg

- *Super Enzyme Capsules* (Twinlab) is a good broad-spectrum enzyme blend, but the quantity of bromelain and papain are listed in milligrams, not units of potency, which is virtually meaningless. Bulk bromelain, for example, can be purchased in up to twelve different strengths. Obviously, 250 milligrams of a very weak strength is not the same as 250 milligrams of a very strong strength. In the Solgar products, above, the same can be said for the pepsin and papain ingredients. Every two capsules of Super Enzyme contain the following:

Pancreatin 4x (quadruple strength) (equivalent to 2,000 mg of pancreatin USP), supplying:	500 mg
—Amylase	50,000 USP units
—Protease (trypsin and chymotrypsin)	50,000 USP units
—Lipase	8,500 USP units
Betaine HCl (betaine hydrochloride)	324 mg (5 grains)
Pepsin NF (1:10,000)	130 mg (2 grains)
Ox Bile	130 mg (2 grains)
Bromelain (pineapple)	250 mg
Papain (papaya)	250 mg

- *Super Enzymes* (NOW) is a comprehensive, balanced formula, properly labeled as to potency. Each tablet contains: Betaine HCl (from beets and molasses), 200 mg; Pancreatin 4X, 200 mg (Supplying—Amylase 20,000 USP units, Protease 20,000 USP, Lipase 3,400 USP units); Papain (70 MCU from papaya), 100 mg; Cellulase (10 FCC units), 10 mg; Ox Bile Extract, 100 mg; Pepsin Enzymes (NF 1:10,000), 50 mg; Bromelain (2,400 GDU from pineapple), 50 mg; Papaya Enzymes, 45 mg; Pineapple Enzymes, 45 mg.
- *Maxi-Zyme* Capsules (Country Life) is a broad-spectrum, high-potency blend of pancreatin 8X, betaine HCL, ox bile, bromelain, and papain, properly labeled.

It should be pointed out that it is okay to list the amount of an enzyme such as bromelain in milligrams as long as the potency of the bromelain is provided, i.e. "2,400 GDU."

Digestive enzymes can also be obtained from nonanimal sources (fungal enzymes). Several examples are provided below:

- *Vegetarian Digestive Aid* (Solgar) lists the potency of its enzyme components only in milligrams, and for this reason we do not recommend the product.
- *Plant Enzymes* (NOW) is a comprehensive blend of vegetarian enzymes active in a broad pH range, properly labeled as to potency. It contains the fungal protease, lipase, and amylase, along with papain and bromelain.
- *Similase* (Tyler) is a popular vegetarian enzyme blend that contains, in addition to the plant enzymes, lactase, sucrase, phytase, and maltase, all properly labeled. I'm not sure who needs "sucrase," but what the heck! You never can tell when something unexpected might come up.
- *Papaya Enzymes, Chewable* (numerous companies) is a product of questionable efficacy. What happens when you eat raw pineapple? The proteolytic enzymes in the pineapple (bromelain) start to digest the protein tissue in your mouth. You may notice some irritation on your tongue and gums. These proteins are used in meat tenderizer. If there was enough proteolytic enzyme content in a chewable tablet, one would expect to end up with similar irritation to the tissues in your mouth.

Energy Support Formulas

Description: "Low energy" is one of the most common complaints heard by doctors and health food store clerks. Usually, the person is looking for some type of miracle pill that will solve the problem. They are not likely to find it.

When they ask us, our response is typically, "Are you taking a good multivitamin? a multimineral? an antioxidant blend?" and perhaps most important, "Have you been to the doctor for a full checkup?" Ideally, you want to look for the underlying cause of the problem, with the help of your doctor, ruling out any medical problems that might be contributing to the condition. If the cause of the lack of energy is stress, suboptimal nutrition, or overexertion, the use of nutritional supplements might actually help.

Ingredients: There are certain nutrients and herbs that are involved with low-energy conditions in a general sense. A deficiency of vitamin B_{12}, for example, can cause fatigue. And taking extra vitamin B_{12} can increase energy, even when there is no deficiency. In the past, it was said that the only way to achieve this was through injection, but we now know that high doses of B_{12} orally will also work. Extra amounts of the entire B-complex family should be taken. Some have found that the amino acid L-carnitine can help, perhaps because it increases the efficiency of cellular energy production. Extra magnesium might help. NADH, a coenzyme involved in the production of cellular energy, might also be helpful. There is a long history of belief in bee pollen and related products as energy enhancers, but a better approach might be to use adaptogenic herbs such as Siberian and American ginseng.

Sample Products:

- *Energy Modulators* (Solgar) is a blend of many of the nutrients and herbs mentioned above. It contains all three types of ginseng, which is quite appropriate for this type of application. In addition, it contains the herb rhodiola, another adaptogenic herb with a history of use in reducing fatigue and enhancing the body's ability to cope with stress. Every two vegicaps contain the following:

Niacin (as niacinamide, niacin)	25 mg
Vitamin B_{12} (as cobalamin)	100 mcg
Creatine Monohydrate	250 mg
Standardized American Ginseng Extract (root) (ginsenosides 10mg [10%])	100 mg
Standardized Siberian Ginseng Extract (root) (eleutheroside E 0.5 mg [0.5%], eleutheroside B 0.3 mg [0.3])	100 mg
Standardized Korean Ginseng Extract (root) (ginsenosides 8 mg [8%])	100 mg
Standardized Rhodiola Extract (root) (salidrozid 1 mg [1%], polyphenols 40 mg [40%])	100 mg
Alpha-Lipoic Acid	60 mg
Coenzyme Q_{10} (as ubiquinone)	60 mg
Octacosanol	1 mg

- *Herb Energizer Liquid Extract* (Nature's Answer) is a product that can be used as a short-term energy supplement, but with caution. It contains ma huang, a source of natural ephedra, along with herbs that contain caffeine, such as guarana and kola nut. It also contains fo-ti, gotu kola, and cayenne. This product, and others like it, certainly can provide an energy boost you can feel, but should not be used by those with high blood pressure, diabetes, thyroid disease, prostate enlargement, heart disease, seizure disorders, or those taking other prescription drugs, including MAO inhibitors.

Some people expect this kind of "kick" when taking ginseng supplements. Ginseng should not produce that type of reaction. The effect is more subtle and pervasive.

- *Balanced Ginseng Liquid Extract* (Nature's Answer) is a blend of three ginsengs, with synergistic herbs (jujube and Chinese licorice), designed to build energy and "chi" (life force), particularly for those feeling tired and debilitated. This product does not contain Siberian ginseng. Instead, it contains American ginseng, and two types of Chinese ginseng, red and white. It is not intended for use during acute illness, pregnancy, or those with hypertension.
- *Cerni-Queen* (Graminex) combines the energy-enhancing benefits of Cernitin Swedish flower pollen extract with royal jelly.

Essential Fatty Acid Blends

Description: Technically, the "essential fatty acids" are linoleic acid, an omega-6 fatty acid, and alpha-linolenic acid, an omega-3 fatty acid. These are the two fatty acids the body needs, but cannot synthesize, or produce on its own. They must be obtained from the diet, as is the case for vitamins. Alpha-linolenic acid is converted in the body to EPA (eicosapentaenoic acid) and DHA (docosahexaenoic acid), which are omega-3 oils found in oily fish. Many believe that today, our diet is too rich in omega-6 fatty acids, which are found in animal protein and vegetable oils, compared to omega-3 oils. Omega-3 oils, EPA and DHA, are also precursors to prostaglandins that exert certain beneficial actions in the body (e.g., reducing inflammation and platelet aggregation). Supplementation with omega-3 oils, therefore, has become popular. The therapeutic benefits are well documented. EPA/DHA-rich oils have been shown to help in cardiovascular disease, asthma, skin diseases, ulcerative colitis, and autoimmune disease.

The term "essential fatty acids" is now used a little more loosely to mean those fatty acids that are therapeutically beneficial, and includes products containing fish oil and olive oil. One mistake that many people now make, after hearing so often that omega-6 oils are "bad" and omega-3 oils are "good," is to start to believe it literally. Not all omega-6 oils are bad per se. Certain omega-6 oils are "essential," and certain others contain fatty acids that lead to the formation of prostaglandins with beneficial actions similar to those derived from EPA and DHA. Examples of these "good" omega-6 oils are evening primrose oil and borage oil. Black currant oil contains both omega-3 and omega-6 fatty acids.

Ingredients: The main "essential fatty acids" found in supplements are as follows: fish oil or EPA and DHA (omega-3); flaxseed or linseed oil, which contains alpha-linolenic acid that can be converted to EPA and DHA; evening primrose oil, borage oil and black currant oil, which contain GLA, or gamma-linolenic acid, which is a precursor to the PG1 series prostaglandins; and olive oil, a monounsaturated fatty acid. The omega-3 oils are precursors to the PG3 series prostaglandins.

Sample Products:

- *MaxEPA/GLA* (Solgar) is a blend of the two major groups of therapeutically beneficial fatty acids, omega-3 (EPA and DHA) and omega-6 (GLA), in their preformed, active form. Every two softgels contain the following:

Vitamin E (as D-alpha tocopherol)	36 IU
EPA (as eicosapentaenoic acid)	360 mg
DHA (as docosahexaenoic acid)	240 mg
GLA (as gamma-linolenic acid)	90 mg

- *Flax Borage Omega-3* (Natrol) is similar to the above product, except it contains flaxseed oil, with smaller amounts of preformed EPA, DHA, and GLA. This is fine for general use, as the body can convert the alpha-linolenic acid in flaxseed oil to EPA and DHA. But for therapeutic purposes, it might not be prudent to rely completely on the efficiency of that conversion, which can be impaired under certain conditions. On the other hand, many people prefer the flaxseed oil over fish oil because they do not like the aftertaste of fish oil. Every one softgel of Flax Borage Omega-3 contains the following:

Essential Fatty Acid	1.2 g
Flaxseed Oil, Borage Oil, Omega-3 Oil (Including alpha-	

> linolenic acid 200mg, linolenic acid 175 mg, oleic acid
> 150 mg, gamma linolenic acid 75, eicosapentanoic acid
> 70 mg, docosahexanoic acid 45 mg)

- *Total EFA* (Health from the Sun) is another good comprehensive blend of the various essential fatty acids. It is available in capsule and liquid form.

Eye and Vision Support

Description: Most eye and vision problems are directly or indirectly related to free radical damage. This includes cataracts and macular degeneration. In cataracts, the damage is to the lens of the eye, and in macular degeneration, the retina is affected. The underlying cause of diabetic retinopathy, obviously, is diabetes and poor blood sugar control, and retinitis pigmentosa results from a genetic disorder. Even though the primary cause of these conditions is not oxidative damage, the use of antioxidant nutrients, capillary-strengthening flavonoids, and essential fatty acids can help control the damage. This includes treatment for glaucoma as well.

A COMMENT FROM DR. ABEL

Macular degeneration can be simply defined as starvation of the retina as a result of poor digestion and weakened circulation. It is a condition that affects the central area of vision, which provides the ability to see small detail such as road signs and print, and aids daytime vision. The cone cells in the macula, a region at the rear of the interior of the eyeball, respond to light and color. They break down in order to send an electrical response through the optic nerve to the brain.

Free radicals are formed during the vision process, which requires rapid neutralization by circulating antioxidants. If your body has a low antioxidant "bank account," degeneration in the macular may result. The cells cannot be rebuilt quickly enough.

There is a yellow-colored pigment, lutein, which is deposited in the retina to help prevent toxicity from ultraviolet and blue light. Symptoms of macular degeneration include: difficulty with small print; missing areas in vision and distortion of the letters on a line. Ninety percent of people who have AMD have the dry, slowly progressive form of macular degeneration. The other 10 percent suffer from the wet form, which may cause a sudden loss of central vision.

Here are some tips to enable you to avoid, or lessen the risk of macular degeneration:

- Wear UV-blocking sunglasses. UV light rays are extremely important as an association to long-term degeneration of the retina.
- Always maintain a positive antioxidant balance. Many investigations have shown certain vitamins confer a protective effect on the retina. Lutein and its isomer zeaxanthin protect some of the delicate cones in the central retina area known as the macula. Other studies have demonstrated that vitamin E and, to a lesser extent vitamin A, are supportive of the sensitive retinal receptors that transmit the light. Glutathione has also been found to be important. These fat-soluble vitamins obviously protect cell membranes, and there is an 80 percent decrease of risk of macular degeneration among people who take 6 mg of lutein daily, or have a cup of spinach four to seven times a week. Recent studies are even indicating that people can reverse the early stages of dry macular degeneration.
- Build retina cell membranes, which have extensive folds and convolutions with DHA. Thirty percent of the brain and retina are composed of docosahexaenoic acid (DHA), which supports the integrity of all cell membranes. Having six double bonds, it is able to handle the onslaught from a great number of free radicals.
- Smoking is another major risk factor for macular degeneration. Be wise in this regard.
- Exercise is important, especially exercising the head and neck muscles and encouraging blood flow in this region.
- Maintain cardiovascular health. Maintain normal cholesterol, blood sugar, and blood pressure.
- Use the Amsler Grid to monitor your eyesight if you do have macular degeneration.
- Postmenopausal females are at the greatest risk of developing macular degeneration and should take preventative steps. People who have low thyroid or are on thyroid supplementation are also at risk, as are light-skinned and light-eyed people. These people should plan ahead and recommend sunglasses for the entire family.

Ingredients: The most important ingredients of all eye and vision support products are the various antioxidants. Of particular importance is glutathione, and glutathione precursors should be a part of any eye formula. This would include vitamin C, methionine, cysteine, n-acetyl-cysteine, and/or glutathione itself. Herbal antioxidants are especially important because they also contribute to the membrane and capillary-strengthening action of the various flavonoids. Bilberry, ginkgo, and eyebright are commonly used for this purpose. Grape seed extract and pine bark extracts, rich in proanthocyanidins, would be appropriate as well, along with the flavonoid quercetin. Lutein is a fat-soluble carotenoid antioxidant compound that is normally present in the central area of the retina. It appears to be important in protecting against macular degeneration. The antioxidant vitamins (vitamins C and E, for example) are clearly indicated to protect against eye and vision problems. Studies have shown that people taking multivitamin supplements for ten years or more have a 60 percent lower incidence of cataract formation.

Sample Products:

- *Ocuguard Plus with Lutein* (Twinlab) is a comprehensive blend of carotenoids, antioxidant vitamins and minerals, glutathione precursors, and bilberry extract. Vitamin B_2 is also involved in glutathione metabolism, and chromium can help to normalize blood sugar levels for those who might be prone to diabetes. Quercetin may also help in that regard, by blocking the accumulation of sorbitol in the eye. Every four capsules of Ocuguard Plus with Lutein contain the following:

Beta-Carotene (pro-vitamin A)	40,000 IU
Lutein	20 mg
Natural Vitamin E (succinate)	400 IU
Vitamin C	1,500 mg
Citrus Bioflavonoid Complex	250 mg
Quercetin (bioflavonoid)	100 mg
Billberry Extract (source of bioflavonoid) standardized for 25% anthocyanosides	10 mg
Rutin (bioflavonoid)	100 mg
Zinc (from zinc picolinate)	25 mg

Selenium (from selenomethionine)	100 mcg
Taurine	200 mg
N-Acetyl-Cysteine (glutathione precursor)	200 mg
L-Glutathione	10 mg
Vitamin B$_2$ (riboflavin)	50 mg
Chromium (GTF)	200 mcg

- *Bilberry Ginkgo Eyebright Complex Plus Lutein* (Solgar) is similar to the above product, except it contains three extremely valuable herbs that are rich in protective flavonoids. Bilberry and eyebright have a long history of use in treating a wide variety of eye problems, including night vision, eye strain, conjunctivitis, and dry or weeping eyes. Every two vegicaps of Bilberry Ginkgo Eyebright Comples Plus Lutien contain the following:

Vitamin A (as palmitate 1000 IU, 80% [4000 IU] as natural beta carotene	5,000 IU
Vitamin C (as calcium ascorbate)	300 mg
Vitamin E (as D-alpha tocopheryl succinate)	100 IU
Zinc (as zinc glycinate)	10 mg
Selenium (L-selenomethionine)	25 mcg
Lutein (from marigold flower)	10 mg
Eyebright Extract [whole-plant] (4:1)	25 mg
Bilberry Extract [berry] (anthocyanosides 2.4 mg [24%])	20 mg
Ginkgo Biloba Extract [leaf] (ginkgoflavoglycosides 5 mg [25%])	10 mg
NAC (N-acetyl-L-cysteine)	100 mg
Taurine	100 mg
Carotenoid Mix (alpha-carotene, lutein, zeaxanthin, cryptoxanthin)	46 mcg

- *Able Eyes* (Carlson) is a new product formulated by Dr. Abel to promote and maintain healthy eyes and lasting vision. It contains antioxidant vitamins, minerals, and DHA, along with lutein and a blend of flavonoids. Every softgel contains:

Vitamin A (from fish liver oil)	5000 IU
Vitamin C (ascorbic acid)	200 mg
Vitamin E (d-alpha tocopherol)	200 IU
Magnesium (from magnesium oxide)	100 mg
Chromium (from chromium amino acid chelate)	120 mcg
Zinc (from zinc citrate)	10 mg
DHA (from fish oils)	100 mg
Lutein (FloraGlo)	2 mg
Bilberry (standardized to 25% anthocyanidins)	100 mg
Citrus Bioflavonoid Complex	60 mg
Quercetin (bioflavonoid)	60 mg
Silymarin Seeds	60 mg

- *Vision Optimizer* (Jarrow) provides higher levels of bilberry, ginkgo, and quercetin than the above products, but does not have any beta-carotene, NAC, or glutathione.

Fiber, Dietary

Description: Fiber is nondigestible carbohydrate. There are two types of fiber, water-soluble and water-insoluble. Each type seems to have unique benefits. The water-soluble fiber is thought to lower cholesterol and modulate blood sugar levels, while insoluble fiber seems to be better at improving bowel function (constipation), lowering the risk of heart disease, and reducing the risk of colon cancer. Recent research seems to indicate that the distinction between the two types of fiber may not be as pronounced as previously thought. For this reason, we prefer the use of mixed fiber blends. An additional use of fiber supplements is as an adjunct to a weight loss program. Taking a dose of fiber, before meals, with ample water, should create a feeling of satiety. Lignan, a type of fiber found in flaxseed, may protect against breast cancer.

Ingredients: Water-soluble fibers include psyllium, oat bran, guar gum, pectin, and fruit. Water-insoluble fiber is usually found in whole grains, such as wheat bran.

Sample Products:

• *Fibersol* (Twinlab) is a water-soluble fiber supplement and is best used for the treatment of high cholesterol and/or blood sugar problems. Every five capsules contain the following:

Fiber Blend Concentrate (from psyllium seed husks, guar gum, apple pectin)	4 g

• *Multiple Fiber Formula* (Solgar) contains five types of fiber, which are mostly water-soluble. Every two vegicaps contain the following:

Oat Bran	200 mg
Apple Pectin	200 mg
Grapefruit Pectin	200 mg
Flaxseed Meal	200 mg
Psyllium Seed Husks	200 mg

• *Colon Care* (Twinlab) adds probiotic supplements and is thus more directed at intestinal function and detox applications. Every serving contains the following:

Psyllium Husk Fiber	5 g
Barley Malt	17 g
Lactobacillus acidophilus (supplying 1 billion live cells at formulation)	107 mg
Bifidobacterium longum (supplying 1 billion live cells at formulation)	136 mg
Buffered Vitamin C (calcium ascorbate)	250 mg

• *Daily Fiber Caps* (Yerba Prima) is a blend of the two types of fiber, though mostly soluble, and is an excellent general-purpose daily supplement. It contains psyllium, acacia gum, soy fiber, oat bran, and apple pectin extract. It is available in capsule and powder forms.

Green Food Concentrates

Description: This category will encompass two types of "green food" concentrates. First, there are concentrates of green foods only. These include spirulina, various other algae concentrates, wheat grass, kamut, barley grass, and chlorella. They are healthy substances, but not "wonder foods" as some of the marketers would like you to believe. They are rich in chlorophyl, carotenoids, and a good source of moderate-quality protein. But when you combine these green food concentrates with concentrates of other vegetables and fruits, you really have something. Few of us eat the recommended quantities of fruits and vegetables, but these foods are rich in powerful, therapeutic phytonutrients with antioxidant and anticancer activity. A broad spectrum green food concentrate, containing a broad range of phytonutrients, should be an integral part of any comprehensive supplement program.

Sample Products:

- **Green Essentials Drink** (Twinlab) is a blend of various green food concentrates, available in tablet and powder form. Every teaspoon contains the following:

Barley Grass	500 mg
Wheat Grass	500 mg
Alfalfa Powder	375 mg
Broccoli Powder	375 mg
Kelp Powder	375 mg
Spinach Powder	375 mg

- *Earth Source Greens and More* (Solgar) is a more comprehensive blend of phytonutrients, green foods, and herbs, available in powder and capsule form. Every teaspoon contains the following:

Vitamin A	1,431 IU
Vitamin C	14 mg
Calcium	32 mg
Iron	2.5 mg

Sodium	81 mg
Lecithin Powder	2 g (2,000 mg)
Hawaiian Blue Green Spirulina	1 g (1,000 mg)
Carrot Powder	400 mg
Orange Juice Crystals	400 mg
Organic Alfalfa Grass Powder	375 mg
Organic Barley Grass Powder	375 mg
Organic Green Kamut Powder	375 mg
Organic Wheat Grass Powder	375 mg
Chinese Chlorella Powder (from broken cell wall)	350 mg
Wheat Sprouts	350 mg
Apple Pectin	300 mg
Brown Rice Bran Powder	300 mg
Flaxseed Meal Powder	300 mg
Oat Bran Powder	300 mg
Red Beet Powder	200 mg
Acerola Extract (berry)	150 mg
Bee Pollen Powder	100 mg
Broccoli Powder	100 mg
Licorice Extract (root)	100 mg
Royal Jelly Powder	100 mg
Maitake Mushroom Powder	75 mg
Organic Reishi Mushroom Mycelia Powder	75 mg
Shiitake Mushroom Powder	75 mg
Astragalus Extract (root)	60 mg
Licorice Powder (root)	60 mg
Milk Thistle Extract (fruit) (48 mg [80%] silymarin)	60 mg
Siberian Ginseng Extract (root)	60 mg
Apple Powder (fruit)	50 mg
Strawberry Powder (fruit)	50 mg
Dulse Powder	25 mg
Bilberry Extract (berry) (5 mg [25%] anthocyanosides)	20 mg

Ginkgo Biloba Extract (leaf) (4.8 mg [24%] ginkgoflavo-glycosides)	20 mg
Grape Seed Extract (10 mg [50%] proanthocyanadins)	20 mg

- **Green Defense** (Jarrow) Contains green foods, botanicals, phytonutrients, and probiotic bacterial metabolites.

Hair, Skin, and Nail Support

Description: Hair, skin, and nails are composed of protein. Specifically, protein rich in sulfur amino acids. The stimulation of collagen synthesis and keratin can result in stronger hair and nails.

Ingredients: Amino acids, especially sulfur-containing amino acids such as cysteine, are the building blocks of hair, skin, nails, and all connective tissue. Protein supplementation may benefit those with borderline protein intake and problems with hair, skin, or nails. Proline works with vitamin C to form collagen, the chief constituent of skin, tendons, and other connective tissue. Antioxidant vitamins and minerals are needed to protect the skin and hair from free-radical damage. Essential fatty acids are important for good skin, hair, and nail health. A slight deficiency of certain nutrients (vitamin A, zinc, iron) can lead to hair loss. For this reason, a broad-spectrum multivitamin-multimineral supplement should always be the first line of defense. Biotin, one of the B vitamins, is especially important, as is the trace mineral silicon.

Sample Products:

- **Skin, Nails and Hair** (Solgar) is a combination of nutrients involved in the synthesis of collagen and keratin, the main building blocks of hair, skin, and nails. Every two tablets contain the following:

Vitamin C (as l-ascorbic acid)	120 mg
Calcium	90 mg
Zinc (as zinc citrate)	15 mg
Copper (as copper glycinate)	2 mg
MSM (as methylsulfonylmethane)	1,000 mg

Silicon (as silica, as L. corallioides [red algae powder])	50 mg
L-Proline	50 mg
L-Lysine (as L-lysine HCl)	50 mg

- **Hair Factors** (Twinlab). Every six tablets contain the following:

L-Cysteine	1,002 mg
Vitamin C (from ascorbic acid)	3,000 mg
Biotin	6,000 mcg
PABA (para-aminobenzoic acid)	1,002 mg
Inositol	2,004 mg

- **Women's Skin Hair Nails** (Natrol). This is a nice, comprehensive formula, and I don't really know what would happen if men took the product! In fact, I think it would work equally well for men as well as women. Every two capsules of Women's Skin Hair Nails contain the following:

Vitamin A (as vitamin A palmitate)	5,000 IU
Vitamin C (as ascorbic acid)	100 mg
Vitamin E (as d-alpha tocopheryl succinate)	50 IU
Thiamine (as thiamin HCl) (vitamin B_1)	10 mg
Riboflavin (vitamin B_2)	10 mg
Vitamin B_6 (as pyridoxine HCl)	20 mg
Vitamin B_{12} (as cobalamin)	50 mcg
Biotin	500 mcg
Zinc (as zinc oxide)	8 mg
Copper (as amino acid chelate)	2 mg
Manganese (as manganese carbonate)	2 mg
MSM (methyl sulfonyl methane)	250 mg
Trace Mineral complex	100 mg
Cysteine (as L-cysteine hydrochloride)	75 mg
PABA (para-aminobenzoic acid)	50 mg
Burdock Root	50 mg

Choline (as choline bitartrate)	25 mg
Inositol	25 mg
Silicon (as colloidal silicon)	20 mg
L-Glutathione	2 mg

Hematinic Formulas

Description: Iron is a mineral that is essential to the blood's ability to provide oxygen to the cells throughout the body. It is essential for growth, energy production, immune system function, and many enzyme systems. Iron deficiency can be caused by loss of blood (excessive menstrual bleeding, gastrointestinal bleeding due to aspirin or similar drugs, ulcers, hemorrhoids) or insufficient dietary intake. For most people, the 10 to 18 milligrams of iron found in multivitamin supplements is sufficient, but there are times when more is needed. This should be determined by a physician. Too much iron can be as bad as too little iron, and the only way to determine if you are in either category is through blood tests (serum ferritin, CBC).

Ingredients: Not all forms of iron are well absorbed, or well tolerated. The types used in the following products were chosen with this in mind. Other nutrients, such as vitamin C, vitamin A, and betaine HCl, can enhance the absorption of iron.

Sample Products:

- *Hematinic Formula* (Solgar) contains a well-tolerated, nonconstipating form of iron. Every three tablets contain the following:

Vitamin C (as calcium ascorbate)	300 mg
Folic Acid	300 mcg
Vitamin B_{12} (as cobalamin)	150 mcg
Calcium (as dicalcium phosphate, calcium ascorbate)	120 mg
Iron (as iron bisglycinate)	45 mg
Desiccated and Defatted Liver Powder	750 mg

- *Hemaplex* (Progressive Labs). This formula contains 32 milligrams of iron, as iron peptonate, which is a very well-tolerated form of iron, along with folic acid and B-complex vitamins.

Immune Support—Cancer Prevention

Description: There are many nutrients that have been shown to enhance or modulate immune system function, and they have been discussed throughout this book. While we still have much to learn about cancer, there is evidence that certain nutrients, or phytochemicals, seem to have a role in preventing certain types of cancer. The exact mechanism may not be known, but if a relationship seems to exist, it would be foolish not to exploit it, especially if there is no downside. No one seems to have a problem recommending an increased amount of fruit and vegetables in the diet as a means of reducing the risk of certain cancers. Why, then, is it not appropriate to take supplemental lycopene, isoflavones, indole-3-carbinol?

It is true that prevention may be one thing, and treatment may be another. There remains some controversy about the advisability of combining nonconventional and conventional cancer therapies. There is concern as to whether using nonconventional remedies, such as elutherococcus, astragalus, or antioxidants, during conventional therapy is advisable. These substances seem to reduce the side effects of chemotherapy and radiation. Does this mean they also reduce their effect? We do not yet know for sure. Fortunately, conventional medicine is now looking more closely at "alternative" treatments.

Ingredients: Most of the ingredients included in these products have been discussed elsewhere in this book. Sometimes the evidence for their value in preventing a certain type of cancer is based on epidemiologial evidence—for instance, women who eat lots of broccoli have the lowest incidence of breast cancer. The evidence can also be in vitro—an extract of I-3-C (found in broccoli) kills cancer cells in a test tube. Much of the evidence is based on animal studies, but there is some research on humans. Regardless of the strength of the evidence, the key, usually, is the benefit-to-risk ratio.

Sample Products:

- *Cell Support* (Solgar). Every three tablets contain the following:

Iron	2 mg
Soy Isoflavone Extract (seed)	400 mg
Beta 1,3 Glucans (from 500 mg yeast cell wall concentrate)	100 mg
D-Limonene	80 mg

Modified Citrus Pectin (average molecular weights 15 KD)	400 mg
Standardized Red Reishi Mushroom Extract (triterpenes 8 mg [4%], polysaccharides 20 mg [10%])	200 mg
LEM Shiitake Mycelia Mushroom Extract	200 mg
Quercetin (from Dimorphandra mollis)	200 mg
Indole-3-Carbinol	5 mg
Lutein (from marigold flower)	5 mg
Lycopene (from tomato)	5 mg

- *Cell-Factors* (Country Life), contains inositol hexaphosphate, grape extract, beta glucans, green tea extract, broccoli sprout extract, knotweed extract, and indole-3-carbinol.

Immune Support—General

Description: The body has many weapons against microorganisms. Healthy, intact skin, mucous membranes, and stomach acid are examples of one type. The thymus gland, bone marrow, spleen, and lymphatic system play a role. And specialized white blood cells (lymphocytes, phagocytes), and antibodies are also involved in immune function. When all of the body's immune system components are working optimally, we can withstand the onslaught of most infectious organisms.

A COMMENT FROM DR. ABEL

Researchers reviewed more than 100 articles trying to determine whether the age-old myth about vitamin C preventing the common cold was valid. (*British Journal of Nutrition,* 1992; 67:3–16). Vitamin C has long been known to contibute to many significant biochemical reactions throughout the body and, as a water-soluble vitamin, could resupply other antioxidants in neutralizing free radicals. Linus Pauling, Ph.D., popularized taking vitamin C on a daily basis. The result of this *British Journal of Nutrition* study was that there was insufficient evidence about vitamin C preventing the common cold because most individuals had not received the vitamin before the study started. However, the majority of the papers they reviewed demonstrated vitamin C was able to shorten the duration and reduce the severity of the colds. The only side effect from their investigation was that large doses of vitamin C could cause diarrhea and stomach discomfort, which stopped when the vitamin C was discontinued. Most people are able to find a comfortable daily level. The studies did not confirm the warning that some doctors have given that large doses of vitamin C could cause calcium oxylate stones, impair vitamin B_{12} status, or create an iron overload. In my experience taking 2,000 to 3,000 mg of vitamin C daily, I have recognized an amazing decrease in my sensitivity to colds, and an increase in my healing of everyday cuts and bruises.

Ingredients: Optimal nutrition, in general, is necessary for optimal immune system function. Certain nutrients, in particular, are known to directly influence the immune system—zinc and vitamins C, A, and E. Other supplements can impact particular aspects of immune function. Probiotic supplements, for example, can influence immune response by optimizing the intestinal flora. Certain herbs and phytonutrients have been shown to boost the number of various white blood cells. Siberian ginseng, astragalus, and various mushrooms (maitake, reishi, shiitake) are good examples. For general immune system support, a blend of these nutrients and herbs can be beneficial. Samples of types of immune-enhancing products are provided below, and your choice depends, in part, on what other supplements you are taking.

Sample Products:

- *Reishi Shiitake Maitake Mushroom Extracts* (Solgar). Every vegicap contains the following:

Vitamin C	70 mg
Certified Organic Reishi Mushroom Mycelia (Ganoderma lucidum)	100 mg
Certified Organic Shiitake Mushroom Mycelia (Lentinula edodes)	100 mg
Maitake Mushroom extract (4:1) (Grifola frondosa)	100 mg
Standardized Red Reishi Mushroom Extract (Ganoderma lucidum) (4% triterpenes, 10% polysaccharides)	30 mg
LEM Shiitake Mycelia Mushroom Extract (Lentinula edodes)	30 mg

• *Immune Protectors* (Twinlab). Every four capsules contain the following:

Dry Vitamin A (from vitamin A acetate)	5,000 IU
Dry Beta-Carotene (pro-vitamin A)	20,000 IU
Total Vitamin A Activity	25,000 IU
Zinc (from zinc gluconate)	50 mg
Copper (from copper gluconate)	2 mg
Dry Vitamin E (d-alpha tocopheryl succinate)	400 IU
Selenium (from selenomethionine and selenite)	200 mcg
CoQ_{10} (coenzyme Q_{10})	5 mg
Vitamin B_6	100 mg
Vitamin C	2,000 mg
Citrus Bioflavonoids	100 mg
Quercetin (non-citrus bioflavonoid)	25 mg
L-Glutathione (reduced)	50 mg
Vitamin B_{12}	250 mcg
Folic Acid	800 mcg
Pantothenic Acid	50 mg
Biotin	100 mcg
Vitamin B_2	10 mg
Manganese (from manganese gluconate)	10 mg
Vitamin B_3 (niacinamide)	10 mg
In a concentrated, specially prepared herbal tea extract base of pau d'arco, onion, garlic, black walnut, echinacea and goldenseal root	

• *Immune CNS* (Willner Chemists). Every three tablets contain the following:

DHA (Neuromins™—Algae & Fish Oil)	30 mg
Standardized Astragalus Root Extract (70% polysaccharides)	75 mg
Standardized Olive Leaf Extract (6% oleuropein)	75 mg

Standardized Deglycyrrhized Licorice Root Extract (1.5% glycyrrhizin)	75 mg
Standardized Korean Ginseng Root Extract (8% ginsenosides)	75 mg
Reishi Mushroom Extract (3:1)	75 mg
Shiitake Mushroom Extract (3:1)	75 mg
Fruit Polyphenols (40% OligoPhenolics from apricot, apple, prune, pomegranate, cherry)	50 mg
NAC (N-acetyl-cysteine)	250 mg
Vitamin C (mineral ascorbates)	200 mg
Selenium (yeast free, I-selenomethionine)	50 mg
Zinc (fully reacted glycinate chelate)	15 mg
Pantothenic Acid	15 mg
Magnesium (fully reacted glycinate chelate)	200 mg

- *Well-Max w/Ester C and NAC* (Country Life). Every three tablets contain the following:

Vitamin A (as retinyl palmitate and 50% as beta-carotene)	5,000 IU
Vitamin C (as calcium polyascorbate)	500 mg
Pantothenic Acid (as d-calcium pantothenate)	125 mg
Calcium (as calcium carbonate)	344 mg
Zinc (as zinc glycinate and zinc citrate)	25 mg
Reishi Mushroom (from 40 mg of a 15:1 extract)	600 mg
Shiitake Mushroom (from 60 mg of a 10:1 extract)	600 mg
Deodorized Garlic (bulb)	500 mg
Echinacea Purpurea (root) (from 125 mg of a 4:1 extract)	500 mg
Astragalus (root)	250 mg
Bee Propolis 2x	250 mg
Echinacea Angustifolia (root) (from 31.5 mg of an 8:1 extract)	250 mg
Pau d'Arco (Bark) (from 50 mg of a 4:1 extract)	200 mg
Golden Seal Extract (root) 5% (hydrastine and berberine)	150 mg

NAC (N-acetyl cysteine)	150 mg
Schizandra Berry (fruit) (from 25 mg of a 4:1 extract)	100 mg
Siberian Ginseng Extract (root) (0.8% eleutherosides)	100 mg
Grape Seed Extract (Vitis vinifera)	30 mg

- *Wellness Formula* (Source Naturals) is primarily a combination of immune-enhancing, adaptogenic, antibacterial, and antiviral herbs, plus vitamins A, C, and zinc.
- *Herbal Immune Complex* (Solgar) is an impressive blend of standardized astragalus extract, cat's claw extract, echinacea extract, deglycyrrhized licorice, elderberry extract, and olive leaf extract in a base of elderberry powder, echinacea powder, licorice powder, olive leaf powder, and astragalus powder. As is the case for many of the Solgar herbal formulas, they combine standardized extracts with powdered concentrates, so that you get the benefit from the whole herb, as well as the concentrated active components. The best of both worlds. This is an excellent herbal immune-enhancing formula.
- *Microbial Modulators* (Solgar). Every two vegicaps contain the following:

Iron	0.7 mg
Standardized Oregano Extract (leaf, oil) (thymol 8 mg [5%])	150 mg
Standardized Blueberry Extract (leaf) (chlorogenic acid 30 mg [20%])	150 mg
Standardized Olive Leaf Extract (leaf) (oleuropein 9 mg [6%])	150 mg
Standardized Cranberry Extract (berry) (organic acids 53 mg [30%])	150 mg
Standardized Elderberry Extract (berry) (polyphenols 45 mg [30%])	150 mg
Standardized St. John's Wort Extract (aerial) (hypericin 0.5 mg [0.3%])	150 mg
Standardized Echinacea Extract (root, leaf) (echinacosides 6 mg [4%], echinacea polysaccharides 23 mg [15%])	150 mg
Standardized Goldenseal/Goldthread Extract (root) (alkaloids 15 mg [10%] as berberine, hydrastine, palmatine)	150 mg

Standardized Basil Extract (leaf) (eugenol 45 mg [30%])	150 mg
Standardized Green Tea Extract (leaf) (polyphenols 75 mg [50%])	150 mg
Organic Garlic Powder (clove)	150 mg
Standardized Fruit Polyphenols (from apple, apricot/ nectarine, cherry, pomegranate, prune) (phenolics 20 mg [40%])	50 mg

- *StayWell* (Nature's Way) is a multisystem defense formula covering seven essential aspects of healthy immunity: (1) epidermal, (2) respiratory, (3) digestive, (4) systemic, (5) circulatory, (6) cellular, and (7) lymphatic. It is similar to Wellness Formula, but adds five mushroom blends.

Lipotropic Formulas

Description: A lipotropic formula is one that is designed to promote the physiological utilization, or metabolism, of fat. It enhances liver and gallbladder function, and can be helpful in detoxification programs.

Ingredients: Products of this type usually contain choline, inositol, betaine (trimethylglycine), and methionine, which are all categorized as "methyl donors." Other complementary ingredients can be vitamin B_6, folic acid, and vitamin B_{12}.

Sample Products:

- *Lipotropic Factors* (Solgar). Every three tablets contain the following:

Choline (as choline bitartrate)	410 mg
Inositol	1 g
L-Methionine	1 g

Some might notice that the amount of choline in this product, and similar products, seems to have changed. Actually, it has not. The choline used to be labeled as choline bitartrate, and is now labeled as choline. One gram (or 1,000 milligrams) of choline bitartrate is equivalent to 410 milligrams of choline.

• *Lipotropic Complex* (Tyler) adds black radish root, beet leaf, dandelion, milk thistle, celandine, chionanthus, and ox bile to the basic ingredients above.

Liver Support Formulas

Description: The liver is a complex organ, protecting us from toxins of all types. It filters the blood, and chemically modifies toxic compounds so they can be neutralized and excreted. The liver is also involved in bile production. Bile is important for detoxification as well as the metabolism of fats.

A COMMENT FROM DR. ABEL

The liver is the most important organ in the body for metabolizing food, detoxifying foreign chemicals, storing essential nutrients, and excreting waste products through the gallbladder into the intestines. Food absorbed through the gastrointestinal tract is directed to the liver. There, it is sorted. Toxins, bacteria, and other particles can be removed from circulation and excreted into the bile (at a rate of one quart daily). The bile and its cholesterol-containing substances are vital for absorption of fat-soluble nutrients, which include vitamins A, D, E, K, and essential fatty acids. Carbohydrates, fat, and protein are broken down in the liver. Vitamins are stored in and activated by the liver, and toxic materials are conjugated or secreted, and strained out of the body via the bile. It is not surprising that a carnivore on the plains of Africa would eat the liver of its prey first, in order to obtain important vitamins that it cannot synthesize itself. In fact, mammals, including us, no longer synthesize a number of these essential nutrients, because of their availability in the past. We have used the space on our chromosomes to develop more sophisticated functions than creating a series of enzymes to make nutrients that our predecessors found readily available.

Ingredients: Liver support formulas will usually contain lipotropic nutrients, along with herbs that support and protect the liver, and enhance bile flow.

Sample Products:

- *Herbal Liver Complex* (Solgar) is an excellent herbal blend of standardized liver-supporting herbs (milk thistle, dandelion, turmeric, schisandra, picrorizha, and phyllanthus, with phosphatidylcholine in a base of milk thistle and dandelion powder.
- *Liver Support Factors* (Country Life) is a complete, broad-spectrum liver formula containing the lipotropic nutrients as well as liver-supporting herbal extracts.
- *Liver Tone* (Nature's Answer) is an excellent alcohol-free liquid combination of sarsaparilla, milk thistle, dandelion root, bupleurum, reishi, ginger, and turmeric.

Meal Replacement Health Formulas

Description: A meal replacement formula is not the same as a protein drink, or an energy drink. To properly function as a meal replacement, the product should contain at least 25 to 35 percent of the recommended daily amounts of vitamins and minerals, in addition to protein and carbohydrate. As the name implies, the product can serve as a meal substitute, either for convenience, or as a way to control calories as part of a weight loss program. When taken between meals, it can help those who want to gain weight. The products listed here are more than mere meal replacement formulas, however, in that they contain a wide array of phytonutrients, herbs, and other health-enhancing ingredients.

Ingredients: In addition to the standard vitamins and minerals, protein, fat, and carbohydrate, these products contain fruit and vegetable concentrates, herbs, and more.

Sample Products:

- *Optein Wellness Beverage* (Solgar). One level scoop contains the following:

  Calories 125, Calories from Fat 10, Total Fat 1 g, 2%DV; Saturated Fat 0.5 g, 3%DV; Cholesterol 5 mg, 2%DV; Total Carbohydrate 17 g, 6%DV; Dietary Fiber 3 g, 12%DV; Sugars 8 g, Protein 12 g, 24%DV; Vitamin A (as [3600 IU] palmitate, 18%DV; [1400 IU] as natural beta-carotene from Dunaliella salina) 5000 IU, 100%DV; Vitamin C (as L-ascorbic acid) 45 mg, 75%DV; Vitamin D (as cholecalciferol) 300 IU, 75%DV; Vitamin E (as D-alpha tocopheryl acetate) 23 IU, 77%DV; Thiamin (as thiamin mononitrate) 1.1 mg, 73%DV; Riboflavin 1.3 mg, 76%DV; Niacin (as niacinamide) 15 mg, 75%DV; Vitamin B_6 (as pyridoxine hydrochloride) 1.5 mg, 75%DV; Folic Acid 300 mcg, 75%DV; Vitamin B_{12} (as cyanocobalamin) 5 mcg, 83%DV; Biotin (as D-biotin) 200 mcg, 67%DV; Pantothenic Acid 7.5 mg (as D-calcium pantothenate) 75%DV; Calcium (as calcium carbonate, calcium from proteinate) 200 mg, 20%DV; Iron (as reduced iron, iron from proteinate) 9 mg, 50%DV; Iodine (as potassium iodide, brown seaweed extract) 115 mcg, 77%DV; Magnesium (as magnesium oxide, magnesium from proteinate) 100 mg, 25%DV; Zinc (as zinc oxide) 11 mg, 73%DV; Selenium (selenium from proteinate, brown seaweed extract) 14 mcg, 20%DV; Copper (as copper gluconate) 1.5 mg, 75%DV; Manganese (manganese from proteinate) 0.4 mg, 20%DV; Chromium (as chromium polynicotinate) 24 mcg, 20%DV; Molybdenum (molybdenum from proteinate) 15 mcg, 20%DV; Sodium 120 mg, 5%DV; Potassium (from malted oat cereal solids) 70 mg, 2%DV; Lecithin (from lecithin oil) 500 mg, Dried Red Beet Powder 50 mg, Dried Broccoli Powder 5 (Brassica aleracea) (aerial) 0 mg, Dried Carrot Powder (Daucus carota) (root) 50 mg, Spirulina Powder 50 mg, Alfalfa Sprouts Powder (Medicago sativa) (aerial) 50 mg, Kamut® Grass Powder (Triticum durham egyptum) (aerial) 50 mg, Wheat Grass Powder (Tritizum vulgare) (aerial) 50 mg, Barley Grass Powder (Hordeum vulgare) (aerial) 50 mg, Reishi Mushroom Extract (Ganoderma lucidum) 20 mg, Maitake Mushroom Extract (Grifola frondosa) 20 mg, Shiitake Mushroom Powder (Lentinus edodes) 20 mg, Brown Seaweed Extract 30 mg, Isoflavones (from soy concentrate) 20 mg, Octacosanol (from wheat germ oil) 250 mcg, Lactoferrins 10 mg, Glutamine Peptides 100 mg, Astragalus Extract (Astragalus membranaceus) (root) 20 mg, Schizandra Extract (Schizandra chinensis) (fruit) 20 mg, American Ginseng Extract (Panax quinquefolium) (root) 20 mg, Siberian Ginseng Extract (Acanthopanax senticosus) (root) 20 mg, Korean Ginseng Extract (Panax ginseng) (root) 20 mg, Rhodiola Extract (Rhodiola rosea) (root) 20 mg, Elderberry Extract (Sambucus nigra, canadensis) (berry) 20 mg, Fruit Polyphenols (from apple, apricot/ nectarine, cherry, prune, pomegranate) 20 mg, Beta-Glucan (from oat fiber) 25 mg, Dried Colostrum Powder 50 mg, Cytidine Monophosphate 5 mg, Adenosine Monophosphate 5 mg, Uridine Monophosphate 5 mg, Guanosine Monophosphate 5 mg, Phosphatidylcholine (from lecithin oil) 100 mg, Phosphatidylinositol (from lecithin oil) 20 mg,

* Percent Daily Values (DV) are based on a 2,000-calorie diet.

• *ProGreens (Allergy Research* Group) ProGreens is an all-natural blended variety of "superfoods" that provide broad-spectrum nutritional support from certified organic grasses and natural food factors not found in isolated vitamins or mineral concentrates. In addition to the green grasses, sea vegetables, and algae, ProGreens contains adaptogenic herbs, active probiotics, fibers, and a variety of nutrient-rich superfoods. It does not exactly fit the definition of "meal replacement" because it does not contain the standard vitamins and minerals, but if taken with a multivitamin-multimineral supplement, is an excellent health- and immune-boosting drink. Every serving contains the following:

Wheat grass powder 350 mg; Barley grass powder 350 mg; Alfalfa grass powder 350 mg; Oat grass powder 350 mg; Spirulina 1,000 mg; Chlorella (cracked-cell) 350 mg; Dunaliella salina 40 mg; Nova Scotia Dulse 30 mg; Licorice root powder 100 mg; Siberian Ginseng 60 mg; Pfaffia paniculata (Suma) 60 mg; Astragalus membranaceus 60 mg; Echinacea purpurea 60 mg; Ginger root powder 5 mg; Lecithin (99% oil-free) 2,000 mg; Wheat sprout powder (gluten-free) 350 mg; Acerola berry juice powder 200 mg; Beet juice powder 200 mg; Spinach octacosanol 150 mg; Royal jelly (5% 10-HDA) 150 mg; Bee pollen 150 mg; Vitamin E (D-alpha-Tocopheryl Acid Succinate) 100 IU; Total count non-dairy probioti cultures 5.0 billion; Lactobacillus group (L.rhamnosus A, L.rhamnosus B, L.acidophilus, L.casei, L.bulgaricus) 3.5 billion; Bifidobacterium group (B.longum, B.breve) 1 billion; Streptococcus thermophilus 500 million; Flaxseed meal 500 mg; Apple pectin and fiber 1000 mg; Fructooligosaccharides (FOS) 500 mg; Milk Thistle extract (80% silymarin) 60 mg; Ginkgo biloba extract 20 mg; Green tea extract (60% catechins) 20 mg; Grape pip extract (92% proanthocyanidins) 20 mg; Bilberry extract (25% anthocyanidins) 20 mg.

• *Glycemic Balance* (Jarrow). This product is a vitamin-and-mineral-enriched meal replacement formula, available in various flavors, designed to have minimal impact on blood sugar levels. It is excellent for those who need help with blood sugar management. It is high in protein and fiber, and can be used for weight loss or weight gain

Menopause Support

Description: During menopause, nutritional needs change. The importance of adequate calcium and magnesium intake is heightened. Hormone balance is altered, and disconcerting symptoms may make life during this period very difficult. These formulas provide vitamin and mineral supplementation tailored to these changing needs, as well as herbs and phytonutrients that can moderate the hormonal changes affecting mood and comfort and increasing the risk of osteoporosis, heart disease, and cancer.

Ingredients: Phytoestrogens are plant-derived compounds that are chemically similar to estrogen, but with very weak estrogen activity. Soy and the soy isolates are a good example. These substances, as well as herbs such as black cohosh, will moderate the effects of changing hormone levels and the symptoms they cause. Calcium, magnesium, vitamin D, boron, and other trace minerals are no more important now relative to their bone supporting properties than they were during the premenopausal years, but at menopause, the effects of a lifetime of inadequate intake of these nutrients becomes apparent, and preventing further loss of bone density becomes a priority. Mood swings and depression can often be controlled with herbs rather than drugs, and kava is a popular option.

Sample Products:

• **Women's MenoPause Formula** (Natrol). Every three capsules contain the following:

Calcium (as calcium carbonate)	250 mg
Magnesium (as magnesium oxide)	125 mg
Soy Isoflavones	100 mg
Genistein (10%)	10 mg

Kava Kava	100 mg
(Kavalactones, 30%)	
Red Raspberry Extract	100 mg
Wild Mexican Yam Extract	50 mg
Licorice Root Extract	50 mg
Red Clover Extract	50 mg
Horse Chestnut Extract	50 mg
Dong Quai Extract	50 mg
Black Cohosh Root	40 mg
Damiana Extract	30 mg
Vitex (agnus-castus) Extract	25 mg
Ginkgo biloba 24:6	25 mg
Gotu Kola Extract	25 mg
Gamma Oryzanol	20 mg

- *Women's Hot Flashex* (Natrol). Every tablet contains the following:

Vitamin E (as d-alpha tocopherol succinate)	50 IU
Licorice Root Extract (Glycrrhiza glabra)	100 mg
Black Cohosh Extract	60 mg
Triterpenes (2.5%)	1.5 mg
Chamomile Extract	50 mg
Kava Kava Extract	30 mg
(Kavalactones, 30%)	

The difference between the two formulas above is that MenoPause Formula is the milder one. Hot Flashex is for the more serious symptoms such as night sweats, hot flashes, insomnia, and irritability. MenoPause Formula might be used when the symptoms have abated.

- *Midlife Ease* (Jarrow Formulas) encourages hormonal balance with soy isoflavones, red clover, dong quai, black chohosh, chaste tree berry, and licorice. In addition, the Chinese herb chai hu supports liver function and wu wei zi tonifies the kidney, while Siberian ginseng functions as a tonic. Valerian is included for its relaxing qualities. Every two capsules of Midlife Ease contain the following:

Isoflavones (from soybean, GMO-free) (Glycine max)	60 mg
Vitex Extract (Vitex agnus castus) (0.5% agnusides)	100 mg
Dong Quai 7:1 extract (Angelica sinensis)	200 mg
Black Cohosh Extract (Cimicifuga racemesa)	80 mg
Red Clover Extract (Trifolium pratene) (8% isoflavone)	50 mg
Siberian Ginseng (Chi Wu Jia) 50:1	100 mg
Valerian Root 6:1 extract (Valeriana officinalis)	200 mg
Licorice Root 4:1 extract (Glycyrrhiza uralensis)	200 mg
Chai Hu 4:1 extract (Bupleureum chinense)	200 mg
Wu Wei Zi 10:1 extract (Schizandra chinensis)	200 mg

- *EstroSoy Plus* (Nature's Way) is a blend of fermented soy, rich in isoflavones, along with black cohosh and red clover blossoms. EstroSoy Plus is a phytoestrogen dietary supplement made from whole soybeans fermented with a natural, proprietary process. Fermentation yields more isoflavones and a diversity of supportive nutrients including beta-glucan and glutathione. EstroSoy Plus delivers soy isoflavones (60 percent genistein/40 percent diadzein) in their "free," unconjugated form for better absorption and more effective use within the body. According to Nature's Way, EstroSoy Plus relieves hot flashes and night sweats, supports breast health, and promotes healthy bones by helping the body retain calcium. Soy, which contains natural phytoestrogens called isoflavones, has been clinically proven to ease hormonal transition. Women with a soy-rich diet report lower incidence of hot flashes and other menopause symptoms. Recent studies also show that women with a soy-rich diet have healthier bones and increased breast health. The diets referred to in these studies involve fermented soy (as in foods like natto, miso, and tempeh).
- *Change-O-Life Formula* (Nature's Way) is a blend containing black cohosh, blessed thistle, false unicorn root, licorice root, sarsaparilla, Siberian ginseng and squaw vine.

Menstrual Cycle Support

Description: There are a number of common problems associated with the menstrual cycle. PMS, or premenstrual syndrome, can involve anxiety, cravings, irritablility, bloating, and depression. Other, more conventional problems include painful menstruation or heavy bleeding.

A COMMENT FROM DR. ABEL

Did you know that birth control pills not only can affect the circulating levels of your vitamins, but also can increase your total lipids and triglycerides. Therefore, your cholesterol levels should be periodically measured. Folic acid is one of the B vitamins that is depleted by the use of oral estrogens. It appears that folate depletion is a factor in human papillovirus infection and cervical dysplasia. Women with abnormal PAP smears should consider folic acid supplementation and perhaps even select an alternative method of birth control. Natural estrogen helps protect women from both heart disease and osteoporosis. This could explain the increased prevalence of these two diseases in the Industrial World among postmenopausal women. It is important to recognize that the estrogens in contraceptive pills are not the same as that which is naturally produced in a woman's body. There are new synthetic postmenopausal estrogen replacement drugs that have been designed to protect against breast cancer while supporting positive effects on heart function and bone mass.

Ingredients: A number of herbal supplements have a hormone-modulating activity that seems helpful during this period (dong quai, chaste tree berry). Magnesium and calcium are thought to exert a certain muscle relaxant action. Mild, calming herbs such as kava, hops, and passion flower may help to counter the anxiety and tension.

Sample Products:

- *MenstraCalm* (Jarrow) contains a blend of both European and Chinese herbs, extra calcium and magnesium, vitamin E, folic acid, and dandelion root. It is recommended that the product be taken from ten days before the period starts through the first two or three days after menstruation begins.

- *Pre-Menses* (Country Life) is a similar formula, but relying more on European herbs. It contains chromium, tyrosine, and milk thistle as well.
- *PMS Formula* (Nature's Way) contains 5-HTP and vitamin B_6, along with the usual herbal hormone modulators. Every three capsules contain the following:

Black Cohosh Root	150 mg
Cramp Bark	250 mg
Dandelion Leaf	150 mg
L-5 Hydroxytryptophan (griffonia bean extract)	5 mg
Lobelia herb	150 mg
Magnesium Amino Acid Chelate	50 mg
Niacin, vitamin B_3	10 mg
Pyridoxine HCL	76 mg
Riboflavin, vitamin B_2	852 mcg
Thiamine, vitamin B_1	750 mcg
Vitamin B_{12}, cyanacobalamin	3 mcg

Migraine Headache Support

Description: Migraine headaches are very painful vascular headaches, which often begin on one side of the head, and can be triggered by various conditions, including certain foods, hormonal fluctuations, and stress.

Ingredients: There are certain nutrients and herbs that have been shown to be beneficial to many with migraine headaches. Magnesium seems to be helpful, as does vitamin B_2 (riboflavin). Studies using vitamin B_2 at dosages in the area of 400 milligrams daily have been very impressive. Some studies have found benefit from 5-HTP supplementation. The herb feverfew is one of the most popular treatments for migraine headaches.

A COMMENT FROM DR. ABEL

Migraine headaches often occur after a visual stimulus. Many individuals who are over fifty years of age will not get the headache, but will notice peripheral flickering lights or a "mirage" effect that is quite disturbing. When it is only in one eye, in one area, one has to eliminate the possibility of a retina or central nervous system problem; however, these possible causes are rare. Migraine tends to have a characteristic pattern in each individual and can be triggered by light, stress, hormone cycles, foods, neck position (high pillow or low bifocal). Light coming from the side, eccentrically, can tickle those eccentric rods. The eye is more than just an organ of sight; it also contributes a great deal of information to the brain in ways which are poorly understood.

Supplements that are excellent for preventing migraines are magnesium, 500 milligrams or more daily, and an herb called feverfew, which has an active ingredient called parthenolide. There are multiple medications that help reduce migraines after they occur.

Turn the flicker rate up on your computer monitor to at least 70 megahertz. You may find this eliminates not only the migraine, but eye irritation as well. And remember that only you can be the medical detective and determine the cause of these migraine headaches. Look at what causes them. Massage any tight muscles at the back of your head.

Sample Products:

- *Herbal Feverfew Complex* (Solgar) contains 250 milligrams of standardized feverfew extract per capsule, along with ginkgo biloba, kava, passion flower, DLPA, white willow powder, and salicin from wintergreen, meadowsweet, and purple willow.
- *Migra-Lieve* (Natural Science Corp of America) combines 200 milligrams of vitamin B_2 (riboflavin), 150 milligrams of magnesium, and 50 milligrams of standardized feverfew extract (0.7% parthenolide).
- *Migra-Profen* (Gaia Herbs) contains concentrated extracts of feverfew, skullcap, kava kava, valerian, Jamaican dogwood, rosemary, and ginger in liquid-filled vegetarian capsules.
- *Headache Relief* (New Chapter) contain "supercritical" and standardized extracts of feverfew, ginger, green tea, wintergreen, and seven other herbs.

Multimineral Formulas

Description: The essential minerals are no less important than vitamins. One of the most common mistakes made by the casual supplement user is to get inadequate calcium and magnesium in their daily vitamin supplement regimen. Those who take a "one-a-day" or "two-a-day" multiple vitamin are certainly not getting enough calcium and magnesium. Some people take a "B-complex" supplement, and mistakenly think it is the same as a "multivitamin." It is not, and among other things, it does not supply minerals. For those who do not get their general mineral supplementation—including the trace minerals such as copper, zinc, chromium, and selenium—in other products, a multimineral supplement may be necessary.

Ingredients: The formulas listed here are not calcium-magnesium supplements. Instead, they contain the full spectrum of essential minerals, including the various trace minerals.

Sample Products:

- *Chelated Solamins Multimineral* (Solgar). Every three tablets contain the following:

Calcium (as tricalcium phosphate, dicalcium phosphate, glycinate amino acid chelate)	500 mg
Iron (as iron bisglycinate amino acid chelate)	10 mg
Phosphorus (as tricalcium phosphate, dicalcium phosphate)	200 mg
Iodine (as kelp)	150 mcg
Magnesium (as glycinate amino acid chelate, oxide)	250 mg
Zinc (as glycinate amino acid chelate)	10 mg
Selenium (as yeast-free L-selenomethionine)	50 mcg
Copper (as glycinate amino acid chelate)	0.25 mg
Manganese (as glycinate amino acid chelate)	10 mg
Chromium (as nicotinoglycinate amino acid chelate)	20 mcg
Molybdenum (as molybdenum amino acid chelate)	60 mcg
Sodium	15 mg
Potassium (as potassium carbonate)	99 mg

- *Full Spectrum Calcium Multimineral Softgels* (Solgar) is a nice formula in that it provides a full 1,000 milligrams of calcium in three softgel capsules, along with decent amounts of magnesium and trace minerals. Extra selenium should be available in an antioxidant blend, and those with carbohydrate metabolism concerns may need more chromium than this formula provides. The calcium is in the form of the carbonate, which means the product should be taken with meals. Every three capsules of Full Spectrum Calcium Multimineral Softgels contain the following:

Calcium (as calcium carbonate)	1,000 mg
Iron (as ferrous fumarate)	18 mg
Magnesium (as magnesium oxide)	400 mg
Zinc (as zinc citrate)	15 mg
Selenium (as L-selenomethionine)	75 mcg
Copper (as copper gluconate)	2 mg
Manganese (as manganese carbonate)	5 mg
Chromium (as amino acid chelate)	100 mcg
Molybdenum (as amino acid chelate)	45 mcg

- *Multi-Mineral Tablets* (Solgar) is an example of a product we do not recommend. Most of the mineral content is from bone meal and dolomite, both of which offer the potential for contaminations with lead and perhaps other undesirable minerals (such as aluminum). The ratio of calcium to magnesium is 5:1 instead of the desired 2:1. The two-tablet serving provides only 0.1 milligram zinc, but has 10 milligrams iron. And those two tablets provide only 374 milligrams of calcium. If you took four tablets, instead of two, you would have closer to the required amount of calcium, 748 milligrams, but already more than the daily requirement of iron, and still almost no zinc. The label lists 10 milligrams of an "herbal blend." Ten milligrams? Why bother?
- *Multi Mineral Capsules* (Twinlab) is a complete four-per-day formula with full potencies of all the minerals. Should be taken with meals.
- *Mineral Balance* (Jarrow) is a six-per-day iron-free formula. Contains hydroxyapatite as the calcium source, and adds vitamins A and D. This formula should also be taken with meals.

Multimineral Formulas, Liquid and Powder

Description: For those who cannot swallow tablets or capsules, and do not want to crush a tablet or empty a capsule, there are liquid mineral supplements available. It is not possible to obtain both minerals and vitamins in the same liquid product because they would interact with each other, and have limited stability.

Sample Products:

- *Mini Quick* (Twinlab). Every two tablespoons contain the following:

Calcium (from calcium gluconate chelate)	300 mg
Magnesium (from magnesium gluconate chelate)	150 mg
Zinc (from zinc gluconate chelate)	15 mg
Manganese (from manganese gluconate chelate)	5 mg
Iron (from ferrous gluconate chelate)	6 mg
Potassium (from potassium gluconate chelate)	10 mg
Selenium (from natural selenite and selenomethionine)	50 mcg
Chromium (from natural trivalent chromium chloride)	50 mcg
Molybdenum (from natural molybdate)	50 mcg

It would take 3 ounces (6 tablespoons) of this product to supply the full daily dose of all the minerals.

Multivitamin Formulas

Description: This section covers those types of multivitamin formulas that include a wide variety of vitamins, trace minerals, and sometimes other nutrients. But they do not contain the recommended amount of calcium and magnesium. There is not enough room in a product designed for one- or two-per-day dosage to accommodate the amount of calcium and magnesium that is necessary.

Ingredients: As explained earlier, the water-soluble nutrients remain in your system for only a limited time before they are excreted. For this reason, it is more beneficial to take a two-per-day product (one in the morning and one in the evening), than it is to take a one-per-day product. But one a day beats nothing!

Sample Products:

- *Daily One Capsules* (Twinlab). Every gelatin capsule contains the following:

Beta-Carotene (pro-vitamin A)	10,000 IU
Vitamin D (from natural form vitamin D_3)	400 IU
Vitamin C	150 mg
Natural Vitamin E (succinate)	100 IU
Vitamin B_1 (thiamine)	25 mg
Vitamin B_2 (riboflavin)	25 mg
Vitamin B_6 (pyridoxine)	25 mg
Vitamin B_{12} (cobalamin concentrate)	100 mcg
Niacinamide	100 mg
Pantothenic Acid	50 mg
Biotin	300 mcg
Folic Acid	400 mcg
PABA (para-aminobenzoic acid)	25 mg
Choline Bitartrate	25 mg
Inositol	25 mg
Calcium (from calcium citrate and calcium carbonate)	25 mg
Magnesium (from magnesium aspartate and magnesium oxide)	7.2 mg
Potassium (from potassium aspartate and potassium citrate)	5 mg
Zinc (from zinc picolinate)	15 mg
Copper (from copper gluconate)	2 mg
Iron (from ferrous fumarate)	10 mg
Manganese (from manganese gluconate)	5 mg
Iodine (from potassium iodide)	150 mcg
Selenium (from selenomethionine and selenate-50/50 mixture)	200 mcg
Chromium (GTF)	200 mcg
Molybdenum (natural molybdate)	150 mcg

• *Daily Two Capsules* (Twinlab). Every two gelatin capsules contain the following:

Beta-Carotene (pro-vitamin A)	25,000 IU
Vitamin D (from natural form vitamin D_3)	400 IU
Vitamin C	500 mg
Natural Vitamin E (succinate)	400 IU
Vitamin B_1 (thiamine)	25 mg
Vitamin B_2 (riboflavin)	25 mg
Vitamin B_6 (pyridoxine)	25 mg
Vitamin B_{12} (cobalamin)	100 mcg
Niacinamide	100 mg
Pantothenic Acid	50 mg
Biotin	300 mcg
Folic Acid	400 mcg
PABA (para-aminobenzoic acid)	25 mg
Choline Bitartrate	25 mg
Inositol	25 mg
Calcium (from calcium citrate and calcium carbonate)	25 mg
Magnesium (from magnesium aspartate and magnesium oxide)	7.2 mg
Potassium (from potassium aspartate and potassium citrate)	5 mg
Zinc (from zinc picolinate)	30 mg
Copper (from copper gluconate)	2 mg
Iron (from ferrous fumarate)	10 mg
Manganese (from manganese gluconate)	5 mg
Iodine (from potassium iodide)	150 mcg
Selenium (from selenomethionine and selenate-50/50 mixture)	200 mcg
Chromium (GTF)	200 mcg
Molybdenum (from natural molybdic acid)	150 mcg

- *MaxiLife Capsules* (Twinlab) is a comprehensive four-per-day formula. It contains levels of niacin high enough to cause flushing and redness of the skin in sensitive individuals. Calcium and magnesium levels are low, so an additional calcium-magnesium supplement might be necessary, but the other mineral levels are adequate.
- *Formula VM-75* (Solgar) is a one-per-day formula. Every tablet contains the following:

Vitamin A (as palmitate 7,500 IU, 50% [7500 IU] as natural beta-carotene from D. salina)	15,000 IU
Vitamin C (as L-ascorbic acid)	250 mg
Vitamin D (as cholecalciferol)	400 IU
Vitamin E (as D-alpha tocopheryl succinate)	150 IU
Thiamin (as thiamin mononitrate)	75 mg
Riboflavin	75 mg
Niacin (as niacinamide)	75 mg
Vitamin B_6 (as pyridoxine HCl)	75 mg
Folic Acid	400 mcg
Vitamin B_{12} (as cobalamin)	75 mcg
Biotin	75 mcg
Pantothenic Acid (as D-Ca pantothenate)	75 mg
Calcium (as calcium carbonate, glycinate amino acid chelate)	20 mg
Iron (as iron bisglycinate)	1.3 mg
Iodine (from kelp)	150 mcg
Magnesium (as glycinate amino acid chelate, magnesium oxide)	10 mg
Zinc (as glycinate amino acid chelate, zinc oxide)	10 mg
Selenium (as L-selenomethionine)	25 mcg
Copper (as glycinate amino acid chelate, copper oxide)	1 mg
Manganese (as glycinate amino acid chelate)	1 mg
Chromium (as niacin amino acid chelate)	25 mcg
Molybdenum (as glycinate amino acid chelate)	25 mcg
Potassium (as potassium amino acid complex)	1.8 mg

Inositol	75 mg
Choline (as choline bitartrate)	31 mg
Betaine HCl	25 mg
Rutin	25 mg
Citrus Bioflavonoids	25 mg
Hesperidin	5 mg
Boron (as boron amino acid complex)	0.5 mg
Carotenoid Mix (alpha-carotene, lutein, zeaxanthin, cryptoxanthin	86 mcg
Natural Powdered Blend (alfalfa [whole-plant], acerola [berry], kelp [whole-plant], parsley [aerial], rose hips [fruit] and watercress [whole-plant])	4 mg

- *Formula VM-2000* (Solgar) is a two-per-day formula. Every two tablets contain the following:

Vitamin A (as palmitate 5,000 IU, 80% [20,000 IU] as natural beta-carotene)	25,000 IU
Vitamin C (as calcium ascorbate)	300 mg
Vitamin D (as cholecalciferol)	400 IU
Vitamin E (as D-alpha tocopheryl succinate)	200 IU
Thiamin (as thiamin mononitrate)	100 mg
Riboflavin	100 mg
Niacin (as niacinamide, niacin)	100 mg
Vitamin B_6 (as pyridoxine HCl)	90 mg
Folic Acid	400 mcg
Vitamin B_{12} (as cobalamin)	100 mcg
Biotin	100 mcg
Pantothenic Acid (as D-Ca pantothenate)	100 mg
Calcium (as calcium carbonate, glycinate amino acid chelate)	50 mg
Iron (as ferrous sulfate, bisglycinate)	10 mg
Iodine (from kelp)	150 mcg
Magnesium (as magnesium oxide, glycinate amino acid chelate)	30 mg

Zinc (as zinc oxide, glycinate amino acid chelate)	15 mg
Selenium (as L-selenomethionine)	25 mcg
Copper (as copper gluconate, glycinate amino acid chelate, copper oxide)	1.5 mg
Manganese (as manganese gluconate, glycinate amino acid chelate)	2 mg
Chromium (as chromium picolinate, yeast-free)	25 mcg
Molybdenum (as glycinate amino acid chelate)	50 mcg
Sodium	12 mg
Potassium (as potassium chloride, glycinate amino acid complex)	10 mg
Inositol	100 mg
PABA (as para-aminobenzoic acid)	100 mg
Choline (as choline bitartrate)	41 mg
Rose Hips (fruit)	40 mg
Rutin	25 mg
Citrus Bioflavonoids	25 mg
Betaine HCl	25 mg
L-Glutamic Acid	25 mg
Pyridoxal-5-Phosphate	20 mg
Hesperidin	5 mg
L-Glutathione	5 mg
Boron (as boron amino acid complex)	1 mg
Carotenoid Mix (alpha-carotene, lutein, zeaxanthin, cryptoxanthin	229 mcg
Whole Food/Herbal blend (alfalfa [whole-plant], lecithin, bee pollen, spirulina, Siberian ginseng [root], Echinacea purpurea [root], Suma, dong quai [root], silica [from horsetail], oat bran, parsley [aerial], and watercress [whole-plant])	260 mg
VM-2000 Soy Protein/Amino Acid Blend (L-glutamic acid, L-aspartic acid, L-leucine, L-arginine, L-lysine, L-phenylalanine, L-serine, L-proline, L-valine, L-isoleucine, L-alanine, glycine, L-threonine, L-tyrosine, L-histidine, L-cysteine, L-methionine, L-ornithine, taurine)	200 mg

- *Multi 1-to-3* (Jarrow) A versatile multivitamin formula with a moderate helping of accessory nutrients and phytonutrients (lutein, bilberry, ginger, MSM, rosemary extract, choline, inositol, and garlic). The label states that you can take from one to three tablets daily, although there is no explanation as to why you would not want to take the full three-tablet dose. Three tablets give a generous amount of B-complex vitamins, and all of the vitamin A you might want. It also provides more calcium and magnesium than most three-a-day formulas (500 mg calcium and 300 mg magnesium), which is good, and would make this an excellent all-in-one product for those who do not feel the need for more calcium and magnesium. On the other hand, an additional antioxidant blend would seem necessary, as the product only supplies 200 IU of natural vitamin E and 100 micrograms of selenium.

- *Daily Two Multiple (Iron Free)* (Nature's Way) is a high-potency tablet that's perfect for those who do not wish to take supplemental iron. All other nutrients are supplied in adequate amounts.

Multivitamin Formulas, Liquid and Powder

Description: Multivitamins are available in liquid and powder form for those who cannot swallow tablets or capsules. Of course, a tablet can be crushed, or the contents emptied from a two-piece gelatin capsule. Due to stability considerations, minerals cannot be mixed with liquid vitamins, and the potencies are usually lower than in tablets and capsules.

Sample Products:

- *Liquid Multiple* (Natrol). Every two teaspoons contain the following:

Vitamin A (as beta-carotene)	10,000 IU
Vitamin C (as calcium ascorbate)	200 mg
Vitamin D (as cholecalciferol)	400 IU
Vitamin E (as d-alpha tocopherol acetate)	100 IU
Thiamin (as thiamin HCl) (vitamin B$_1$)	7.5 mg

Riboflavin (vitamin B$_2$)	8.5 mg
Niacin (as niacinamide)	20 mg
Vitamin B$_6$ (as pyridoxine HCl)	17 mg
Folate (as folic acid)	400 mcg
Vitamin B$_{12}$ (as cyanocobalamin)	50 mcg
Biotin	300 mcg
Calcium (as calcium ascorbate, d-pantothenate)	28 mg

• *Liquid Antioxidant* (Natrol). Every two teaspoons contain the following:

Vitamin A (as beta-carotene)	10,000 IU
Vitamin C (as calcium ascorbate)	500 mg
Vitamin E (as d-alpha tocopherol)	200 IU
Calcium (as calcium ascorbate)	25 mg
Selenium (monomethionine)	90 mcg
G.P. Flavonoids (hesperidin, acerola, rutin, quercetin, billberry, milk thistle, hawthorn berry, rose hips, grapeskin, turmeric)	34 mg

• *Vita Quick* (Twinlab) is a pineapple-orange-flavored combination of vitamins in liquid form.

Multivitamin Formulas for Men

Description: Just as there are multivitamins designed specifically for women, there are products designed for men. Most men, as we have already indicated, will do just fine with regular multivitamin supplements. But older men, especially those with early prostate concerns, might find these products of interest.

Ingredients: A multivitamin supplement intended for men will differ in several ways from a standard multivitamin product. It will typically contain a higher level of zinc, and a lower level of iron. These products will also usually contain herbs designed to support prostate health. There is some question, however, as to whether taking such herbs prophylactically, in the absence of signs of prostate problems, is advisable.

Sample Products:

• *Male Multiple* (Solgar) is a three-a-day formula high in the homo-cysteine reducers (folic acid, vitamin B_6, and vitamin B_{12}). It also contains 400 milligrams each of calcium and magnesium, full levels of the other minerals and almost no iron. Every three tablets of Male Multiple contain the following:

Vitamin A (as palmitate 5,000 IU, 75% [15,000 IU] as natural beta-carotene)	20,000 IU
Vitamin C (as L-ascorbic acid)	400 mg
Vitamin D (as cholecalciferol)	400 IU
Vitamin E (as D-alpha tocopheryl succinate)	400 IU
Thiamin (as thiamin mononitrate)	50 mg
Riboflavin	50 mg
Niacin (as niacinamide, niacin)	60 mg
Vitamin B_6 (as pyridoxine HCl)	75 mg
Folic Acid	800 mcg
Vitamin B_{12} (as cobalamin)	500 mcg
Biotin (as D-biotin)	300 mcg
Pantothenic Acid (as D-Ca pantothenate)	80 mg
Calcium (as calcium carbonate, glycinate, citrate)	400 mg
Iron	0.5 mg
Iodine (as kelp)	150 mcg
Magnesium (as magnesium oxide, glycinate, citrate)	400 mg
Zinc (as zinc glycinate, histidinate)	50 mg
Selenium (as L-selenomethionine)	200 mcg
Copper (as copper glycinate)	1.5 mg
Manganese (as manganese glycinate)	2 mg
Chromium (as chromium nicotinoglycinate)	200 mcg
Molybdenum (as molybdenum glycinate)	50 mcg
Sodium	25 mg
Potassium (as potassium glycinate complex)	99 mg
Citrus Bioflavonoids	100 mg

Choline (as choline bitartrate)	100 mg
Inositol	100 mg
Pantethine	7 mg
Cocarboxylase	6 mg
Pyridoxal-5-Phosphate	6 mg
Riboflavin-5-Phosphate	6 mg
Dibencozide	21 mcg
Boron (as boron glycinate complex)	250 mcg
Siberian Ginseng Extract (4:1) (root) (Eleutherococcus senticosus)	25 mg
Standardized American Ginseng Extract (root) (Panax quinquefolium) ginsenosides 3 mg [10%])	25 mg
Standardized Korean Ginseng Extract (root) (Panax ginseng) (ginsenosides 2 mg [8%])	25 mg
Saw Palmetto Extract (4:1)(berry) (Serenoa repens)	25 mg
Stinging Nettles Extract (4:1)(leaf) (Urtica dioica)	25 mg
Pygeum Extract (bark) (Pygeum africanum)	25 mg
Standardized Soy Isoflavone Extract (seed)	25 mg
Lycopene (from tomato)	1 mg
Carotenoid Mix (alpha-carotene, lutein, zeaxanthin, cryptoxanthin	172 mcg

- *MaxiLife Men's Protector* (Twinlab) is a four-a-day formula, including phytosterols and high-potency saw palmetto. More suitable for men with specific prostate risk factors.

Multivitamin Formulas for Women

Description: A so-called women's multivitamin supplement is a multivitamin designed for women.

Ingredients: A multivitamin designed for women will usually contain the full recommended amount of iron, if not more, along with extra folic acid (800 mcg). The presence of iron and extra folic acid should make it clear that these products are designed primarily for premenopausal women. In addition, they often contain herbs that are involved with modulating women's unique hormonal variations. They also contain all of the bone-building factors as well, such as boron and vitamin K, along with calcium and magnesium. None of these products, however, supply the total requirement for calcium and magnesium, so an additional calcium-magnesium supplement is necessary unless the dietary intake is unusually high.

Sample Products:

- *Female Multiple* (Solgar). Every three tablets contain the following:

Vitamin A (as palmitate 5,000 IU, 75% [15,000 IU] as natural beta-carotene)	20,000 IU
Vitamin C (as L-ascorbic acid)	400 mg
Vitamin D (as cholecalciferol)	400 IU
Vitamin E (as D-alpha tocopheryl succinate)	400 IU
Vitamin K (as phytonadiione)	20 mcg
Thiamin (as thiamin mononitrate)	50 mcg
Riboflavin	50 mg
Niacin (as niacinamide, niacin)	60 mg
Vitamin B$_6$ (as pyridoxine HCl)	50 mg
Folic Acid	800 mcg
Vitamin B$_{12}$ (as cobalamin)	200 mcg
Biotin (as D-biotin)	300 mcg
Pantothenic Acid (as D-calcium pantothenate)	80 mg
Calcium (as calcium carbonate, glycinate, citrate)	400 mg
Iron (as iron bisglycinate)	18 mg
Iodine (as kelp)	150 mcg
Magnesium (as magnesium oxide, glycinate, citrate)	400 mg
Zinc (as zinc glycinate, histidinate)	30 mg
Selenium (as L-selenomethionine)	200 mcg
Copper (as copper glycinate)	1.5 mg
Manganese (as manganese glycinate)	2 mg
Chromium (as chromium nicotinoglycinate)	200 mcg
Molybdenum (as molybdenum glycinate)	50 mcg

Sodium	25 mg
Potassium (as potassium glycinate complex)	99 mg
Citrus Bioflavonoids	100 mg
Choline (as choline bitartrate)	100 mg
Inositol	100 mg
Pantethine	7 mg
Cocarboxylase	6 mg
Pyridoxal-5-Phosphate	6 mg
Riboflavin-5-Phosphate	6 mg
Dibencozide	21 mcg
Boron (as boron glycinate complex)	500 mcg
Dong Quai Extract (4:1) (root) (Angelica sinensis)	25 mg
Uva Ursi Extract (4:1) (Arcostaphylos uva ursi)	25 mg
Chaste Extract (4:1) (berry) (Vitex agnus-castus)	25 mg
Standardized American Ginseng Extract (root) (Panax quinquefolium) (ginsenosides 3 mg [10%])	25 mg
Milk Thistle Extract (4:1) (aerial) (Silybum marianum)	25 mg
Black Cohosh Extract (4:1) (root) (Cimicifuga racemosa)	25 mg
Standardized Soy Isoflavone Extract (seed)	25 mg
Carotenoid Mix (alpha-carotene, lutein, zeaxanthin, cryptoxanthin)	172 mcg

- *Maxine* (Country Life) is one of three multivitamin products designed by Country Life for women. All contain those vitamins and herbs generally considered necessary for women. The regular Maxine formula contains raw ovary concentrate, whereas the vegetarian formula, Maxine Vegetarian, obviously does not. There is also an iron-free version of the product available.

Multivitamin Formulas with Calcium and Magnesium

Description: As previously explained, it is impossible to include the daily requirement of calcium and magnesium in one or two tablets or capsules. This makes it necessary to take at least two separate products, a multivitamin along with a calcium-magnesium supplement, to get a full dosage of vitamins, trace minerals, calcium, and magnesium.

An alternative is to take one product that contains that amount of calcium and magnesium. To accommodate this, the daily dose must be a minimum of four tablets or six capsules. The advantage is that a full day's requirement of all essential vitamins and minerals can be obtained from only one product.

Ingredients: These products are intended to serve as a balanced, broad-spectrum basic multivitamin-multimineral supplement, and are an ideal foundation product upon which a personalized program can be designed.

Sample Products:

- *Willvite* (Willner Chemists). Every four tablets contain the following:

Vitamin A (acetate)	5,000 IU
Natural Beta-Carotene (D. salina)	15,000 IU
Vitamin C (ascorbic acid/calcium ascorbate)	1,000 mg
Vitamin D_3 (cholecalciferol)	400 IU
Vitamin E (d-alpha tocopheryl succinate)	300 IU
Vitamin K (phytonadione)	60 mcg
Vitamin B_1 (thiamine)	25 mg
Vitamin B_2 (riboflavin)	25 mg
Niacin (as niacinamide)	50 mg
Vitamin B_6 (pyridoxine)	25 mg
Folic Acid (folacin)	400 mcg
Vitamin B_{12} (hydroxo-cobalamin)	100 mcg
Biotin	300 mcg
Pantothenic Acid (d-calcium pantothenate)	50 mg
Calcium (carbonate and citrate)	1,000 mg
Iron (chelated ferrous fumarate)	9 mg
Iodine (from Norwegian kelp)	150 mcg
Magnesium (oxide and aspartate)	500 mg
Zinc (amino acid chelate)	30 mg
Selenium (L-selenomethionine and selenite)	200 mcg

Copper (chelated copper gluconate)	2 mg
Manganese (chelated manganese gluconate)	5 mg
Chromium (as picolinate)	200 mcg
Molybdenum	150 mcg
Potassium (amino acid chelate)	37.5 mg
Betaine Hydrochloride	50 mg
Choline Bitartrate	50 mg
Glutamic Acid Hydrochloride	50 mg
Inositol	25 mg
PABA (para-aminobenzoic acid)	10 mg
Boron	1 mg
Silicon (from horsetail)	350 mcg
Vanadium (sulfate)	10 mcg

- *Dualtabs* (Twinlab). Every four tablets contain the following:

Pro-Vitamin A (beta-carotene)	15,000 IU
Vitamin A (from palmitate)	10,000 IU
Total Vitamin A Activity	25,000 IU
Vitamin D_3 (cholecalciferol)	400 IU
Vitamin E (d-alpha tocopheryl succinate)	200 IU
Vitamin K (phytonadione)	50 mcg
Vitamin C	1,000 mg
Vitamin B_1 (thiamine)	75 mg
Vitamin B_2 (riboflavin)	75 mg
Niacin (from niacinamide)	100 mg
Pantothenic Acid (from D-calcium pantothenate)	150 mg
Vitamin B_6 (pyridoxine)	75 mg
Vitamin B_{12} (hydroxo-cobalamin)	100 mcg
Folic Acid	400 mcg
Biotin	300 mcg
Choline Bitartrate	50 mg

Inositol	25 mg
PABA (para-aminobenzoic acid)	10 mg
Calcium (from calcium carbonate and calcium citrate)	1,000 mg
Magnesium (from magnesium oxide and magnesium aspartate)	500 mg
Potassium (from potassium citrate, potassium chloride, and potassium aspartate)	37.5 mg
Zinc (from chelated zinc gluconate)	30 mg
Copper (from chelated copper gluconate)	2 mg
Iron (from chelated ferrous fumarate)	10 mg
Manganese (from chelated manganese gluconate)	5 mg
Iodine (from Norwegian kelp)	150 mcg
Selenium (from L-selenomethionine and selenite)	200 mcg
Chromium (from natural trivalent chromium chloride)	200 mcg
Molybdenum (from natural molybdate)	500 mcg
Silicon (from natural vegetable silica)	10 mcg
Vanadium (natural food source)	10 mcg
Betaine HCl	100 mg
Glutamic Acid HCl	100 mg

- *My Favorite Multiple* (Natrol) comes in both tablet and capsule form. The daily dose for the tablet (below) is four per day, and the dose for the capsule is six per day. A greater nutrient density can be achieved in a compressed tablet. Every four tablets contain the following:

Vitamin A (as retinyl palmitate and 50% beta-carotene [D. salina])	10,000 IU
Vitamin C (as calcium ascorbate)	250 mg
Vitamin D (as cholecalciferol)	400 IU
Vitamin E (as d-alpha tocopheryl succinate)	400 IU
Thiamin (as thiamin HCl) (vitamin B_1)	50 mg
Riboflavin (vitamin B_2)	50 mg
Niacin (as niacin, niacinamide)	50 mg

Vitamin B_6 (as pyridoxine HCl)	50 mg
Folic Acid	400 mcg
Vitamin B_{12} (as cyanocobalamin)	50 mcg
Biotin	300 mcg
Pantothenic Acid (as d-calcium pantothenate)	50 mg
Calcium (as calcium carbonate, citrate, ascorbate)	1 g
Iron (as ferrochel amino acid chelate)	18 mg
Iodine (from kelp)	150 mcg
Magnesium (as magnesium oxide, citrate)	400 mg
Zinc (as zinc amino acid chelate)	25 mg
Selenium (as selenium amino acid chelate)	200 mcg
Molybdenum (as molybdenum amino acid chelate)	50 mcg
Potassium (as potassium chloride)	99 mg
Betaine (as trimethylglycine [TMG])	300 mg
MultiEnzyme Blend (amylase, papain, protease, bromelain, lipase)	110 mg
G.P. Flavonoid Complex Extracted from (rose hips [fruit], turmeric [root], acerola [berries], hawthorn [berries], grape [skin], milk thistle [seed])	100 mg
PABA (as para-aminobenzoic acid)	50 mg
Choline (as choline bitartrate)	50 mg
Inositol	50 mg
Hesperidin	25 mg
Rutin	25 mg
Siberian Ginseng 4:1 Extract (root)	15 mg
Boron (as amino acid chelate)	200 mcg

Multivitamins Formulas with Calcium and Magnesium, Powder

Description: These products are not meal replacements, as they do not contain protein, carbohydrate, and fats. They are, instead, the equivalent of a multivitamin-multimineral supplement in powder form.

Ingredients: While dry, the vitamins do not interact with minerals, so they can be combined in one product. After the dose is dissolved in liquid, it should be consumed quickly.

Sample Products:

* *MaxiLife Pure Nutrient Powder* (Twinlab). This product has more than adequate levels of just about all the vitamins and minerals, plus some extra antioxidants. However, be aware that the niacin content is high and will probably cause a flush if used as directed. It does not contain iron. Every three teaspoons of Maxi-Life Pure Nutrient Powder contain the following:

Vitamin A Acetate	5,000 IU
Beta-Carotene (pro-vitamin A)	50,000 IU
Natural Vitamin E (succinate)	500 IU
Natural Vitamin E (mixed tocopherols)	500 IU
Total Vitamin E Activity	1,000 IU
Organic Selenium (selenomethionine)	100 mcg
Inorganic Selenium (selenate)	100 mcg
Total Elemental Selenium	200 mcg
Zinc (from zinc picolinate)	25 mg
Zinc (from zinc histidine complex)	25 mg
Total Elemental Zinc	50 mg
Choline Bitartrate	500 mg
Vitamin B_{12}	250 mcg
Vitamin B_1 (thiamine)	100 mg
Vitamin B_2	100 mg
Vitamin B_3 (niacin)	1,000 mg
Pantothenic Acid (from calcium pantothenate)	505 mg
Vitamin B_6	100 mg
N-Acetyl-Cysteine	250 mg
Vitamin C (buffered ascorbic acid)	3,250 mg
PABA (para-aminobenzoic acid)	50 mg
Ascorbyl Palmitate	250 mg

Citrus Bioflavonoid Complex	100 mg
Inositol	250 mg
Calcium (from calcium citrate and calcium carbonate)	1,000 mg
Vitamin D_3	400 IU
Magnesium (from magnesium aspartate and magnesium oxide)	500 mg
Potassium (from potassium citrate and potassium aspartate)	500 mg
Biotin	300 mcg
Folic Acid	800 mcg
Manganese (from chelated manganese gluconate)	10 mg
Iodine (from potassium iodide)	150 mcg
Chromium (from yeast-free GTF)	200 mcg
Molybdenum	300 mcg
L-Glutathione	25 mg
Copper (from chelated copper gluconate)	2 mg
CoQ_{10} (coenzyme Q_{10})	30 mg
Pantetheine (biologically active form of pantothenic acid)	5 mg

- *All One Powders* (Nutritech). The All One product line consists of vitamins, minerals, and amino acids in powder form, plain ("original"), or in a "green phyto base" or a "rice base." They also have a formula designed for "active seniors."
- *Multi E-Z* (Jarrow) is a vanilla-flavored blend of vitamins and minerals with an added antioxidant-rich rice bran concentrate.

Multivitamin Formulas with Phytonutrients

Description: These products combine the benefits of the basic vitamins and minerals with phytonutrients.

Ingredients: Phytonutrients are powerful antioxidant and anticancer substances found in various plants. Adding these extracts and concentrates to the vitamins and minerals usually found in a basic multivitamin supplement adds a great deal of additional activity to the product. These products can fall into one of two categories. Some add food concentrates, or dehydrated plant substances. Another term used is "food-based." In general, the more food-based material, the better. The products in this section, however, employ food extracts rather than concentrates.

Sample Products:

- *Omnium* (Solgar) is Solgar's high-end phytonutrient-rich multi containing a wide array of phytonutrient extracts and accessory nutrients. Every two tablets contain the following:

Vitamin A (as palmitate 5,000 IU, 75% [15,000 IU] as natural beta-carotene from D. salina)	20,000 IU
Vitamin C (as calcium, magnesium, zinc ascorbates)	300 mg
Vitamin D (as cholecalciferol)	200 IU
Vitamin E (as D-alpha tocopheryl succinate)	300 IU
Vitamin K (as phytonadione)	20 mcg
Thiamin (as thiamin mononitrate)	30 mg
Riboflavin	35 mg
Niacin (as niacinamide, niacin)	60 mg
Vitamin B_6 (as pyridoxine HCl)	50 mg
Biotin (as D-biotin)	100 mcg
Pantothenic acid (as D-Ca pantothenate)	80 mg
Calcium (as glycinate amino acid chelate)	25 mg
Iron (as iron bisglycinate)	9 mg
Iodine (from kelp)	150 mcg
Magnesium (as glycinate amino acid chelate)	25 mg
Zinc (as glycinate amino acid chelate)	15 mg
Selenium (as L-selenomethionine)	70 mcg
Copper (as glycinate amino acid chelate)	1.5 mg
Manganese (as glycinate amino acid chelate)	2 mg
Chromium (as chromium picolinate)	100 mcg
Molybdenum (as glycinate amino acid chelate)	50 mcg
Sodium	7 mg
Potassium (as potassium glycinate amino acid complex)	10 mg
Choline (as choline bitartrate)	75 mg

Inositol (as myo-inositol)	75 mg
Standardized Soy Isoflavone Extract (seed)	50 mg
Standardized Turmeric Extract (curcuminoids 47.5 mg [95%])	50 mg
Broccoli Cruciferous Extract	50 mg
Phosphatidylserine Complex (phosphatidylserine 10 mg [20%])	50 mg
Tocotrienol Complex (tocotrienols 3.8 mg [7.5%])	50 mg
N-Acetyl-L-Cysteine	50 mg
Citrus Bioflavonoids	50 mg
D-Limonene (from citrus)	25 mg
Quercetin (as dimorphandra)	10 mg
Proanthocyanidins (from pine bark and grape seed extracts)	10 mg
Alpha-Lipoic Acid	10 mg
Coenzyme Q_{10}	10 mg
Pyridoxine-5-Phosphate	1 mg
Riboflavin-5-Phosphate	1 mg
Alpha-Carotene	344 mcg
Cryptoxanthin	84 mcg
Zeaxanthin	69 mcg
Lutein	54 mcg
Nickel (as nickel sulfate)	5 mcg
Vanadium (as vanadyl sulfate)	5 mcg
Dibencozide	0.6 mg
Boron (as boron animo acid complex)	0.5 mg

- *MaxiLife Phytonutrient Protector* (Twinlab). Maxilife Phytonutrient Protector (Twinlab) is a six-a-day capsule formula providing very generous amounts of phytonutrients. It also supplies high levels of antioxidants, adequate amounts of all the vitamins, but the calcium and magnesium levels are low.

Osteoporosis and Bone Support Formulas

Description: These products are designed to support bone growth and maintain bone density. Some are intended for routine use, to prevent osteoporosis, as part of a regular supplement program. Others are intended for use as a treatment for osteoporosis. The latter-type product would typically contain isoflavone extracts such as ipriflavone.

Ingredients: The primary ingredients would be the minerals involved in bone support, including calcium, magnesium, silica, boron, copper, and zinc. Vitamin D may be included, as it is necessary for absorption of calcium. Vitamin K facilitates the action of calcium as well. Some of the products may contain sources of soy isoflavones, and those designed for therapeutic purposes may also contain ipriflavone. In most instances, these products are designed to be used in addition to your regular multivitamin-multimineral supplements. Look at the total amount of calcium and magnesium in each of the products, and take enough of both to reach a total of from 1,200 to 1,500 milligrams calcium per day.

Sample Products:

- *Advanced Calcium Complex* (Solgar). Every four tablets contain the following:

Vitamin D (as cholecalciferol)	200 IU
Vitamin K (as phytonadione)	65 mcg
Calcium (as calcium carbonate, citrate, malate, glycinate)	800 mcg
Iron (naturally occurring)	3 mg
Magnesium (as magnesim glycinate, citrate, oxide)	500 mg
Zinc (as zinc glycinate)	5 mg
Copper (as copper lysinate)	0.5 mg
Manganese (as manganese glycinate)	2 mg
Sodium	60 mg
Silica (from red algae Lithothamnium corallioides)	15 mg
Boron (as boron glycinate complex)	2 mg

- *Tri Boron Plus* (Twinlab). Every four capsules contain the following:

Boron (from boron citrate, boron aspartate, and boron glycinate)	3 mg
Calcium (from calcium citrate and calcium carbonate)	1,000 mg
Magnesium (from magnesium aspartate and magnesium oxide)	500 mg
Vitamin D$_3$	400 IU
Zinc (from zinc picolinate and histidine complex)	15 mg
Manganese (from manganese gluconate)	5 mg
Copper (from copper gluconate)	500 mcg
Betaine HCl (betaine hydrochloride)	324 mg

- *Bone Complex* (Willner Chemists) is designed for use in addition to a regular calcium supplement, especially for those at high risk of osteoporosis. Every four tablets contain the following:

Calcium (from MCHC, citrate, carbonate)	800 mg
Magnesium (from oxide, citrate)	400 mg
Ipriflavone	600 mg
Soy Isoflavone Concentrate	300 mg
Vitamin D (cholecalciferol)	200 mg
Zinc (as glycinate)	10 mg
Copper (as lysinate)	0.5 mg
Manganese (as citrate)	5 mg
Horsetail Extract (4:1)	25 mg
Boron (as glycinate)	1.5 mg
Vitamin K (as phylloquinone)	80 mcg

- *Bone Support* (Solgar). Every four tablets contain the following:

Vitamin D (as cholecalciferol)	400 IU
Vitamin K (as phytonadione)	80 mcg

Calcium (as calcium carbonate, glycinate, citrate)	800 mg
Iron	0.7 mg
Magnesium (as magnesium glycinate, citrate, oxide)	400 mg
Zinc (as zinc glycinate, histidinate)	10 mg
Copper (as copper lysinate)	0.5 mg
Sodium	20 mg
Ipriflavone (as 7-isopropoxyisoflavone)	600 mg
Soy Isoflavone Concentrate (seed)	400 mg
Boron (as boron glycinate complex)	1.5 mg

• *Bone support with Ostivone* (Twinlab). Every four tablets contain the following:

Ostivone (Ipriflavone) (7-Isopropoxy Isoflavone)	600 mg
Calcium (from calcium citrate and carbonate)	1,500 mg
Magnesium (from magnesium aspartate and oxide)	750 mg
Vitamin D (from cholecalciferol)	800 IU
Boron (from boron citrate, glycinate, and aspartate)	3 mg
Novasoy Phytoestrogen Extract (containing 40 mg of soy isoflavones)	100 mg

• *Women's Bone and Joint Care* (Natrol). Every three capsules contain the following:

Vitamin D (as cholecalciferol)	200 IU
Vitamin K (as phytonadione)	10 mcg
Calcium (as calcium carbonate and calcium citrate)	250 mg
Magnesium (as magnesium oxide)	125 mg
Zinc (as zinc citrate)	5 mg
Copper (as copper gluconate)	100 mcg
Glucosamine Sulfate	250 mg
MSM (methylsulfonylmethane)	250 mg
7-Isopropoxy Isoflavone	100 mg

Sea Cucumber (monopolysaccharides 26%)	100 mg
Mucopolysaccarides (26%)	26 mg
Horsetail Grass (Silica, 8 mg)	100 mg
Bamboo Extract	100 mg
Salicylic Acid	10 mg
Boron	2 mg

- *MaxiLife Women's Bone Protector* (Twinlab) is similar to Tri-Boron Plus, but contains twice as much Vitamin D, which may be necessary for those who have little exposure to sunlight and do not eat much dairy. The calcium is present as calcium citrate. Another difference is that it contains soy phytoestrogen concentrate.
- *Ultra Bone-Up* (Jarrow) is a six-per-day tablet supplying 1,000 milligrams of calcium as hydroxyapatite plus ipriflavone, MSM, and glucosamine, along with the usual bone support nutrients. Designed for those at risk for or having osteoporosis.
- *Bone-Up* (Jarrow) is a six-per-day capsule that's very similar to the above formula but does not contain MSM or ipriflavone. It is an excellent general bone support combination.

Prenatal Formulas

Description: The need for optimal nutrition during pregnancy is obvious. Supplementation with certain nutrients has been shown to reduce the incidence of birth defects and miscarriage and increase birthweight. Requirements for certain nutrients, such as calcium, are estimated to be doubled during pregnancy. Adequate intake of calcium is associated with reduced risk of preeclampsia and pregnancy-induced hypertension.

Ingredients: A prenatal supplement will provide higher amounts of folic acid, and perhaps more zinc, iron, and calcium. Some feel that additional DHA is beneficial. The amount of preformed vitamin A should be kept below 5,000 IU. Carotenoids have not been shown to be a problem. Too little vitamin A can lead to birth defects, as can too much vitamin A.

Sample Products:

- *Prenatal Nutrients* (Solgar). Every four tablets contain the following:

Vitamin A (as palmitate 3,000 IU, 63% [5000 IU] as natural beta-carotene from D. salina)	8,000 IU
Vitamin C (as L-ascorbic acid)	100 mg
Vitamin D (as cholecalciferol)	400 IU
Vitamin E (as D-alpha tocopheryl succinate)	30 IU
Thiamine (as thiamine mononitrate)	1.7 mg
Riboflavin	2 mg
Niacin (as niacinamide)	20 mg
Vitamin B_6 (as pyridoxine HCl)	2.5 mg
Folic Acid	800 mcg
Vitamin B_{12} (as cobalamin)	8 mcg
Biotin	300 mcg
Pantothenic Acid (as D-Ca pantothenate)	10 mg
Calcium (as calcium citrate, calcium carbonate)	1,300 mg
Iron (as iron bisglycinate)	45 mg
Iodine (from kelp)	150 mcg
Magnesium (as magnesium citrate, magnesium oxide)	450 mg
Copper (as copper chelate, copper gluconate)	2 mg
Zinc (as zinc chelate, zinc oxide)	15 mg
Selenium (as L-selenomethionine)	25 mcg
Manganese (as manganese chelate, manganese gluconate)	2 mg
Chromium (as chromium picolinate [yeast-free])	25 mcg
Potassium (from potassium amino acid complex, potassium gluconate)	50 mg
Inositol	10 mg
Choline (as choline bitartrate)	4 mg
PABA (as para aminobenzoic acid)	2 mg
Alpha-Carotene	114 mcg
Cryptoxanthin	28 mcg
Zeaxanthin	23 mcg
Lutein	18 mcg

Soy Protein Isolate/Amino Acid Blend (L-glutamic acid, L-aspartic acid, L-leucine, L-arginine, L-lysine, L-phenylalanine, L-serine, L-proline, L-valine, L-isoleucine, L-alanine, glycine, L-theonine, L-tyrosine, L-histidine, L-cysteine, L-methioine, L-ornithine, taurine)	160 mg

• *Pre-Natal* (Twinlab). Every four capsules contain the following:

Vitamin A (as palmitate 3,000 IU, 63% [5000 IU] as natural beta-carotene	8,000 IU
Vitamin C (as L-ascorbic acid)	100 mg
Vitamin D (as cholecalciferol)	400 IU
Vitamin E (as D-alpha tocopheryl succinate)	30 IU
Thiamine (as thiamin mononitrate)	1.7 mg
Riboflavin	2 mg
Niacin (as niacinamide)	20 mg
Vitamin B_6 (as pyridoxine HCl)	2.5 mg
Folic Acid	800 mcg
Vitamin B_{12} (as cobalamin)	8 mcg
Biotin	300 mcg
Pantothenic Acid (as D-Ca pantothenate)	10 mg
Calcium (as calcium citrate, calcium carbonate)	1,300 mg
Iron (as iron bisglycinate)	45 mg
Iodine (from kelp)	150 mcg
Magnesium (as magnesium citrate, magnesium oxide)	450 mg
Copper (as copper chelate, copper gluconate)	2 mg
Zinc (as zinc chelate, zinc oxide)	15 mg
Selenium (as L-selenomethionine)	25 mcg
Manganese (as manganese chelate, manganese gluconate)	2 mg
Chromium (as chromium picolinate [yeast-free])	25 mcg
Potassium (from potassium amino acid complex, potassium gluconate)	50 mg
Inositol	10 mcg

Choline (as choline bitartrate)	4 mg
Carotenoid Mix (alpha-carotene, lutein, zeaxanthin, cryptoxanthin)	57 mcg
Soy Protein Isolate/Amino Acid Blend (L-glutamic acid, L-aspartic acid, L-leucine, L-arginine, L-lysine, L-phenylalanine, L-serine, L-proline, L-valine, L-isoleucine, L-alanine, glycine, L-threonine, L-tysosine, L-hisitidine, L-cysteine, L-methionine, L-ornithine, taurine)	160mg

- *Preg-Natal + DHA* (Jarrow) is a balanced prenatal multivitamin supplement with additional DHA. DHA is the omega-3 fatty acid (part of the EPA-DHA omega-3 fish oil complex) that has been shown to be essential for normal brain development in the fetus and infant. It also supplies the necessary amount of calcium (1,200 mg), magnesium (500 mg), and extra iron (25 mg). The product consists of packets, each containing six tablets and one softgel capsule. Take one packet daily.
- *Women's PreNatal Care* (Natrol) adds ginger, red raspberry, rosemary, squaw vine, and DHA to the basic prenatal formula. Additional calcium and magnesium would be required as the formula provides 250 milligrams of calcium. Also, the presence of the herbs in this product may be of some concern. Check with your nutritionist or physician if you are unsure as to whether you should take herbs during pregnancy.

Prostate Formulas

Description: When the prostate gland enlarges, it contricts the urethra, causing a number of potentially serious symptoms, including increased frequency of urination, difficult urnination, and increased risk of urinary tract infection and kidney damage. It is estimated that about one-half of men over 50 years of age have this condition, referred to as benign prostatic hyperplasia. Other conditions affecting the prostate include prostatis, which is caused by a microbial infection, and prostate cancer. The symptoms of each type of problem can be similar. It is important to get a medical examination to determine the exact nature of the problem.

Ingredients: Perhaps the most impressive nondrug agent for treating BPH is the herb saw palmetto. This herb has now been well researched, and has been shown to be perhaps as effective as the popular prescription drugs, with fewer side effects. Other herbs, also shown to be helpful, are pygeum, nettle roots, and pumpkin seed oil. Beta-sitosterol, found in various plants, has been shown to be effective. Beta-sitosterol is a plant sterol, and is also effective in lowering cholesterol levels. Zinc is important, and there is evidence that rye pollen extract is effective in treating BPH. Three amino acids—alanine, glutamic acid, and glycine—have also been used to alleviate the symptoms of BPH.

Sample Products:

- *MaxiLife Prostate Protector* (Twinlab). Every two softgels contain the following:

Saw Palmetto Berry (*Serenoa repens*) Extract (standardized for 85–95% fatty acids)	320 mg
Beta Sitosterol (from 120 mg of soy phytosterol complex)	60 mg
Natural Vitamin E	800 IU
Lycopene	10 mg
Vitamin D	400 IU
Zinc (from zinc picolinate)	30 mg
In a base of soy isoflavones	

- *Prostate Support* (Solgar). Every two vegicaps contain the following:

Calcium	25 mg
Zinc (as zinc glycinate)	10 mg
Selenium (as L-selenomethionine)	25 mcg
Sodium	15 mg
Modified Citrus Pectin (average molecular wt. 15 KD)	200 mg
Standardized Pygeum Africanum Extract (bark) (phytoesterols 3 mg–5 mg [2%-3%])	150 mg
Standardized Saw Palmetto Extract (berry) (free fatty acids 68 mg–75 mg [45%-50%])	150 mg
Standardized Stinging Nettles Extract (leaf) (silic acid 2 mg [1%])	150 mg

Pumpkin Powder (seed)	100 mg
Soy Isoflavone Concentrate (seed)	100 mg
Lycopene (from tomato)	7 mg

• *ProstatExcell* (Natrol). Every two tablets contain the following:

Vitamin E (as d-alpha tocopheryl succinate)	60 IU
Calcium (as dicalcium phosphate)	130 mg
Zinc (as gluconate)	10 mg
Selenium (as yeast-bound selenium)	200 mcg
Saw Palmetto Extract	300 mg
Pygeum 2.5% Extract	200 mg
Stinging Nettles Extract	150 mg
Secale Cereale Extract (pollen extract)	100 mg
Panax Ginseng Extract	100 mg
Soy Extract (isoflavones 10%)	150 mg
Flax Seed Powder (lignin 4.6%)	100 mg
Tomato Powder (lycopene 1.5%)	200 mg

• *Lycopene Carotenoid Complex* (Solgar). Lycopene has been shown to possibly protect against prostate cancer. A number of well-designed studies have shown that a high intake of tomatoes (containing lycopene) was associated with a low incidence of prostate cancer. Lycopene is more bioavailable in cooked tomatoes, or supplements, than in fresh raw tomatoes. Every vegicap of Lycopene Carotenoid Complex contains the following:

Vitamin A (100% as natural beta-carotene)	2,500 IU
Lycopene (from tomato)	15 mg
Carotenoid Mix (alpha-carotene, lutein, zeaxanthin, cryptoxanthin	29 mcg

• *Palmetto Complex II with Lycopene* (Allergy Research Group) provides the highest-quality standardized saw palmetto extract, together with other active nutrients that complement its action. In addition to the recommended 320 milligrams of palmetto extract, this formulation provides 60 milligrams of beta-sitosterol, the major active principle in pygeum. Also included is a generous portion of pumpkin seed oil (from Eastern Europe), zinc, and vitamin B_6. Lycopene is an antioxidant carotenoid that has been shown in recent studies to support the prostate gland. The studies revealed low levels of lycopene in abnormal prostate tissue. Every two softgels of Palmetto Complex II with Lycopene contain the following:

Zinc (as zinc citrate)	10 mg
Pumpkin Seed Oil	1.5 g
Saw Palmetto (Serenoa repens) Berry extract (standardized to 85–95% fatty acids)	320 mg
Beta-Sitosterol	120 mg
Lycopene	15 mg

- *Saw Palmetto Pygeum Lycopene Complex* (Solgar) contains 4 milligrams of lycopene, but relatively low amounts of standardized saw palmetto and pygeum, along with 10 milligrams of zinc, 25 micrograms of selenium, and 50 milligrams of cactus flower. It would be a good product to add to others, if they do not contain lycopene.
- *PC Care Prostate Formula* (Natrol) is an example of a product we do not recommend. This is because quantitative information is not provided for the eight herbs listed as active ingredients. Instead, it contains a "proprietary blend 960 mg" of these herbs. There is no valid reason for listing the ingredients in this manner.
- *Comprehensive Prostate Formula* (Doctor's Best) contains saw palmetto, pygeum, stinging nettle root, lycopene, and the amino acids alanine, glutamic acid, and glycine, together with antioxidant minerals in a three-per-day tablet. An excellent combination.

Stress Formulas

Description: Stress is unavoidable. It is important that our bodies are capable of coping with stress. Stress puts an additional burden on the adrenal glands. Providing nutritional and herbal support of the adrenals is one way to enhance our ability to handle stress.

Ingredients: Certain B vitamins have been shown to be associated with adrenal gland function, including vitamin C, vitamin B$_6$ and pantothenic acid. The minerals zinc and magnesium are important. Adaptogenic herbs, such as Siberian ginseng and Asian ginseng (Panax) are thought to be helpful in stress. When possible, the cause of the stress, that is, anxiety, fatigue, should be addressed.

Sample Products: :

B-Complex with C Stress Formula Tablets (Solgar). Every two tablets contain the following:

Vitamin C (as L-ascorbic acid)	500 mg
Thiamin (as thiamin mononitrate)	10 mg
Riboflavin	10 mg
Niacin (as niacinamide)	100 mg
Vitamin B$_6$ (as pyridoxine HCl)	10 mg
Folic Acid	100 mcg
Vitamin B$_{12}$ (as cobalamin)	25 mcg
Biotin (as D-biotin)	25 mcg
Pantothenic Acid (from D-Ca pantothenate)	100 mg
Inositol	100 mg
Choline (as choline bitartrate)	41 mg

A COMMENT BY DR. ABEL

The simple ways to deal with stress should be kept in mind and should be part of your daily protocol for successful living. The body has essentially two nervous systems. One is under your direct control and governs your body movements. The other, the autonomic nervous system, is indirect because it is controlled by processes that you may not even think about. For instance, you don't usually think about your heart rate, your breathing rate. . . . If you did, who would be managing your breathing and heart beats while you were sleeping? The autonomic nervous system has two components-a speed-up and a slow-down. The sympathetic nervous system speeds up the body, and causes the well-known fight-or-flight phenomena. It increases blood pressure, heart rate, pupil dilation, and sweating; it also stimulates your adrenal gland to produce the "stress hormones." The parasympathetic nervous system slows down your heartbeat and many of your metabolic processes. The goal in reducing stress is to stimulate your parasympathetic pathways, and neutralize you sympathetic pathways. Yes, you can be taking things like pantethine, Siberian ginseng, MSM, CoQ_{10}, or NADH in order to improve energy. But directly stimulating your relaxation pathways is the real trick. This can be done as simply as taking a deep breath. Rhythmic breathing, stretching, regular exercise, and your own form of meditation are ways of slowing down. Haven't you noticed if you take a deep breath, you are able to think a little more clearly?

Appendix A

Vitamins: Historical Comparison of RDIs, RDAs, and DRIs, 1968 to Present

VITAMIN	RDI*	1968 RDA**	1974 RDA**	1980 RDA**	1989 RDA**	DRIs***
Vitamin A	5,000 IU	5,000 IU	1,000 RE (5,000 IU)	1,000 RE	1,000 RE	900 mcg (3,000 IU)
Vitamin C	60 mg	60 mg	45 mg	60 mg	60 mg	90 mg
Vitamin D	400 IU (10 mcg)	400 IU (10 mcg)	400 IU (10 mcg)	10 mcg (400 IU)	10 mcg (400 IU)	15 mcg (600 IU)
Vitamin E	30 IU (20 mg)	30 IU (20 mg)	15 IU (10 mg)	10 mg (15 IU)	10 mg (15 IU)	15 mg #
Vitamin K	80 mcg	—	—	70–140 mcg	80 mcg	120 mcg
Thiamine	1.5 mg	1.5 mg	1.5 mg	1.5 mg	1.5 mg	1.2 mg
Riboflavin	1.7 mg	1.7 mg	1.8 mg	1.7 mg	1.8 mg	1.3 mg
Niacin	20 mg	20 mg	20 mg	19 mg	20 mg	16 mg
Vitamin B_6	2 mg	2 mg	2 mg	2.2 mg	2 mg	1.7 mg
Folate	0.4 mg (400 mcg)	400 mcg	400 mcg	400 mcg	200 mcg	400 mcg food, 200 mcg synthetic ##
Vitamin B_{12}	6 mcg	6 mcg	3 mcg	3 mcg	2 mcg	2.4 mcg ###
Biotin	(300 mcg)	150–300 mcg	100–300 mcg	100–200 mcg	30–100 mcg	30 mcg
Pantothenic	10 mg	5–10 mg	5–10 mg	4–7 mg	4–7 mg	5 mg
Choline	—	—	—	—	—	550 mg

* The Reference Daily Intake (RDI) is the value established by the Food and Drug Administration (FDA) for use in nutrition labeling. It was based initially on the highest

1968 Recommended Dietary Allowance (RDA) for each nutrient, to assure that needs were met for all age groups.

** The RDAs were established and periodically revised by the Food and Nutrition Board. Value shown is the highest RDA for each nutrient, in the year indicated for each revision.

*** The Dietary Reference Intakes (DRI) are the most recent set of dietary recommendations established by the Food and Nutrition Board of the Institute of Medicine, 1997–2001. They replace previous RDAs, and may be the basis for eventually updating the RDIs. The value shown here is the highest DRI for each nutrient.

Historical vitamin E conversion factors were amended in the DRI report, so that 15 mg is defined as the equivalent of 22 IU of natural vitamin E or 33 IU of synthetic vitamin E.

It is recommended that women of childbearing age obtain 400 mcg of synthetic folic acid from fortified breakfast cereals or dietary supplements, in addition to dietary folate.

It is recommended that people over 50 meet the B_{12} recommendation through fortified foods or supplements, to improve bioavailability.

Reprinted by permission of the Council for Responsible Nutrition.

Minerals: Historical Comparison of RDIs, RDAs and DRIs, 1968 to Present

NUTRIENT	RDI*	1968 RDA**	1974 RDA**	1980 RDA**	1989 RDA**	DRIs***
Calcium	1,000 mg	1,300 mg	1,200 mg	1,200 mg	1,200 mg	1,300 mg
Phosphorus	1,000 mg	1,300 mg	1,200 mg	1,200 mg	1,200 mg	1,250 mg (700 adult)
Iron	18 mg	18 mg	18 mg	18 mg	15 mg	18 mg
Iodine	150 mcg	150 mcg	150 mcg	150 mcg	150 mcg	150 mcg
Magnesium	400 mg	400 mg	400 mg	400 mg	400 mg	420 mg
Zinc	15mg	10–15 mg	15 mg	15 mg	15 mg	11 mg
Selenium	70 mcg	—	—		70 mcg	55 mcg
Copper	2 mg	—	—	2–3 mg	1.5–3 mg	0.9 mg
Manganese	2 mg	—	2.7–7 mg	2.5–5 mg	2–5 mg	2.3 mg
Chromium	120 mcg	—	—	50–200 mcg	50–200 mcg	35 mcg
Molybdenum	75 mcg	—	45–500 mg	150–500 mcg	75–250 mcg	45 mcg

* The Reference Daily Intake (RDI) is the value established by the Food and Drug Administration (FDA) for use in nutrition labeling. It was based initially on the highest 1968 Recommended Dietary Allowance (RDA) for each nutrient, to assure that needs were met for all age groups.

** The RDAs were established and periodically revised by the Food and Nutrition Board. Value shown is the highest RDA for each nutrient, in the years indicated for each revision.

*** The Dietary Reference Intakes (DRI) are the most recent set of dietary recommendations established by the Food and Nutrition Board of the Institute of Medicine, 1997–2001. They replace previous RDAs, and may be the basis for eventually updating the RDIs. The value shown here is the highest DRI for each nutrient.

Reprinted by permission of the Council for Responsible Nutrition.

Resource List

Following are the companies whose products are mentioned in this book. Please note that many additional high-quality products are available from other reputable companies.

Advanced Medical Nutrition
2247 National Avenue
Hayward, CA 94540-5012

America's Finest
140 Ether Road West
Piscataway, NJ 08854

Alacer
19631 Pauling
Foothill Ranch, CA 92610

Amino Acid & Botanic Supply
31 Oakridge Road
Parsippany, NJ 07034

Allergy Research
30806 Santana Street
Hayward, CA 94544

Arkopharma
432 Fairfield Ave.
Stamford, CT 06902

Alta Health
2137 East Summersweet Drive
Boise, ID 83716

Atkins
185 Oser Avenue
Hauppauge, NY 11788

American Lecithin
15 Hurley Road, Unit 2B
Oxford, UT 06478

Barlean
4936 Lake Terrell Road
Ferndale, WA 98248

Bioplex Nutrition
150 West Axton Road
Bellingham, WA 98226

Carlson
15 College
Arlington Heights, IL 60004

Country Life
180 Motor Parkway
Hauppauge, NY 11788

Da Vinci
20 New England Drive
Essex Junction, VT 05453-1504

Desert Essence
27460 Avenue Scott
Valencia, CA 91355

Doctor's Best
1120 Calle Cordillera #101
San Clemente, CA 92673-6238

Douglas Labs
600 Boyce Road
Pittsburg, PA 15205

EAS Labs
555 Corporate Circle
Golden, CO 80401

Eclectic Institute
36350 Industrial Way
Sandy, OR 97055-7377

Ecological Formulas
1061-B Shary Circle
Concord, CA 94518

Enzymatic Therapy
825 Challenger Drive
Green Bay, WI 54311

Essential Phytosterolins
4 Commerce Crescent
Acton, Ontario
Canada L7J2X3

Essiac International
P.O. Box 6013
Pompano Beach, FL 33060

Ethical Nutrients
100 Avenida La Pata
San Clemente, CA 92373

European Reference Lab
P.O. Box 131135
Carlsbad, CA 92103

Flora
805 East Badger Road
Lynden, WA 98264-0073

Gaia Herbs
108 Island Ford Road
Brevard, NC 28712

Gary Null
11272 East Central Avenue
Del Ray, CA 93616-0249

Graminex
95 Midland Road
Saginaw, MI 48603

Green Foods
320 North Graves Avenue
Oxnard, CA 93030

Green Kamut
1542 Seabright Avenue
Long Beach, CA 90813

Health from the Sun
53 Shore Road
Winchester, MA 01890

Herb Pharm
P.O. Box 116
Williams, OR 97544

Herbs Etc.
1340 Rufina Circle
Sante Fe, NM 87501

Japanese Health
251 Carolina Drive
Tryon, NC 28782-3657

Jarrow
1824 South Robertson Blvd.
Los Angeles, CA 90035

JHS Natural Products
P.O. Box 50398
Eugene, OR 97405

Klaire Labs
140 Marine View Avenue
Solana Beach, CA 92075-2122

Klamath
2625 Toqua Road
Chiloquin, OR 97624

Kwai (Lichtwer Pharma)
2 Industrial Way West
Eatontown, NJ 07724-2265

Kyolic (Wakunaga)
23501 Madero
Fullerton, CA 92691-2744

Lane Labs
25 Commerce Drive
Allendale, NJ 07401-1600

Lily of the Desert
1887 Geesling Road
Denton, TX 76208

Longevity Science
c/o Klabin Marketing
2067 Broadway, Suite 700
New York, NY 10023

Maitake Products
222 Bergen Turnpike
Ridgefield Park, NJ 07660-2320

Medical Research Institute
1001 Baynill Drive
San Bruno, CA 94066-4037

Menuco
350 5th Avenue, Suite 7509
New York, NY 10118

Metabolic Response Modifiers
2633 West Pacific Coast
Highway, #B
Newport Beach, CA 92663

Metagenics
100 Avenida La Pata
San Clemente, CA 92373

Natren
3105 Willow Lane
Westlake Village, CA 91361

Natrol
21411 Prairie Street
Chatsworth, CA 91311

Natural Science Corp of America
17401 Ventura Boulevard
Encino, CA 91316

Naturally Vitamins
4404 East Elwood
Phoenix, AZ 85040

Nature's Answer
75 Commerce Drive
Hauppauge, NY 11788-3943

Nature's Herbs
47444 Kato Road
Fremont, CA 94538

Nature's Life
7180 Lampson Avenue
Garden Grove, CA 92841

Nature's Plus
548 Broad Hollow Road
Melville, NY 11747

Nature's Way
10 Mountain Springs Parkway
Springville, UT 84663

Natureworks
207 East 94th Street
New York, NY 10128

New Chapter
22 High Street
Brattleboro, VT 05301

North American Herb and Spice
(NAH)
212 Willow Parkway
Buffalo Grove, IL 60089

NOW Foods
395 South Glen Ellyn Road
Bloomingdale, IL 60108

Nutraceutical Research
1400 Kearns Boulevard
Park City, UT 84060

Nutrex Hawaii
73-4460 Queen Kaahumanu
Highway, #102
Kailua-Kona, HI 96740

Nutribiotic
865 Parallel Drive
Lakeport, CA 95453

Nutricia
6111 Broken Sound Parkway
NW
Boca Raton, FL 33487-3693

Nutrition Supply Corp.
3107 North Deer Run Road
Carson City, NV 89701

Olympian Labs
1600 Mid Atlantic Court
Martinsberg, WV 25401

Orjene
5-43 48th Avenue
Long Island City, NY 11101

Pharmanex
75 West Center Street
Provo, UT 84601

Pharmaton
900 Ridgebury Road
Ridgefield, CT 06877

Phytotherapy
P.O. Box 555
Franklin Lakes, NJ 07417

Pines
1992 East 1400 Road
Lawrence, KS 66044-9303

Premier One
1500 Kearns Boulevard,
Suite B-200
Park City, UT 84060

Prince of Peace
3536 Arden Road
Hayward, CA 94545-3908

Progressive Labs
1701 West Walnut Hill Lane
Irving, TX 75038

Pure Encapsulations
490 Boston Post Road
Sudbury, MA 01776

R Pur Aloe
P.O. Box 787
Yucaipa, CA 92399

Root to Health
P.O. Box 509
Wausau, WI 54402

Scandinavian Natural
13 North Seventh Street
Perkasie, PA 18944

Scientific Botanicals
8003 Roosevelt Way Northeast
Seattle, WA 98115

Seagate (Gold)
c/o First Fisheries Development
11097 Via Temprano
San Diego, CA 92124

Smithkline Beecham
Consumer Healthcare, LP
Pittsburgh, PA 15230

Solaray
1500 Kearns Boulevard
Suite B-200
Park City, UT 84060

Solgar
500 Willow Tree Road
Leonia, NJ 07605

Sonne
705 McGee Street
Kansas City, MO 64106

Source Naturals
23 Janis Way
Scotts Valley, CA 95066

Sun Chlorella
3914 Dale Amo Boulevard
Torrance, CA 90503

Symbiotics
2301 West Highway 89A,
Suite 107
Sedona, AZ 86336

TE Neesby
9909 North Meridian Avenue
Fresno, CA 93720

Thorne
25820 Highway 2 West
Dover, ID 83825

Thursday Plantation
c/o Natural Organics
548 Broad Hollow Road
Melville, NY 11747

Twinlab
150 Motor Parkway, Suite 210
Hauppauge, NY 11788

Tyler
2204-8 NW Birdsdale
Gresham, OR 97030

Vita Carte
c/o Phoenix Bio Logics
Carlsbad, CA 92008

Vitaline
385 Williamson Way
Ashland, OR 97520

Willner Chemists
100 Park Avenue
New York, NY 10017

Yasoo Health
1425 Russ Boulevard,
Suite T-107A
San Diego, CA 92101

Yerba Prima
740 Jefferson Avenue
Ashland, OR 97520-3743

For More Information

For additional information on any of the subjects discussed in this book, go to www.bestsupplementsforyourhealth.com.

Books

Abel, Robert. *The DHA Story: How Nature's Supernutrient Can Save Your Life*. New Jersey: Basic Health Publications, 2002.

———. *The Eye Care Revolution*. New York: Kensington Publishing, 1999.

Blumenthal, Mark, et al. *Herbal Medicine: Expanded Commission E Monographs*. Austin, TX: American Botanical Council, 2000.

Brown, Donald J. *Herbal Presciptions for Better Health*. Rocklin, CA: Prima Publishing, 1996.

Bruneton, Jean. *Pharmacognosy, Phytochemistry, Medicinal Plants*. Paris, France: Lavoisier Publishing, 1995.

Duke, James A. *Handbook of Medicinal Herbs*. Boca Raton, Fl: CRC Press, 1985.

Duke, James A. *The Green Pharmacy*. Emmaus, PA: Rodale Press, 1996.

Ebadi, Manuchair. *Pharmacodynamic Basis of Herbal Medicine*. Boca Raton, Fl: CRC Press, 2002.

Ensminger, Audrey H., et al. *The Concise Encyclopedia of Food and Nutrition*. Boca Raton, Fl: CRC Press, 1995.

Evans, W.C. *Trease and Evan's Pharmocognosy*, 14th Edition. London: W.B. Saunders Co., Ltd., 1996.

Germano, Carl, et al. *The Osteoporosis Solution*. New York: Kensington Publishing, 1999.

Guyton, Arthur C. *Textbook of Medical Physiology*, 8th Edition. Philadelphia, PA: W.B. Saunders Co., 1991.

Hendler, Sheldon Saul, et al. *PDR for Nutritional Supplements*. Montvale, NJ: Medical Economics Co., 2001.

Institute of Medicine. *Dietary Reference Intakes for Vitamin C, Vitamin E, Selenium, and Carotenoids*. Washington, DC: National Academy Press, 2000.

Institute of Medicine. *Dietary Refernce Intakes for Thiamine, Riboflavin, Niacin, Vitamin B_6 Folate, Vitamin B_{12}, Pantothenic Acid, Biotin, and Choline*. Washington, DC: National Academy Press, 1998.

Institute of Medicine. *Dietary Reference Intakes for Calcium, Phosphorus, Magnesium, Vitamin D, and Fluoride*. Washington, DC: National Academy Press, 1997.

Lieberman, Shari, et al. *The Real Vitamin and Mineral Book*. Garden City Park, NY: Avery Publishing Group, 1997.

Lombard, Jay, et al. *The Brain Wellness Plan*. New York: Kensington Publishing, 1997.

Mahan, L. Kathleen, et al. *Krauses Food, Nutrition, and Diet Therapy*. Philadelphia, PA: W.B. Saunders Co., 2000.

Marderosian, Ara Der. *Natural Product Medicine: A Scientific Guide to Foods, Drugs, Cosmetics*. Philadelphia, PA: George F. Stickley Co., 1988.

McCaleb, Robert S., et al. *The Encyclopedia of Popular Herbs*. Rocklin, CA: Prima Publishing, 2000.

Murray, Michael, et al. *Encyclopedia of National Medicine*, 2nd Edition. Rocklin, CA: Prima Publishing, 1998.

Murray, Michael. *Encyclopedia of Nutritional Supplements*. Rocklin, CA: Prima Publishing, 1996.

National Research Council. *Diet and Health: Implicatons of Reducing Chronic Disease Risk*. Washington, DC: National Academy Press, 1989.

Papas, Andreas. *Antioxidants Status, Diet, Nutrition, and Health*. Boca Raton, FL: CRC Press, 1999.

Papas, Andreas. *The Vitamin E Factor*. New York: HarperPerennial, 1999.

Samuelson, Gunnar. *Drugs of Natural Origin: A Textbook of Pharmacognosy*. Stockholm: Swedish Pharmaceutical Press, 1992.

Shils, Maurice E., et al. *Modern Nutrition in Health and Disease*, 9th Edition. Baltimore: Lippincott Williams and Wilkins, 1999.

Somer, Elizabeth. *The Essential Guide to Vitamins and Minerals*. New York: HarperPerennial, 1992.

Stipanuk, Martha H. *Biochemical and Physiological Aspects of Human Nutrition*. Philadelphia, PA: W.B. Saunders Co., 2000.

Tillotson, Alan Keith et al. *The One Earth Herbal Sourcebook*. New York: Kensington, 2001.

Tyler, Varro. *Herbs of Choice*. Binghamton, NY: Pharmaceutical Products Press, 1994.

Tyler, Varro, et al. *Pharmacognosy*, 9th Edition. Philadelphia: Lea and Febiger, 1988.

Wildman, Robert E. C., et al. *Handbook of Nutraceuticals and Functional Foods*. Boca Raton, FL: CRC Press, 2001.

Websites

American Medical Association, Ethics
http://www.ama-assn.org/ama/pub/category/2416.html

Council for Responsible Nutrition
http://www.crnusa.org

Dietary Supplement Education Alliance
http://www.suplementinfo.org

National Institutes of Health, Office of Dietary Supplements
http://dietary-supplements.info.nih.gov

Index